INSANELY EASY!
SEVENTH EDITION

Loretta Manning, MSN, RN, GNP
President, I CAN Publishing®, Inc.

Sylvia Rayfield, MN, RN, CNS

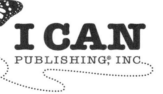

I CAN Publishing®, Inc. ◆ Duluth, GA
www.icanpublishing.com

I CAN Publishing®, Inc., Duluth, GA 30097
2650 Chattahoochee Dr., Suite 100
Duluth, GA 30097
www.icanpublishing.com

Editorial Assistants: Lydia R. Zager, Columbia, SC; Kathy Gallum, Tampa, FL; Teresa R. Davidson, Greensboro, NC
Cartoon Illustrations: Teresa R. Davidson, Greensboro, NC; Eileen Burke, Pass Christian, MS; Paulina Hanson, Words & Pictures; Jeanne Woods, Design Master, New Orleans, LA; Mitch Rubin, Rubin Art, Albuquerque, NM; John Sheppard, Shep Art Studios, Alpharetta, GA
Cover Design: Teresa R. Davidson, Greensboro, NC
Design and Technical Director: Mary Jo Zazueta, Traverse City, MI
Publishing Service Managers: Jennifer Robinson and Kelly Cain

© 2014 by I CAN Publishing®, Inc.

All rights reserved. No part of this book may be used or reproduced or transmitted in any form or by any means, electronic or mechanical, including photocopying, recording, or by an information storage and retrieval system without written permission from I CAN Publishing®, Inc., except for the inclusion of brief quotations in a review.

ISBN-13: 978-0-9842040-8-3
Library of Congress Catalog Control Number: 2013921047

Nursing procedures and/or practice described in this book should be applied by the nurse or healthcare practitioner under appropriate supervision according to established professional standards of care. These standards should be used with regard to the unique circumstances that apply in each practice situation. Every effort has been taken to validate and confirm the accuracy of information presented and to describe generally accepted practices. However, the authors, editors, and publisher cannot accept any responsibility for errors or omissions or for consequences from application of the information in this book and make no warranty, express or implied, with respect to the contents of this book.

Every effort has been exerted by the authors and publisher to ensure that drug selection and dosage set forth in this text is in accord with current recommendations and practice at the time of publication. However, in view of ongoing research, the constant flow of information relating to governmental regulations, drug therapy, and drug reactions, the reader is urged to check the manufacturer's information on the package insert of each drug for any change in indications and dosage and for added warnings and precautions. This is particularly important when the recommended agent is a new or infrequently used drug.

This book is written to be used as a memory tool (A Visual Approach to Memory) for students, graduates, and faculty. It is not intended for use as a primary resource for procedures, treatments, medications, or to serve as a complete textbook for nursing care. Copies of this book may be obtained directly from I CAN Publishing®, Inc. at www.icanpublishing.com.

In discovering new ways of thinking about nursing concepts and creative ways of helping learners to remember was the reason for writing this book. This is our 7th edition of a book that has sold internationally and helped thousands of learners "get it." We are grateful to our contributors.

Karen E. Alexander, RN, PhD, CNOR
A.D.N Program Director LVN/Paramedic to A.D.N. Mobility Program
San Jacinto College South
Houston, Texas

Julia Aucoin, DNS, RN-BC, CNE
Chief Knowledge Officer
Practical Success
Durham, NC

Marie Bremner, DSN, RN, CS
Professor of Nursing
Kennesaw State Univ.
Kennesaw, Georgia

Pam Chally, PhD, RN
Dean of the College of Health
Univ. of North Florida
Jacksonville, Florida

J. Chris Chandler, BA, BSN, RN
Nursing ADP Coordinator
Atlanta VA Hospital
Decatur, Georgia

Judy J. Duvall, EdD, RN
Assistant Professor
Whitson-Hester School of Nursing
Tennessee Technological University
Cookeville, Tennessee

Darlene Franklin, RN, MSN
Assistant Professor of Nursing Emeritus
Whitson-Hester School of Nursing
Tennessee Technological University
Nursing Consultant
Cookeville, Tennessee
I CAN Publishing®, Inc.
Duluth, Georgia
Sylvia Rayfield & Associates
Pensacola, Florida

Kathy Gallun, MSN, RN
Educational Consultant
Tampa, Florida
I CAN Publishing®, Inc.
Duluth, Georgia
Sylvia Rayfield & Associates
Pensacola, Florida

Melissa J. Geist, APRN, BC, EdD
Assistant Dean
Tennessee Technological University
Cookeville, Tennessee

Cieanna Hairston, RN, MSN, MHA
Director of Clinical Practice and Education
Morehead Memorial Hospital
Eden, NC

Alita R. Maddox, APRN, MSN, PNP-C
In Memory

Sylvia McDonald, RN, MEd, MSN
Consultant
Jefferson, Georgia
I CAN Publishing® Inc.
Duluth, Georgia
Sylvia Rayfield & Associates
Pensacola, Florida

Jackie McVey, PhD, RN
University of Texas-Tyler
Tyler, Texas

Tina Rayfield, RN, BS, PA-C, MSN
President
Sylvia Rayfield & Associates
Pensacola, Florida

Jessica Roberts, MSN, RN, FNP-BC
Sounding Provider
Physicians Express Care, LLC.
Johns Creek & Towne

Lake Georgia
Sylvia Rayfield & Associates
Pensacola, Florida

Vanice W. Roberts, DSN, RN
Dean of Nursing
Berry College
Rome, Georgia

Barbara Rhine, MSN, RN
Nursing Instructor
Ranger College
Brown County Campus
Early, Texas

Bedelia H. Russell, PhD(c), MSN, RN, CPNP-PC, CNE
Interim Dean
Whitson-Hester School of Nursing
Tennessee Technological University
Cookeville, Tennessee

Martha Sherman, MSN, MA, RN
Retired

Mayola Villarruel, DNP, ANP-BC, NEA-BC
Director Patient Care Services
Community Hospital
Munster, Indiana

Lydia R. Zager, MSN, RN, NEA-BC
Clinical Professor
College of Nursing
University of South Carolina
Columbia, SC

JoAnn Zerwekh, EdD, MSN, RN
President/CEO
Nursing Education Consultants
Chandler, Arizona

Also Published By
I CAN PUBLISHING®, INC.

NCLEX-RN® 101: How to Pass

NCLEX-PN® 101: How to Pass

Nursing Made Insanely Easy!

Pharmacology Made Insanely Easy!

Pathways to Teaching Nursing: Keeping it Real

The Eight-Step Approach to Teaching Clinical Nursing

The Eight-Step Approach For Student Clinical Success

We Do Not Die Alone: "Jesus is Coming to Get Me in a White Pickup Truck"

Pharmacology: NCLEX® Reviews

Contents

Preface xv
Acknowledgments xvii

MANAGEMENT

Prioritizing 2
Prioritization Strategies For Test Questions 4
Priorities 7
"Trending" Helps Prevent Complications (Trending) 8
"Infor Matics" 10
Provide and Receive Report On Assigned Clients: What is SBAR? (SBAR) 12
Informed Consent (Consent) 14
HIPAA Privacy Rule (HIPAA) 16
Legal Aspects (The 4 Ds) 18
Delegation (Delegator) 20
Ancillary Personnel Limitations (Part, Can't) 22
Tasks to Be Delegated to the UAP (Bart) 24
Nurses Who Float Between Units (Float) 26
Tasks That Can Be Delegated to the New Graduate (Grad) ... 28
Do Not Delegate What You "Teach!" (Teach) 30
Cost Effectiveness (Save) 32
Management: Safety 34
Accuracy of Orders (Drip) 36
Cover Your Assets (Mess) 38
Standard of Care (Standards) 40
Recognize the Need For Referrals (Discharge) 42

How To Decide Which Client Should Be Discharged Early
(Stable) 44

Priority Topics For Teaching (Educates) 46

The 8 Rights to Medication Administration 48

SAFETY & INFECTION CONTROL

Proper Identification 52

Assignment of Rooms (Risk) 54

Hand Hygiene (Hands) 56

Standard Precautions (Gloves) 58

Standard Precautions For The Care of All Clients in All
Healthcare Settings 60

Categories of Transmission-Based Precautions 62

Airborne Precautions (AIIR) 64

Viral Infections (Simplex and Zoster) 66

Plan For Clients With Varicella (Chicken Pox) (Isolate) 68

DroPlet Precautions (Patty the Pathogen) 70

Priority Nursing Plan For Clients With Clostridium
Difficile (Private) 72

Clostridium Difficile (Bad) 74

Methicillin-Resistant Staphylococcus Aureus (MRSA) 76

Infection Prevention: Positive Pressure (Positive Paul) 78

Sequence For Donning PPE 80

Sequence For Removing PPE 82

Fever 84

Beta Strep 86

Fall Risk (ABCs) 88

Anaphylactic Reactions: Priority Nursing Care That
"Limits Dyspnea" (Limits & Dyspnea) 90

Safe Use of Equipment (Safe) 92

Priority Plan Regarding Restraints (Restraint) 94

Applications of Heat and Cold (Burn/Cold) 96
Disaster Plan (ABC) 98
Triage (Stop Light). 100

CARDIAC SYSTEM

Tools of Physical Assessment 104
Stethoscope 106
Vital Signs 108
Vital Sign Values 110
Cardiac Sounds 112
Diagnostic Procedures (Act Now) 114
Diagnostics For The Cardiac System 116
Priority Care Prior to a "Gram" (Dyes) 118
Priority Care After a "Gram" (Hard) 120
Cyanotic Heart Defects (Four Ts) 122
Tetralogy of Fallot (Drop) 124
Assessments for Congenital Heart Disease (Hearts) 126
Symptoms of Hypoxia In An Infant (Grunts) 128
Kawasaki Disease (Strawberry) 130
System-Specific Assessments For Heart Failure
(Dyspnea/Edema) 132
Reduce Cardiac Workload (Spare) 134
Cardiac Management (OANM) 136
Ace Inhibitors (Pril Sisters) 138
Beta Blockers 140
Calcium Channel Blockers............................. 142
Loop Diuretics (Lou La Bell). 144
Atrial Dysrhythmias 146
Defibrillate or Cardiovert? 148
Heart Blocks. 150

Hemodynamics: A New Approach to Values! (The 6s) 152
Hemodynamics: A New Approach to Values! (The 12s) 154
Peripherally Inserted Central Catheter Care (Peripheral) 156
Peripheral Vascular Disease: Arterial Versus Venous 158
Priority Plan For Clients With Inadequate Peripheral
Artery Perfusion (Pain) 160
Raynaud's Phenomenon: Prevention of Vasospasms (Stress) . 162

RESPIRATORY /ACID BASE

Breath Sounds 166
Transmitted Voice Sounds 168
Diagnostics For The Respiratory System 170
Priority Care For a "Centesis" 172
Assessments After Any Test That Ends in "Scopy" (Scope) . . 174
Pulmonary Edema (Dog Mad) 176
Acid-Base (Red Van) 178
Acid-Base Status (Rome) 180
Compensatory Mechanisms 182
Acid-Base (Calling the Shots) 184
Shock 186
Help Stamp Out Shock 188
Lung Sounds 190
Chronic Obstructive Pulmonary Disease (COPD) 192
Interventions For COPD (ABCs) 194
Asthma 196
Beta$_2$-Adrenergic Agonists (Max Air) 198
Cystic Fibrosis (Sicker Kid) 200
Water-Sealed Chest Drainage (Pleur-evac) 202
Ventilator Care (Vents) 204
Tuberculosis (Ina) 206

FLUID VOLUME / RENAL SYSTEM

Fluid Volume Status.................................. 210
Fluid Shifts.. 212
Hypernatremia...................................... 214
Hyponatremia....................................... 216
Hyperkalemia (Death)............................... 218
Hypokalemia (Weak)................................. 220
Hypercalcemia (The Fat CA^{++}T: The Ds) 222
Hypocalcemia (The Skinny CA^{++}T: Twitch).............. 224
Renal Pathology.................................... 226
Drugs That Can Cause Nephrotoxicity................ 228
Diagnostics For The Renal System................... 230
Lab Changes With Chronic Renal Failure............. 232
Chronic Kidney Disease (Chronic Renal Failure/CRF)..... 234
Dialysis... 236

ENDOCRINE

Diagnostics For The Endocrine System 240
SIADH (Soggy Sid) 242
Diabetes Insipidus (Dilute) 244
Hyperthyroidism (Go Getter Gertrude)............... 246
Thyroidectomy (Bow Tie) 248
Hypothyroidism (Morbid Matilda) 250
Diabetes Mellitus (Fido) 252
Insulin (Peak Times for Insulin) 254
Hypoglycemia (Tired) 256
Cushing's Disease/Syndrome (Cushy Carl) 258
Addison's Disease (Anemic Adam) 260

GASTROINTESTINAL SYSTEM

Diagnostics For The Gastrointestinal System 264
Priority Plans For Infant With Severe Diarrhea
(Weight) 266
Peptic Ulcer Disease (Pud) 268
Gastric Reflux (Reflux) 270
Anticholinergics 272
Antacids 274
Treatment of Ulcerative Colitis and Crohn's (Cramps) 276
Colostomy (Connie Colostomy) 278
Dumping Syndrome (Dump Truck) 280
Tubes 282
Post-Operative GI Assessment (Drapes) 284
Diverticular Disease (Fiber) 286
Diagnostics For The Hepatic And Biliary System 288
Elevated Liver Enzymes (ABC) 290
Cirrhosis (Ascites) 292
Tylenol (Acetaminophen) Overdose 294
Pancreatitis (Ases High) 296

MUSCULOSKELETAL SYSTEM

Diagnostics For the Musculoskeletal System 300
Osteoporosis (Josephine Bone-A-Part) 302
Arthritis (Arthur Itis) 304
Nonsteroidal Anti-Inflammatory Drugs (NSAIDs) 306
Gout 308
Care of Client in Traction (Fractures) 310
Adverse Effects of Immobility (Awful) 312
Crutch Walking (Part/One) 314

Crutch Walking (Good/Bad) 316
Cane Walking (Cane) 318
Walking With a Walker (Walk) 320

NEUROLOGICAL SYSTEM

Diagnostics For The Neurological System 324
Meningocele/Omphalocele (Seals) 326
Hydrocephalus (PIES) 328
Glasgow Coma Scale 330
Cranial Nerves (3, 4, 6, and 8) 332
Cranial Nerves 334
Neurological Checks (Perl Mae) 336
Vital Signs For Shock vs. IICP. 338
Nursing Care For Increased Intracranial Pressure
(Heads) 340
Priority Clinical Assessment Findings For
Meningitis (Necks) 342
Priority Nursing Interventions For Meningitis (Meninges) .. 344
Seizures (Caesar) 346
Dilantin (Dial at Ten). 348
Parkinson's Disease (Park Dark) 350
Myasthenia Gravis (Time) 352
Bell's Palsy (Image) 354
Trigeminal Neuralgia (Tic Douloureux) (Paine). 356
Botox 358
Care of the Spinal Cord Client (Paralyzed) 360
Anticoagulants 362
Autonomic Dysreflexia 364
Stroke (Fast) 366

SENSORY PERCEPTION

Diagnostics For Ophthalmic and Hearing 370
Visual Changes. 372
Symptoms of Open Angle Glaucoma (Open) 374
Medications For Open Angle Glaucoma (Bahm). 376
Miotics (Constrict Eyes: Glaucoma) 378
Ear Drops (Up/Down) 380
Priority Plan For Client With Hearing Impairment
(Hearing) 382

INTEGUMENTARY SYSTEM

Diagnostics For The Integumentary System 386
Impetigo (Honey Bees) 388
Parasitic Infestations: Pediculosis (Lice) 390
Priority Care For Decreasing Altered Skin
Integrity (Pressure Ulcers) 392
Basal Cell Carcinoma (Pit) 394
Malignant Melanoma (ABCDE) 396
Burns 398

HEMATOLOGY

Diagnostics For Hematology 402
Sickle Cell Anemia (Hops) 404
Polycythemia (Red) 406
Priority Assessments For Leukemia (Nat) 408
Multiple Myeloma (Bone) 410

MEN & WOMEN'S CARE / CANCER

Benign Prostate Hypertrophy (Turps) 414
Care of Client After Mastectomy (Breast) 416
Safety With Radium Implants 418

HEALTH PROMOTION

Levels of Prevention................................ 422
Client Education (Teach Back) 424
Growth and Development Throughout the Life
Span (Spine)...................................... 426
Obesity (Small) 428
Infancy 430
Toddler—1 to 3 years (Praise) 432
Poison Control (Tommy Toxin) 434
Preschool—4 to 5 Years (Magic) 436
School Age—6 to 12 Years (Dimple) 438
Adolescent—13 to 18 Years (Pairs) 440
Young Adulthood—19 to 40 Years (Intimacy) 442
Middle Adulthood—40 to 60 years (Sandwich).......... 444
Older Adulthood—60 to 85 Years (Accept) 446
Geriatrics—85 Years and Over (Geriatric) 448
Priority Nursing Care For Geriatrics (Fan Capes) 450
Immunizations (Immunized) 452
Diagnostics For The Maternity Client 454
Normal Discomforts During Pregnancy (Backaches)...... 456
Danger Signs in Pregnancy (Cabs) 458
Pregnancy-Induced Hypertension (Peace) 460
Magnesium Sulfate Toxicity (Burp) 462
Gestational Diabetes (Fetal)......................... 464
Decelerations (Veal Chop) 466

Fetal Heart Decelerations: Early
Detections (Head Compression) 468

Fetal Heart Decelerations: Variable Decelerations
(Cord Compression) 470

Fetal Heart Decelerations: Late Decelerations
(Uteroplacental Insufficiency)......................... 472

Late Decelerations (Uncoil) 474

Pitocin 476

Regional Anesthesia (Region) 478

Postpartum Assessment (Bubble) 480

Neonate Assessments: "The 4 Hs"..................... 482

DIETS

Foods High in Folic Acid............................ 486

Foods High in Iron................................. 488

Foods High in Protein 490

Foods High in Potassium 492

Foods High in Sodium.............................. 494

Low-Residue Diet 496

Celiac Disease Diet 498

PSYCHOSOCIAL INTEGRITY

Therapeutic Communication (Trust) 502

Communication Strategies For Test Questions 504

Conditions That Must Be Reported As Required By
The Law (Cage) 506

Documentation Guidelines For Suspected Abuse 508

Anorexia (Starve) 510

Bulimia (Stuff) 512

Interventions For Anxiety (Calmer) 514

Anti-Anxiety Medications (Bats) 516

Symptoms of Depression (In Sad Cages) 518

Management of Depression (Suicide) 520

Antidepressant Medications: Tricyclic
Antidepressants (Tina Tricycle) 522

Monoamine Oxidase (MAO) Inhibitors 524

Bipolar Disorder (Manic) 526

Lithium 528

Schizophrenia (Hard Time) 530

Undesirable Effects of Antipsychotic Drugs (Stance) 532

Alcoholism (Copes) 534

Abstinence Maintenance Following Detoxification by
Way of Revia (Beat) 536

Abstinence Maintenance Following Detoxification
Antabuse (Ant-Abuse: Barfs)........................ 538

Difference In Delirium And Dementia 540

Dementia 542

Combative Client (Combat) 544

Post-Traumatic Stress Syndrome (Nite) 546

Cultural Aspects (Spirit) 548

LABORATORY VALUES

The Magic 2s 552

The Magic 4s 554

References 557

Index 559

Belief

is the knowledge that we CAN do something.
It's the inner feeling that what we undertake,
we CAN accomplish.
For the most part, all of us have the ability
to look at something and know
whether or not we CAN do it.
We CAN do only what we think we CAN do.
We CAN be only what we think we CAN be.
What we do, what we are, what we accomplish,
all depend on what we think.
So, in belief there is power: our eyes are opened;
our opportunities become plain;
our visions become realities.

I CAN Publishing®, Inc. has selected the butterfly for our logo since our mission is to help transform your learning from complexity to simplicity! Just as the caterpillar changes into a cocoon, and then emerges as a brilliant butterfly, our mission is to assist you from being overwhelmed to having confidence in your ability to remember and understand nursing and how to remember and understand nursing concepts. Our name, "**I CAN**" is the mnemonic for Creative Approaches to Nursing! We know with "I CAN" you **CAN** learn, have fun, and be successful all at the same time!

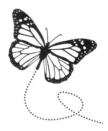

Preface

A MESSAGE TO OUR LEARNERS

Nursing Made Insanely Easy, first edition was developed to make learning and life easier for student nurses and teachers in registered and practical nurse programs, graduating nursing students preparing for exit exams, new graduate nurses preparing for NCLEX-RN® and NCLEX-PN® exams, experienced international graduates preparing for the CGFNS® exam and other medical and allied health students that will find it useful. The common denominator that each of these groups have is the struggle to review an overwhelming volume of complex nursing information, and then to remember it after the struggle! Recall of information must occur prior to experiencing success on exam items, NCLEX®, or clinical practice.

Nursing Made Insanely Easy continues to use the visual approach to learning while linking the concepts to the current NCLEX® Standards. We are so pleased that you have enjoyed the mnemonics and images over the years. We are excited to bring you the 7th edition! Each of the tools and techniques has been written and designed based on current NCLEX® Standards. Many of our images and tools have been updated and added to reflect changes in current practice. In this 7th edition, we have also reorganized the concepts, so that the most important (according to National Council of State Boards of Nursing research) come first in the book. Our goal is to assist you in working "Smarter" versus "Harder".

Our experience with thousands of learners each year has helped us develop images and strategies that accelerate the learning process. The format is insanely easy! On the left page is the "bottom line information" about the concept. The "image or memory tool" is on the right page. This format incorporates both the principles of Accelerated Learning and Cognitive Learning Theory by using visual images and/or mnemonics to simplify and transfer volumes of complex information into the long-term memory.

A little background on Accelerated Learning may be useful as you proceed forward and learn how you can optimize your learning and memory by engaging both the left and right side of your brain. The left side of your brain is analytical, logical, linear, and includes rote memory. The right side of your brain involves images, visual, imagination, and is musical. *Nursing Made Insanely Easy, 7th Edition* uses several techniques to engage the whole-brain to learn and think about concepts. These tools and techniques will help you with associations to assist in transferring the information into the long-term memory. As you review the tools, remain active in the process and write down ideas you may also have. Remember, color activates the brain activity and the right brain activity is increased with music. Let's get the colored pencils or crayons out, and get active with our learning! *Remember, if the body isn't moving, the brain isn't grooving!* Turn on some soft music, preferably music at a beat of 60/min. This will also assist with retention of newly reviewed information.

The outcome for Cognitive Learning Theory focuses on transferring information from the working memory to the long-term memory for retrieval when answering questions or involved in direct nursing care. The key to finding the right file in your long-term memory is to review the simple but clever tools and techniques such as acronyms, diagrams, jingles, sayings, images, etc. that we have developed to assist you in remembering complex information. After simplifying the complex concepts or information, then this information can be applied to complex clinical decision-making. Information that is read or heard, but not learned is only filed superficially, if at all, and will soon be lost.

We hope you enjoy the book as much as we have loved and enjoyed working on this. With the use of accelerated learning tools linking the concepts to the current NCLEX® Standards, there are two powerful words that describe the outcome when you apply the tools used in this book, NCLEX® SUCCESS! Enjoy your journey!

Loretta Manning and Sylvia Rayfield

Acknowledgments

We wish to express our appreciation to both our families for their never ending support and love, while we developed this book.

- A special thank you to my husband for his tolerance, support, and love as we continue to juggle family, business, travel, and creating.

- A special thank you to my precious daughter, Erica Manning, who remained flexible and supportive during this project.

- A special thank you to my wonderful mother, Juanita Shera, who inspires me daily.

- A special thank you to Teresa Davidson, our dear friend, artist, computer guru, and the genius who takes our words and ideas and interprets them into meaningful and sometimes hilarious images. She has been with me from the first edition of each of our books. She is always calm and very supportive, even when I make the last-minute change prior to sending to the printer.

- Jennifer Robinson, Project Director of I CAN Publishing®, Inc., who is our friend and lifeline in our project development and distribution center. Thank you for keeping me laughing and your ongoing support.

- Kelly Cain, Administrative Director of I CAN Publishing®, Inc., who is our friend and keeps us organized as we juggle creating books and managing a business at the same time.

- Mary Jo Zazueta, our dear friend and book designer, who takes our sloppy drafts and transforms them into a book.

- Our associates in Sylvia Rayfield and Associates, Inc., who make the words and images come to life when they present them in NCLEX® reviews

- Our contributors (students, teachers, and friends) who see worth in our work and want to be a part of it.

*Dedicated with love to nursing students, educators,
and practicing nurses in the United States and abroad.*

*What we ARE communicates
far more eloquently than anything
we can say or do.*

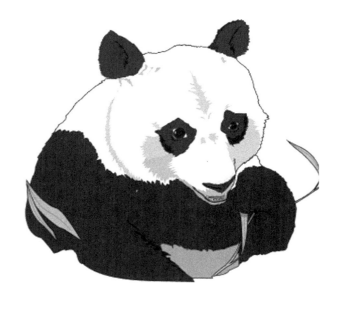

MANAGEMENT

"Managing your time without setting priorities is like shooting randomly and calling whatever you hit the target."

PETER TURLA

Prioritizing

We want to introduce you to "MERRY MANAGER," a nurse manager, that will accompany you on your journey throughout these first two chapters. As you can see by looking at her, she is positive both in her management style as well as in her thinking. She is outcome oriented and always attempts to understand the concerns of her nursing staff. "MERRY" is indeed a nurse leader that every nurse wants to emulate. Thank you for joining us as we begin our journey through this "INSANELY EASY" and FUN book!

The role of the RN has continued to develop and expand, and the management of care has become more important. New concepts have been added to this chapter because of the increased emphasis with management on the NCLEX®. Each of these management tools has been developed within the structure of the NCLEX® Standards and with a focus on client safety.

A major part of providing safe nursing care is to be competent at prioritizing. Nurses are faced daily with the challenge of which client should be assessed first or which nursing action should be implemented first. The keys to this process are to identify which client is most unstable and changing and/or which client is at a higher risk for developing complications. Another component of prioritizing may be that the NCLEX® presents you with a client situation, and you have to decide what would be the first nursing action. Most nurses will agree that the NCLEX® is full of priority questions. There may be several ways questions are worded to evaluate nursing priorities. Here are some examples:

"What is the priority nursing action?"
"What is the best nursing action?"
"What should the nurse implement first?"

The sole purpose of the NCLEX® is to determine that the nurse can provide safe care for the clients by identifying the most important nursing action to be implemented. You will find the options all look correct in these questions, but one of these actions should be initiated prior to the others. Critical thinking is so important in answering these questions!

A tool to simplify this process and help you learn effective prioritization strategies for test questions can be found on pages 4-7. The mnemonic "**PRIORITIES**" will assist you with the process of prioritizing.

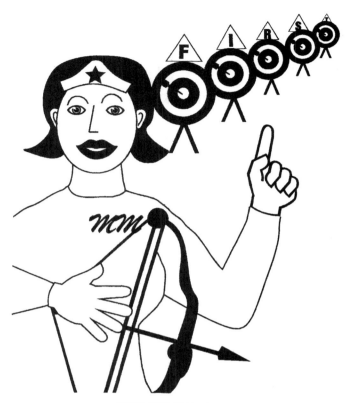

©2002 I CAN Publishing, Inc.

MERRY MANAGER is our STAR manager, because she has the qualities that we believe are so important in any manager.

    S STRENGTH to grow, help and allow others to grow

    T THE "HAPPINESS FACTOR" (comfortable in her own shoes, is not a victim and does not blame)

    A A VISIONARY that can think "out of the box"

    R REACTIVE LAST, proactive first

PRIORITIZATION STRATEGIES FOR TEST QUESTIONS

The definition of prioritizing is to select the client who is most likely to experience problems or ill effects if not taken care of first. The question that nursing graduates are faced with is, *"How can I prioritize when all of the clients need to be assessed FIRST?"* We have organized several strategies below using the mnemonic **"PRIORITIES"** to assist with answering test questions.

- **P** **Prioritize: Assess, the first step in the Nursing Process.** The nursing process provides a basis for your decisions on test questions just like it does in clinical. The first step in the Nursing Process is to *assess*; however, Do NOT jump on the answer of *assessment*! If *assessments* were given already in the stem of the question, the answer would *not be to assess*! If there were no *assessments* given in the stem, then indeed the priority would be to *assess*.

- **R** **Review if Maslow's Hierarchy of basic needs is the priority.** Remember, physiologic needs is a higher priority than teaching or psychosocial. The ABCs (airway, breathing, circulation) are the critical physiologic needs which are also at the base of Maslow's Hierarchy. This also applies to questions evaluating the psychosocial need. While these needs have not changed, do remember that The American Heart Association has changed the sequence of CPR from "ABC" to "**CAB**"; External **C**ardiac compressions, **A**irway, **B**reathing.

- **I** **Identify the client who is unstable or highest risk for developing complications.** When the nurse has several clients to provide care for, the ABCs are critical physiologic needs. Oxygenation is an immediate concern if physiological changes (i.e., vital signs, skin color, O_2 saturation, or change in the client's mental status such as confusion) indicate hypoxia. Selecting "airway", however, is NOT always the best answer. For example, if a client has been depressed, and starts presenting with more energy, giving away favorite possessions, and has a plan to hurt self, the priority of care is **SAFETY** due to the risk for suicide. Let's say the alternative option in this question is to select a client with COPD who is asymptomatic; the answer is still the client who is at risk for suicide. This is an acute safety issue, and the client with COPD is chronic with no new symptoms. *(Note, this strategy went back to Maslow's hierarchy of basic needs.)* Do NOT read into the question, and give client an airway problem if this is NOT an issue!

O **Organize priority nursing interventions based on the key concepts.** If the stem of the question provides you with assessment data, then it will be important to analyze and determine what is the priority concept or issue of concern. The key concept or issue will help you decide what the priority actions are to implement. Is the question about Maslow's hierarchy of needs, or the ABCs, or Physiological or Psychosocial needs, and/or Management of Care **"RISK"**?

- **R** Recognize limitations of staff members
- **I** Infection control
- **S** Safe medication administration
- **K** Keep client/environment safe *(falls, equipment, etc.)*

R **Remember to think about what is the desired outcome.** If a nursing action has already been implemented in the stem of the question, then the question may be asking you to determine if the desired outcome was met, or to evaluate the effectiveness of the care or action (i.e., desired outcome of a medication given). Always connect the desired outcomes to the information in the stem of the question. For example, if a client with CHF has bilateral rales and receives Lasix, the desired outcome is the lungs will be clear on auscultation. Urine output > 30 mL/hour is not the desired outcome.

I **Identify standard of practice (scope of practice, wrong orders, interactions, etc.).** Scope of practice and standards of practice are often the focus of the questions. The question may be asking if the standard of practice was met. It may be asking if the nurse needs to intervene, or what care is appropriate to delegate, or did the administration of medications follow "The 8 Rights to Medication Administration" (i.e., lack of appropriate client identification), or the need to question an order (i.e., an order for a nonselective beta blocker for a client with asthma).

T **Trend, compare and contrast client's response (interventions, medications, etc.).** Information in the stem of the question or in the distractors (options) may require you to compare and contrast current assessments to previous ones. You may need to determine if there is a trend, and if it is trending towards the desired outcome. For example, B/P was 176/89 and is now 135/78 after receiving a beta-blocker indicating there is a trend to the desired outcome. In contrast to this, another trend may be indicating a potential complication for a post-op client such as the HR was 70 BPM, RR was 14/min, and now the HR is 104 BPM and the RR is 24/min. This may be indicating a problem with bleeding requiring an intervention to prevent further complications from occurring. *Anyone can recognize clients are in trouble after they have crashed and present with a low blood pressure, cyanosis, etc.; however, the goal is to PREVENT this through excellent assessment skills and wise clinical decision-making.*

I **Infection control.** This is very important to the safety of clients and healthcare personnel. The test questions may ask the following: *What are the necessary infection control precautions for prevention and spread of the disease, to include how to avoid communicable diseases or even activities such as room placement, hand washing, steps to donning personal protective equipment (PPE), etc.*

E **Environmental safety "RISK."** As the nurse manager of care, you must manage the "RISK" to help ensure client SAFETY. *(Refer to "O" above for review of "RISK".)* Reduction of hazards in the environment may include fall/accident prevention such as bed position, use of assistive devices, rugs, cords, etc., or could include identifying a client who is at risk for suicide. Questions may ask about safety situations in both the home and the acute care setting. See "SAFE EQUIPMENT" on p. 92-93.

S **Synthesize all the information and review.** Here are some more helpful strategies. **ACUTE before CHRONIC** (i.e., is the client actively bleeding or does client have a chronic pulmonary condition and presenting with normal symptoms for their condition?) **EARLY versus LATE** is another strategy to use when you are saying to yourself, *"All of these clients are bleeding or have pre-eclampsia or have an infection. How do I prioritize these?"* It is very easy! Ask yourself, *"If the client is bleeding, is he/she experiencing early or late symptoms of bleeding? Early or late signs of shock?"* (OR) *"If the obstetrical client is presenting with hypertension, peripheral edema, and proteinuria, would this be a concern: are these early or late signs of preeclampsia? Yes, but the second client has a headache, blurred vision, and epigastric pain!"* You know these are LATE, and require an immediate intervention! Another priority strategy is if all of the clients are vomiting or having diarrhea, remember the **"IC"** clients will be the priority, "Geriatr**IC** or Pediatr**IC**"! If they are both included, then the lab values, vital signs, time period for vomiting/diarrhea, would assist in the decision making process.

PRIORITIES

P rioritize: Assess, the first step in the Nursing Process

R eview if Maslow's hierarchy of basic needs is the priority; review ABCs

I dentify the client who is unstable or highest risk for developing complications

O rganize priority nursing interventions based on the key concepts

R emember to think about what the desired outcome is

I dentify standard of practice (scope of practice, wrong orders, interactions, etc.)

T rends, compare and contrast client's response (interventions, medications, etc.)

I nfection control

E nvironmental safety—"RISK" (equipment, risk for falls, suicide, etc.)

S ynthesize all the information and review

©2014 I CAN Publishing, Inc.

"Trending" Helps Prevent Complications

BODY SYSTEM	TRENDS TO MONITOR FOR PREVENTING COMPLICATIONS
Cardiovascular (CV)	Vital signs, hemodynamics, O_2 saturation, sounds, EKG
Respiratory	RR, breath sounds, cough, secretions, O_2 saturation
Neurological/Psychosocial	Neuro checks, Glasgow coma scale, emotional/social changes
Neurovascular	Pulse, pain, pallor, paralysis, paresthesia
Elimination	I & O; specific gravity, weight; drainage from tubes*, wounds
Integumentary	Skin breakdown (Braden Scale); healing (PUSH Tool)
Drug	System changes (i.e., CV, Respiratory, Neurological, I&O); labs
Disease	System changes specific to disease (i.e., angina-ECG changes)
Diagnostic Test	O_2 saturation, EKG; Electrolytes; Serum glucose
Gastrointestinal	Bowel sounds, constipation/diarrhea, N/V, abdominal girth

*Several trends you may consider to monitor with drainage are the "**COLOR**":

Color and consistency of drainage
Output changes in amount of ↑ or ↓
Look at vital signs/hemodynamics to evaluate for loss of fluid
Odor of Drainage
Review if equipment is working and operated appropriately

I CAN TESTING HINTS: The key to answering questions evaluating your understanding of when to intervene with trends and complications is to compare and contrast all the options. During this process, always ask yourself, *"Is this assessment or clinical finding an expected or an unexpected outcome (s)?"* For example, if the urine output is orange after taking Rifampin, this is not a trend/complication and is an expected outcome. If the client complains of a headache after taking nitroglycerin, this is not a trend/complication, but an expected outcome. Another question to ask yourself, *"Is the client presenting with early or late signs of a complication, such as shock, ICP, etc.?"* Do NOT wait for the urine output to be < 30 mL/hr or RR to be < 12/min. Monitor the "**TRENDING**" and intervene! This is a must for SAFE nursing care! You CAN do this!

TRENDING

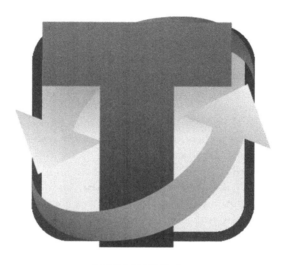

T he vital signs; hemodynamic values

R espiratory assessments

E valuate cardiac assessments; emotional

N eurological; neurovascular

D rainage, intake and output

I ntegumentary

N ote: trending with any assessments or changes related to a specific drug, disease, diagnostic test, diagnostic procedure

G astrointestinal assessment

"Infor Matics"

Confidentiality is one priority when documenting electronically. It is important to **log off when the nurse walks off**. It is important to **click "submit" when entering data** and to **hide the screen when the nurse is working**. Healthcare professionals are responsible to maintain confidentiality of client's health information in accordance with the HIPAA regulations.

When the nurse is utilizing information resources to enhance the care provided to a client, the facts should only come from **approved digital resources and e-books**. "INFOR" on the right page will summarize "The DO's" to documentation.

"MATICS" on the right page will assist you in organizing "THE DON'TS" to documentation. It is important **not to delay** this process and keep current with the documentation. **All data is confidential**, so no breaching of confidentiality is ever appropriate. The **social networking site or any online format should NEVER have client data entered**. It is **NEVER acceptable to take pictures of the client** with the smart phone. *(Only if the client provides consent.)* **Copying or pasting data is out**. It is **never appropriate to share your password**.

When applying this standard to test questions, remember the importance of intervening when confidentiality has been breached by staff members. Client confidentiality is a nursing legal and ethical responsibility. "**INFOR MATICS**" will assist you in organizing *"The Do's and Don'ts"* for providing care within the legal scope of practice regarding computer documentation and the use of information technology when enhancing the care provided to a client.

INFOR MATICS

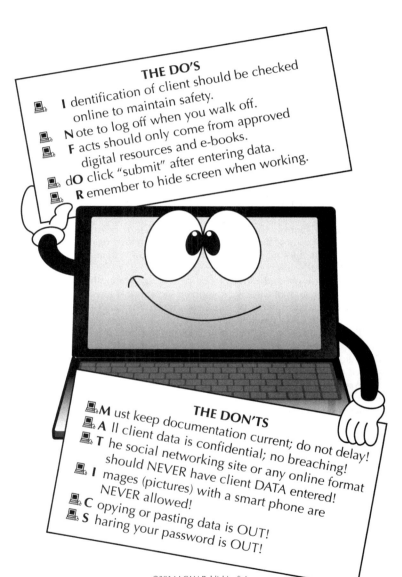

THE DO'S
- **I**dentification of client should be checked online to maintain safety.
- **N**ote to log off when you walk off.
- **F**acts should only come from approved digital resources and e-books.
- d**O** click "submit" after entering data.
- **R**emember to hide screen when working.

THE DON'TS
- **M**ust keep documentation current; do not delay!
- **A**ll client data is confidential; no breaching!
- **T**he social networking site or any online format should NEVER have client DATA entered!
- **I**mages (pictures) with a smart phone are NEVER allowed!
- **C**opying or pasting data is OUT!
- **S**haring your password is OUT!

©2014 I CAN Publishing®, Inc.

Provide and Receive Report On Assigned Clients: What is SBAR?

"**SBAR**" is a standardized communication technique for today's healthcare professional. The standardized communication tool helps ensure client safety by using a structured format for healthcare providers to communicate with one another. The outcome of using the SBAR tool is efficiency and accuracy in communication.

"**SBAR**" was developed by the US Navy as a communication technique that could be used on nuclear submarines. SBAR was introduced into healthcare settings in the late 1990s as part of its Crew Resource Management training curriculum. Since that time, SBAR has been adopted by hospitals and care facilities around the world as a simple and effective process to standardize communication between healthcare providers.

Here is an example of a call from the nurse to a healthcare provider using the SBAR: *(Let's see if this sounds familiar to you!)*

Introduction: HCP's name, this is *Nurse's name, RN*; I am calling from the medical/surgical unit at Hospital Success.

Situation: Here is the situation: *Client's name* is having complaining of increased shortness of breath. The O_2 sat has decreased from 97% to 91%, the respiratory rate has increased from 18 to 26/min at rest, and the temperature is 100.5° F orally. The pulse is 88 bpm and her B/P is 135/76. There are scattered rales throughout the lower lobes of the lungs bilaterally, and she now has a productive cough of thick yellow-green secretions. I have started O_2 at 4L/min, raised the head of the bed, and encouraged the client to cough and deep breathe at least every two hours.

Background: The supporting background information is that she came to the hospital with complaints of shortness of breath with activity. She is reporting that she has had a bad cold for several weeks. The current symptoms started this morning when she got up to the bathroom.

Assessment: My assessment of the situation is that client may be developing a respiratory infection.

Recommendation: I recommend that *Client's name* may need a chest x-ray for diagnosis along with a sputum culture. We also need a CBC because one has not been ordered since admission.

HCP Response: Thank you for the call. I hear that your *Client's name* is experiencing some respiratory distress. I agree with your recommendation to get a chest x-ray. I am also writing an order for the CBC and the sputum culture. Please keep the O_2 on to keep the O_2 sat above 95%. Call me when you have the results of the chest x-ray.

Read back: You would then read back the orders to the HCP for accuracy. If it was a phone order, you would need to follow the institution's policy for phone orders (it usually requires a second person on the phone).

Hand-offs or the process of passing on specific information about clients from one caregiver or one team member to another has been identified in the past as being a major factor in causing harm to clients. This harm can be prevented by effective communication. The Joint Commission on Accreditation of Hospitals has added, "standardized communication" to the Patient Safety Goals and recommends SBAR as a best practice.

SBAR

Situation—What is going on with the client? A concise statement of the problem.

Background—What is the background information that is pertinent to the situation?

Assessment—What did you find? Analysis and considerations of options.

Recommendation—What action/recommendation is needed to correct the problem? What do you want to happen for this client?

Adapted From *The Eight-Step Approach To Teaching Clinical Nursing*
Original Author: Michael Leonard, Physician Coordinator of Clinical Informatics at Kaiser Permanente

©2014 I CAN Publishing®, Inc.

I CAN TESTING HINT: While you study for the NCLEX® and/or practice in clinical, the strategy for safe reporting is to commit this process to memory. It is as simple as 1, 2, 3, but the key is to practice this until it becomes a habit. "SBAR" is to team communication as CPR is to the life of a client!

Informed Consent

This informed consent is the process where the client is informed of the benefits, adverse effects, and the options for certain procedures and provides consent for a procedure to be done. When answering questions about this concept, the right page will assist you in organizing this information. It is important for the **nurse to witness** the client's signature to determine the **client competency, validate the client signature, and verify that the consent is voluntary.**

The nurse should **not witness the signature if the client does not have all the information to make an informed decision.** The client must **understand the benefits, risks,** and alternatives to the procedure. Since this is a legal document, the client **must be free from mind-altering drugs or conditions when signing the consent.** The client must be informed about who the **healthcare provider is that will be performing the procedure.** The client is **educated about the procedure** in terms the client can understand.

The consent can be withdrawn verbally or in writing. This can take place any time, even after the procedure has been started.

There are exceptions for obtaining an informed consent. One exception is when there are life-threatening emergencies or urgent situations. An informed consent may not be the priority due to the immediate urgency. Another example is when clients are 18 years of age and under, the consent typically requires a parent's signature. **The emancipated minor, however, would be an exception.** Definitions may vary, but typically this is a minor who is self-supporting and does not live at home. Mentally incapacitated individuals mandate the signature of the consent from a legal guardian or person specified in medical power of attorney.

I CAN TESTING HINT: The strategy for answering questions regarding this concept is to ensure the client has been provided an informed consent for treatment. The nurse is responsible for participating in obtaining the informed consent. It is NOT the nurse's role to educate the client regarding the surgical procedure or the steps to a diagnostic procedure because this is not within the scope of practice for the nurse.

CONSENT

Client competency is why the nurse witnesses signature, validates the signature, ensures consent is voluntary

Omit witnessing if client does not have all of the information to make an informed decision

Note, client understands the benefits and risks of the procedure

Signed while client is free from mind-altering drugs or conditions; consent is a legal document

Educated on alternatives to procedure; Emancipated minor: Definitions may vary, but usually this is a minor who is self-supporting and living away from home

Notes the healthcare provider performing the procedure

Taught procedure to the client in terms she/he can understand

SIGNED _____

HIPAA Privacy Rule

The Hippo looking around the privacy fence will assist you to remember the most common standards utilized by nurses to comply with the HEALTH INSURANCE PORTABILITY AND ACCOUNTABILITY ACT (HIPAA). While not all inclusive, the reminders on the next page affect hospitals, physicians and other provider offices, pharmacies, and many other entities that are privy to private information. These entities must, according to federal law, implement standards to protect and guard against the misuse of individually identifiable health information. Compliance with HIPAA standards allows nurses to provide care within the legal scope of practice.

THE HIPAA Privacy Rule provides federal protection for personal health information held by cover entities and gives clients an array of rights with respect to that information.

The Privacy Rule gives these rights over their health information? Health insurers and providers must comply with the client's right to:

- Ask to review and get a copy of health records.

- Have corrections added to health information.

- Receive a notice that tells the client how the health information may be used and shared.

The Privacy Rule sets rules and limits on who can look at and receive client health information. *The fence (Rule) is there to protect the Hippo. Our responsibility as a client advocate is to reinforce the rule and protect our clients.*

Reference: *Understanding HIPAA Privacy* (n.d.). U.S. Department of Health & Human Services. Retrieved from http://www.hhs.gov/ocr/privacy/hipaa/understaning/consumers/index.htm

HIPAA

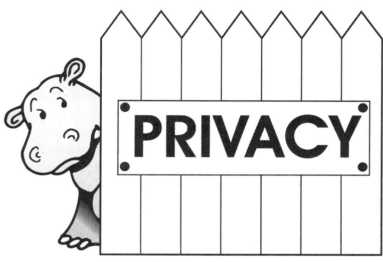

H ow to release information to health care workers that "need to know"

I mpermissible uses and disclosures result in lawsuits

P rotect privacy of individually identifiable health information

A rrange for sharing information with families in a discreet manner

A ccess by clients to medical records including the right to see and copy

Legal Aspects

DUE PROCESS–Hospitals, nursing homes, and other institutions where nurses practice have policies and procedures. For example, the little old lady climbs over her bedrail and falls on the floor. Due process is to pick her up, take her to x-ray, evaluate if anything is broken, complete and file an incident report, and notify her physician and family. If any of the steps identified as "the due process" are skipped, covered up, not charted or reported, there is a legal issue of negative proportions.

DECISION/ARBITRARY–The nurse's decision to refuse a family member visiting rights because she doesn't like their pierced nose and motorcycle jacket may be arbitrary and cause a legal issue.

DEPRIVATION OF PROPERTY–Nursing faculty that choose to give course outlines to all students during the first day of class, but refuse to share with the student who shows up the next day may be dealing with "deprivation of property".

DEPRIVATION OF CONFIDENTIALITY–The nurse that discusses one client with another may be dealing with a deprivation of confidence.

INTEGRITY TAKES US A LONG WAY
IN KEEPING US OUT OF COURT!

LEGAL ASPECTS

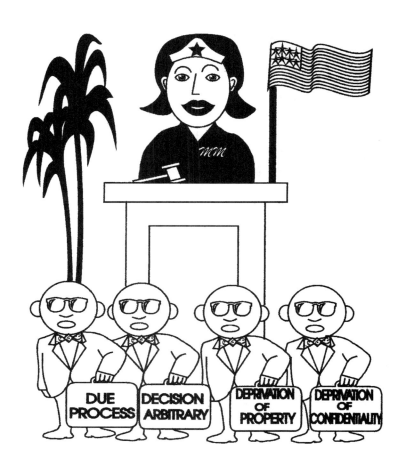

Delegation

The "DELEGATOR" delegates tasks but NOT responsibility. He tells his colleague how to be helpful to him. *(It is important to practice excellent communication skills or the colleague may become "stinky" like a skunk!)* Management issues are a part of the NCLEX® Test Plan. Delegating has always been a part of management, but the scope of practice laws vary from state to state regarding the meaning of delegation. These facts are a generalization and should generally keep the DELEGATOR out of trouble on the NCLEX®. Before we **TELL** someone to do something we know that we're usually legally responsible for the outcomes. These are the facts we need to know.

T **TAUGHT**–Has the individual been taught the skill, treatment or service?

E **EVALUATE**–Just because they have been taught how to do something doesn't mean they are competent to do it. Has their return demonstration been performed and documented?

L **LICENSE**–Does the individual have or need a license to do this task? Is it within their scope of practice?

L **LISTS**–What lists of standards of care (agency policies) are written regarding this task?

Remember–The DELEGATOR delegates the task
NOT THE RESPONSIBILITY!

DELEGATOR

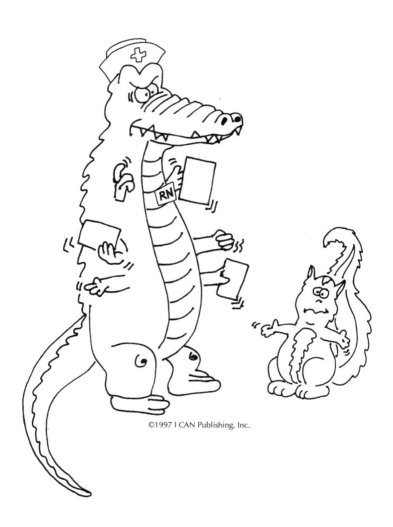

Ancillary Personnel Limitations

LPNs and UAPs are key players in the current healthcare team. In order to delegate appropriately, the RN must be aware of their scope of practice. Since it will take more space than we have to review what both of these groups can do, let's review the **PART** of care the LPNs cannot do and the UAPs **CAN'T** do. This is based on our interpretations of the various Nurse Practice Acts as reflected across the United States of America.

LPN

P **PLAN IN ISOLATION OF RN**–LPNs plan in collaboration with the RN. They will not do this in isolation of the RN.
PUSH IV MEDICATIONS–The current LPN standard is not to push IV medications.

A **ASSESS INITIALLY**–LPNs will participate in ongoing data collection; however, the RN is responsible for the initial assessment.
ANALYZE–LPNs do not make nursing diagnosis or analyze the nursing care.

R **REVIEW–EVALUATE IN ISOLATION OF RN**–The LPN is responsible for collaborating with the RN during the evaluation process.

T **TEACH INITIALLY**–While LPNs may be involved in the teaching process, they are not responsible for initiating the teaching process. This is the responsibility of the RN. The LPN may reinforce teaching.

UAP

C **CAN'T IRRIGATE A FOLEY**–The UAP should not conduct this intervention.
CAN'T MAKE CLINICAL DECISIONS–UAPs can make observations, but are not responsible for clinical decisions.

A **ANTICIPATE CLINICAL CHANGES**–UAPs should never be accountable for anticipating client's clinical changes.

N **NO INVASIVE PROCEDURES**–UAPs should not be accountable for any invasive procedures or specialized procedures.

T **TEACH**–UAPs are not responsible for teaching.

ANCILLARY PERSONNEL LIMITATIONS

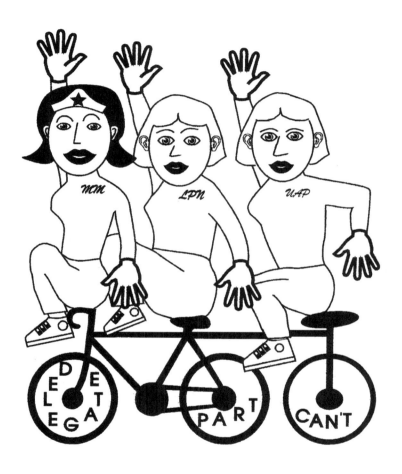

Tasks to Be Delegated to the UAP

"**BART**" (on the next page) will assist you in remembering what tasks can be delegated to the UAP (Unlicensed Assistive Personnel).

"**BART**" will assist you in also remembering that UAPs are a link to the strength and success of any nursing team. Nurses need to remember that nursing consists of many tasks that require critical decision-making, so this must be considered when delegating tasks to the UAP. For example, it is acceptable for the UAP to **bathe** a client; however, if the client is in acute distress or has any complications such as a decubitus ulcer, then the nurse may implement the bath due to the need for ongoing clinical assessments.

Ambulation that is routine can also be delegated to the UAP. Of course, if there are any complications, such as with hypotension, syncope, and/or post-op implications, then the nurse must be present for this intervention.

Routine tasks that do not require **critical thinking** such as obtaining a urine specimen, stool for blood, etc. are acceptable to delegate to the UAP. It will be the nurse who will make clinical judgments and decisions based on the data. A great rule to follow for delegation is to delegate tasks that have identified guidelines. Tasks that are unchanging, have systematic guidelines, and are used for stable clients can typically be safely delegated. Feeding, bathing, collecting urine specimens, and assisting with ambulating are a few examples of these tasks.

TASKS TO BE DELEGATED TO THE UAP

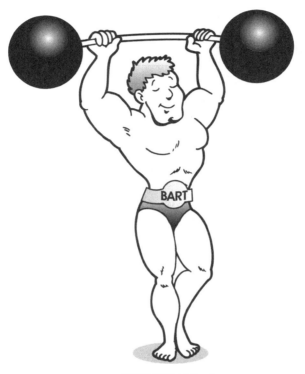

B aths (Routine and uncomplicated)

A mbulation

R outine tasks

T asks that do not require critical thinking

Nurses Who Float Between Units

The *"nurse float"* will assist you in remembering how to decide which nurse to send to a unit for a designated shift due to shortages in staffing. When making a decision on who to send to another unit, it is important to consider the **functions** of the unit such as the type of client who will be requiring assessment, planning, and evaluating. Nursing judgment cannot be delegated. The nurse must **look** for expected outcomes with assignments which indicate that it would be safe to send a nurse to provide care for this stable client. In addition to the outcomes, it is important to evaluate the clinical condition. **Omit** delegating **specialized care** to nurses who float to a new unit to assist when staffing is short. For example, if a medical surgical nurse floats to the Pediatric Unit, it would not be appropriate to delegate an infant who is in Bryant's traction to this nurse since this traction is specific to pediatrics. The **acuity** of the client must also be considered. The more unstable a client is with numerous medications, numerous systems involved in the medical condition, and unexpected outcomes, the less likely it will be that this is who will be delegated to the floating nurse. The **age** of the client is another consideration when delegating to a nurse coming in from another floor. The younger and older a client is, the quicker the clinical findings can change. If a medical surgical nurse is being pulled to the Pediatric unit, then the appropriate age of client for this nurse would be an older child versus a newborn or infant. This developmental stage has very specific clinical assessment findings that are unique to this group. If the nurse had not worked with this young stage of development, then it is a possibility that they may not remember the specific information. Always consider the **accountability** an issue when delegating. One of the major considerations when delegating is to make certain that the nurse has appropriate knowledge to implement the **tasks** that are delegated. It is a great idea to be knowledgeable of your institution's orientation clinical check off sheet. This will provide you with a compass to guide you in the appropriate direction when it comes to delegating to a nurse who is floating from another unit.

NURSES WHO **FLOAT** BETWEEN UNITS

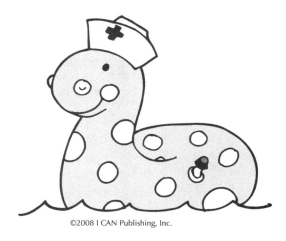

F unctions of assessment; planning, evaluating nursing judgment cannot be delegated

L ook for expected outcomes with assignments
ook at clinical condition of client

O mit specialized care

A cuity, accountability and age must be considered

T asks (knowledge required)

Tasks That Can Be Delegated to the New Graduate

The new graduate can provide safe care to the client who has **expected outcomes and is stable**. The new graduate must have the **skills and knowledge necessary** to provide safe care. The new graduate should **not be assigned a new admission** or should not be responsible for the **initial assessments** for a new client until a baseline has been established. The new graduate should **not have to coordinate many disciplines, services, agencies,** etc. during an admission, transfer, or discharge.

I CAN TESTING HINT: This strategy will assist you in answering a question that evaluates how to *"Assign and supervise care provided by others (e.g., LPN/VN, assistive personnel, new graduate, etc.")* or *"Provide care within the legal scope of practice".*

The strategy for answering questions regarding what can be delegated to the new graduate is to remember **"expected outcomes"** and the **"skills and knowledge"** the new graduate has currently. Any new client or clients who require a lot of coordination with a multidisciplinary team would not be appropriate for the new graduate!

GRAD

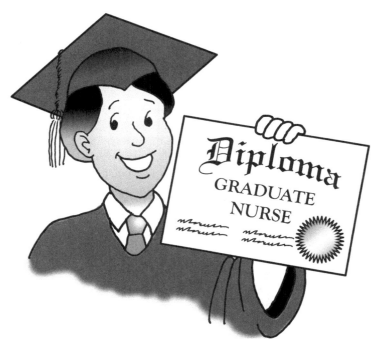

G ive assignment to the client who has expected outcomes and is stable

R eady with necessary skills and knowledge

A dmission and assessments that are NOT new or initial

D o NOT have to coordinate many disciplines, services, agencies, etc.

Do Not Delegate What You "Teach!"

We have reviewed *"The Scope of Practice"* by reviewing the nursing care that is appropriate to delegate to the UAP, LPN, GRAD, and Floating Nurses. We also reviewed the exceptions of care for the LPN, and the care that cannot be provided by the UAP. "BART" was a review for the care the UAP can provide.

Now, we want to summarize and review an easy strategy to assist you in remembering the care that should NOT be delegated by the RN. Remember, **DO NOT DELEGATE WHAT YOU "TEACH"**! Refer to the right page to review CONTRAINDICATIONS TO DELEGATION. The principles of teaching, "A PIE", are the scope of practice for the RN. The activities of *assessing*, *planning*, reviewing physical and psychological comfort, *implementing*, and *evaluating the teaching plan* are an integral part of **client teaching and should NOT be delegated.**

Critical thinking, clinical decision-making, and judgment should NEVER be delegated. The RN is the one with the knowledge and critical thinking skills to analyze a situation, prioritize the appropriate information, move forward with a clinical decision, evaluate the outcome, and revise the plan as necessary.

The RN should also be the one to help coordinate interdisciplinary personnel due to the complexity involved. **Interdisciplinary coordination should NOT be delegated** to the LPN, GN, or UAP, since this process usually involves a client whose care is complex. This process of coordinating involves teaching, assessing, planning, implementing, evaluating, collaborating and coordinating numerous disciplines to provide the optimum level of care for the client.

I CAN TESTING HINT: The key to answering these questions successfully is to delegate stable clients with the most predictable outcome and clients who are least likely to have changes in condition requiring critical nursing judgments. Tasks that have specific guidelines are the best ones to delegate.

The RN is the one to lead the "TEACHING" and "DELEGATING"! The RN has the critical thinking skills to provide care for clients who are unstable and have changes in their clinical presentation with unpredictable outcomes. **DO NOT DELEGATE UNSTABLE CLIENTS**, and **"DO NOT DELEGATE WHAT YOU TEACH"**!

TEACH

DO NOT DELEGATE WHAT YOU "TEACH"!

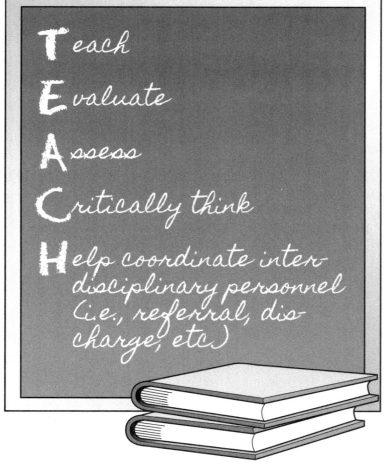

Cost Effectiveness

"MERRY MANAGER" is responsible for managing both the quality of nursing care as well as the financial budget. It is imperative for her as well as all nurses to be cost effective. **SAVE** will assist you and "MERRY" in reviewing some strategies to achieve the outcome of cost effectiveness.

S **STAFF**–When making assignments, the selection of the appropriate nursing personnel is a key component in being cost effective. If an LPN is able to provide the nursing care safely and efficiently, it is not financially wise to assign the RN to the same client.

A **AVOID DUPLICATION**–This will also assist in providing cost effective care. For example, if a department has an unlicensed nursing personnel scheduled to run arterial blood gases to the lab, but the individual is only busy during the morning; it is wise to share this staff member with another unit and share in the cost.

V **VIEW INFECTION**–"AN OUNCE OF PREVENTION IS WORTH A POUND OF CURE". Infections are expensive! Wash those hands and practice standard precautions.

E **EDUCATE**–Discuss the budget with the nursing staff. *(An informed consumer is a smart shopper.)* AN INFORMED STAFF MEMBER CAN BE A SMART MANAGER!

COST EFFECTIVENESS

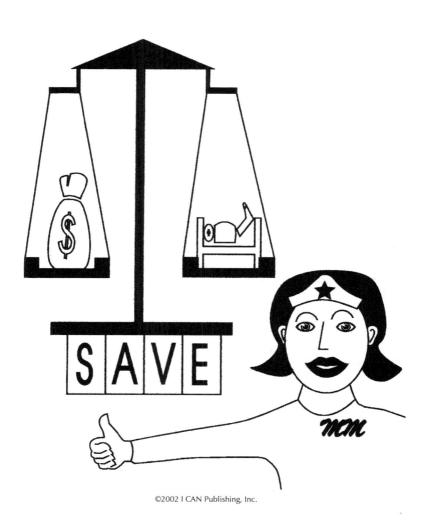

Management: Safety

Management is currently the largest piece of the NCLEX-RN® Exam and further points can be found in the National Council of State Boards of Nursing's *Detailed Test Plan* under Safe Effective Care. We have used the word **SAFETY** as an acronym to help you remember these key concepts. Each client must have a **system-specific assessment** before decisions are made regarding their care. We have placed these assessments at the beginning of each chapter. The manager is responsible for evaluating the staff and determining their skill in this area. **Accuracy of orders and assignments** will not be accurate without a client assessment.

Due to the complexity of the healthcare needs of clients today, it is imperative that the nurse knows what to do **first**. The setting of **priorities** contributes to the safe effective care of the client. We must diligently **evaluate the pharmaceutical products** that we administer. Many of our clients are taking medications for many years instead of many days. For this reason, we are responsible for teaching about the interactions of their drugs, foods and alternative complimentary agents. We must also be concerned about cost control. Why administer a high cost medication if it is not going to have the desired effect?

Speaking of cost containment-infection has a devastating effect on cost. This is not just dollar cost, but cost in well-being, family dynamics, length of time to recover, and the list goes on and on. **Teach** and practice **infection control** tops the list of hospital nightmares and the NCLEX-RN® Test Plan.

Most of us know what c**Y**a means. In this instance, we are meaning to cover your assets. The things listed under the last heading of SAFETY are the reasons for law suits. Managers are responsible for safe effective care of their clients and their staff and must be unremitting and constant in preventing these issues.

MANAGERS

S ystem-specific, focused assessment

A ccuracy of orders/assignments

F irsts—prioritize, especially in emergencies

E valuate pharmacology

T each and practice infection control

c**Y**a–cover your assets—identification, confidentiality, privacy, falls, suicide, drugs, electrical hazards, malfunctioning equipment, malfunctioning staff

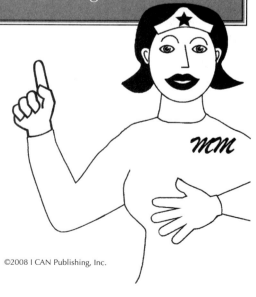

©2008 I CAN Publishing, Inc.

Accuracy of Orders

Just because a healthcare provider writes an order or gives a verbal order does not mean that we as nurses should carry out the order. We are professionals and must stand on our own two feet to determine if the order is right. We are legally responsible for our mistakes and our client if we administer the wrong medication or perform any treatment that is harmful to any person. For this reason, we must determine the accuracy of the order.

Our responsibility is to think critically and always be alert for potential errors. We want the client to receive safe care that will assist in maintaining great blood flow to our client versus reducing circulation which may reduce it to a "**DRIP**." "**DRIP**" will assist you in remembering information about *"accuracy of orders."*

For example, is the **diagnostic test** appropriate for the client? If a client had diabetes mellitus for twenty years, along with renal impairment, then any diagnostic tests ordered requiring dyes should be questioned. If a client has an order for liver biopsy, but is currently bleeding due to alteration in coagulation studies, then this order would also be questioned. With this data, the order should be contraindicated. This is why it is so very important to ALWAYS assess the client or evaluate labs prior to any intervention.

A question the nurse always has to ask, "Is this procedure **right** for the client?" When the nurse **interprets the order**, it is imperative that the questions consistently asked include: "Is this order correct for this client? Are the abbreviations correct? Is the order clear?"

Pharmacology is a top reason for alterations in client safety during hospitalization. In order to understand the accuracy of orders, nurses must understand the action of the drug, the priority in nursing care, and the desired outcomes of the medication. Nurses must have an understanding of drug-drug, food-drug interactions, and medical conditions that may result in complications from specific medications.

Our client must be able to trust us to think about every incident. Put yourself in your client's place. If you suffered from the same disease, would the ordered medication be safe for you to take? Is the dose correct? Should you receive a medication if you have had a previous allergic reaction? Should your right leg be cut off if your left leg is the one with gangrene? Should you be given a breathing treatment if you have a broken finger?

The most important gift that we can give to our client is our full attention and our brain power. Think about what you are doing! The accuracy of orders will likely determine the client's well-being. Remember, it is one thing to be a critical thinker, but the key to delivering quality, safe, client care is to have the courage to clarify and verify any orders that may be inaccurate.

ACCURACY OF ORDERS

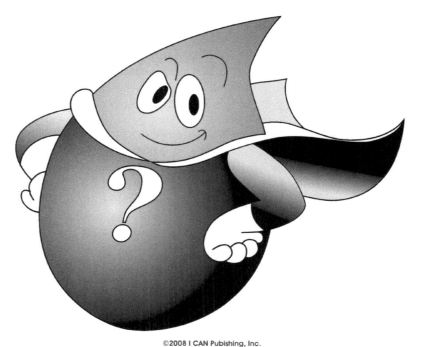

D iagnostic tests

R ight procedure

I nterpretation of order

P harmacology

Cover Your Assets (CYA)

Most of us have an idea what CYA means. For the purpose of this book, we are going to call it "COVER YOUR ASSETS"!

One of the most important assets that we have as a nurse is our nursing license. We cannot work as a nurse and take care of sick people unless we have this credential. Consequently, we must CYA to make sure we keep it.

Things that will cost our license include mistakes such as medication errors. If a client needs restraints, then it is imperative to manage these appropriately by having an order from the provider of care. It is also important for the nurse to document neurovascular checks. It is also important to document when the restraints were removed to allow for mobility and skin assessment. If a client falls, we can be sued for neglect and our license removed. Lack of confidentiality is a big problem that the nurse might be blamed for. Assigning clients to impaired staff (involved with drugs or alcohol) can turn into a crisis! Equipment that is broken and allows the client to be injured is serious trouble.

Being very present, paying attention to everything, caring, and CYA can keep us out of a "**MESS**."

CYA

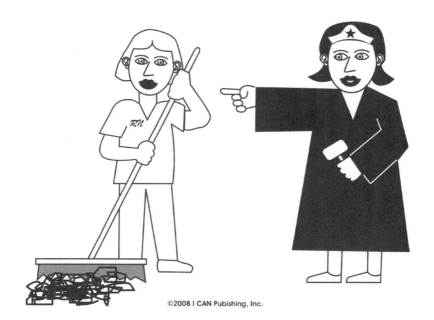

M edication errors
anage restraints

E nsure confidentiality, and identity

S afe equipment (prevent falls)
afe staff

S afe delegation
uicide assessment

Standard of Care
"Report Unsafe Care of Healthcare Personnel and Intervene as Appropriate"

Graduates have been asking us, *"How do we answer questions evaluating when to intervene with an LPN, UAP or any healthcare personnel who is performing care, and what exactly does this mean?"* This means that the nurse must intervene with the healthcare personnel if and when care is UNSAFE and not consistent with the "**STANDARD**" OF CARE. The standards of nursing include protecting the client from anyone in the healthcare setting who engages in unethical, illegal, or incompetent practices. Examples can include issues such as unreported medication errors; the nurse gives the wrong medication to the client and does not fill out an incident report; not administering necessary treatment to a client; lack of informed consent; differences in belief system involving abortion, organ procurement, and/or donation. A brief description of several of these unsafe clinical situations is outlined on the right page, and will be reviewed below.

- **S** **S**tandard of Care is not being followed: A client gets up to go to bathroom following a cardiac catheterization. The UAP limits fluids for a client after a procedure requiring dye.
- **T** **T**he position is incorrect for procedure/care: The nurse elevates the head of the bed for a client who is in hypovolemic shock. Client is positioned on left side after liver biopsy.
- **A** **A**ssessments indicate trend or complication not identified: A client with a T6 or higher spinal cord injury has not had a bowel movement for 3 days, and this assessment was ignored. (leading to autonomic dysreflexia)
- **N** **N**ot focusing on the lab data specific to meds, care, etc.: A client has an order for digoxin (Lanoxin) and furosemide (Lasix). When the nurse begins to administer meds, the client complains of leg cramps. The nurse gives medications with no action.
- **D** **D**ietary/fluid and electrolyte needs are being ignored: Client is taking furosemide (Lasix), but diet does not include foods high in potassium.
- **A** **A**cute vs. chronic: inappropriate prioritizing: After shift report, the nurse assesses the client with chronic lung disease who is stable before assessing the client who is 30 min post op following a coronary artery bypass grafting surgery.
- **R** **R**eviewing client identity prior to providing care; Reviewing and verifying inappropriate orders for meds, treatment, etc., are not done. The nurse does not identify client prior to administering a medication or going for a diagnostic test.
- **D** **D**oes not focus on client SAFETY: infection control, room placement, meds, etc. Client who is immunocompromised is placed in a room with a client who has varicella.
- **S** **S**cope of practice is not being followed: The nurse delegates discharge teaching to the LPN.

Substance abuse: The nurse comes to work after drinking alcohol.

STANDARDS

S tandard of Care is not being followed

T he position is incorrect for procedure/care

A ssessments indicate a complication not identified

N ot focusing on the lab data specific to meds, care, etc.

D ietary/fluid and electrolyte needs are being ignored

A cute vs. chronic: inappropriate prioritizing

R eviewing client identity prior to providing care; reviewing and verifying inappropriate orders for meds, treatment done or not done, etc.

D oes not focus on client SAFETY: infection control, room placement, meds, etc.

S cope of practice is not being followed; Substance abuse

©2014 I CAN Publishing®, Inc.

I CAN TESTING HINT: The NCLEX® and clinical practice are all about SAFE nursing care. The nurse is the leader of care and must intervene to promote **"STANDARDS"** versus allowing unsafe care to be practiced.

Recognize the Need For Referrals
Collaborate With Healthcare Members in Other Disciplines When Providing Care

"**DISCHARGE**" will assist you when answering questions or coordinating care for clients when they are discharged to home, rehab, long-term care, etc. This planning needs to begin with the admission of the client so timely referrals can be made. Many clients in the hospital today are older with chronic multiple-system complications and they require multiple medications, etc.

Let's simplify this process by beginning with: "**Do refer/collaborate if there are any physiological complications**". What do we mean by this? For example, these complications may include the 12 B's: "**B**reathing, **B**leeding, **B**lue (cyanotic), **B**lood clots, **B**owel, **B**ladder, **B**lood sugar, **B**rain (ICP/LOC ↓), **B**alance of fluid and electrolyte may be altered, **B**lanching of the skin may be altered, **B**othersome (pain), and/or **B**ruising. Now of course, as you make your assessment, it is important that you understand the clinical findings for each of these B's so you can recognize the need for intervention and/or referrals. *Referring and collaborating as necessary are a part of the standard, "Recognize signs and symptoms of complications and intervene appropriately when providing care"*. For example, if a post-op client was to present with an immediate clinical change that included a new onset of tachypnea, dyspnea, decrease in the O_2 saturation, and circumoral pallor, then it would be imperative to intervene, and notify the provider of care. Of course, we would reposition and focus on the client initially, and then collaborate with the provider of care.

"**Interdisciplinary care**" is an important component of referral/collaboration. Respiratory therapy, social services, dieticians, chaplains, counselors, and/or occupational therapists may need to be involved in the care, requiring a referral based on clinical needs. "**Safety**" for the client may create a need for an additional referral for home health if the client is going to be discharged and needs an environmental assessment at home. "**Equipment Education**" may result in a need for a referral regarding safe use and maintenance of the medical equipment (e.g. O_2, MDI, nebulizers, ventilators, etc.). If the client is being discharged on IV medications, dressing changes, etc., this may require further education and/or nursing support to optimize safe care. "**Community Resources**" may also be necessary referrals for clients and/or family members who are in need of CPR classes, a support group and/or use of additional community resources.

"**Health Promotion Activities**" may require collaboration/referrals to community healthcare nurses if there is a need for primary health prevention such as an up-to-date immunization(s), referrals for secondary health prevention i.e. a mammogram or colonoscopy and referrals for rehab for tertiary health prevention plans.

The need for "**Activity**" or an alteration in activity may also create a need for a referral for physical therapy or occupational therapy. "**Routine follow-up**" may also require referrals for regular primary healthcare visits.

"**Guidelines for meds and notifying the healthcare provider**" will facilitate the process for referrals and discharge teaching. Signs and symptoms of infection, respiratory distress, and/or characteristics of pain must be reported due to a potential complication, etc. It is important to collaborate with the provider of care to ensure the client has all the needed prescriptions and referrals to assist with the safe continuity of care of care when the client is "**DISCHARGED**".

DISCHARGE

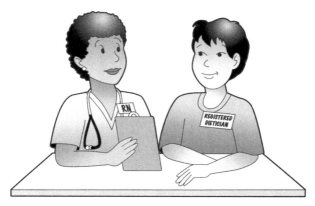

D o refer/collaborate if there are any physiological complications

I nterdisciplinary care

S afety

C ommunity resources

H ealth Promotion activities

A ctivity

R outine follow-up

G uidelines for meds, and notifying HCP, etc.

E quipment Education

How To Decide Which Client Should Be Discharged Early
From the Hospital When a Bed is Needed For an Emergency

CRITERIA	YES-DISCHARGE	NOT-DISCHARGE
Scheduled surgery in a.m. for stable client	X	
Telemetry, Diagnostic Tests, Clinical findings		
• Within Normal Limits (WNL)	X	
• Scheduled in AM	X	
• Dysrhythmias, Abnormal results		X
Acutely ill with new presenting symptoms		X
Chronic condition who is stable	X	
B's		
• Breathing issues		X
• Bleeding		X
• Bruising (New symptom)		X
• Blue (cyanosis)		X
• Balance of fluid and electrolytes	X	
• Balance of fluid and electrolytes altered		X
• Blood clots		X
• Blood sugar irregular		X
• Brain (LOC ↓)		X
Bothersome (Pain-new symptom)		X
Bladder		
(New symptom of incontinence, dysuria, etc.)		X
Bowel (New symptom of constipation)		X
Lab Values for medical condition and meds currently taking		
• Lab Values within normal range	X	
• Lab Values out of normal range		X
Evaluation of medications		
• Therapeutic level	X	
• Desired outcomes	X	
• Meds can be administered at home	X	
• New symptom of undesirable effect		X

"STABLE" *will assist you in making a decision on discharging early when a bed is needed.*

STABLE

S cheduled surgery for a client who is stable, and who is not acute can be discharged early

T elemetry, Diagnostic Tests, Any Data—if these clinical findings are WNL, then client can be discharged early

A cute versus chronic! A chronic client who is stable can be discharged early; an acute client CANNOT!

B leeding, bladder, bowel, blood clots, breathing, bothersome symptoms (pain)–NOT discharged early

L ab Values within normal range for client's medical condition

E valuation of meds indicate NO adverse effects; therapeutic levels, desired outcome; ELIMINATE discharging elderly client(s) if presenting with a NEW symptom; discharge normal developmental changes (i.e., presbyopia, keratosis, etc.)

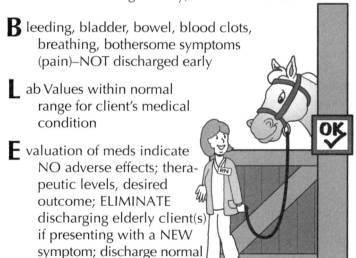

©2014 I CAN Publishing®, Inc.

Priority Topics For Teaching

This mnemonic on the right page has been developed to assist you in successfully answering NCLEX® questions regarding priority topics for teaching. For example, you may need to answer a question about a nurse going to an inservice to learn about a new piece of equipment. After returning to the nursing unit, the nurse is responsible for teaching the staff about this new piece of equipment. As you study, review equipment such as ventilators, Pleur-evac for chest tubes, a new ECG monitor, etc. Some other examples that may need to be taught include: a new drug, an infection control standard, or a new protocol for fall reduction. *(Refer to right page for other examples.)*

It is also very important for you to be able to apply the principles for education when you are answering questions about teaching. To simplify this, let's think of "**A PIE**" that is sweet and how much we enjoy the flavor after a nice meal. "**A PIE**" will assist you in recalling these principles and assist in making the teaching successful.

Assess–What do the staff need to know and do they perceive the need to learn the information? Are there any learning barriers? Assess the staff's readiness to learn and understand their learning preferences and barriers to learning.

Planning–The nurse needs to develop a plan to teach the staff this new information. This may include a demonstration, and then provide the staff with the opportunity to return a demonstration. Other strategies may include a short video with hands on practice; written material for review; an interactive presentation including the equipment or any of the topics outlined on the right page.

Physical and Psychological Comfort–It is important for the nurse who is leading the teaching to always consider the physical comfort of the learner(s). For example, if the teaching session takes place prior to lunch, and the staff are hungry then minimal learning will take place. If there are distractions within the environment, then this will also affect the learning process. Many staff experience anxiety and fear when presented with new information. Always attempt to start the teaching session by identifying or assessing what the staff knows about the topic. This will also decrease the anxiety prior to teaching.

Implementation–The information should be presented in a manner the staff will understand. Provide opportunities for discussion, feedback, demonstrations, etc. The more active the learner is the more they are likely to learn. Repetition is the mother of learning. Plan short sessions.

Evaluation–Return demonstrations are an excellent strategy for evaluating if a skill was accurately learned. Of course, a written quiz or verbal feedback includes additional strategies that may be used for evaluation.

EDUCATES

E quipment

D rugs

U se of new procedures

C reative management strategies

A new standard of care

T he appropriate infection control procedures

E ducate on safety and resources after discharge

S elf care; interdisciplinary support; Client SAFETY

©2014 I CAN Publishing®, Inc.

The 8 Rights to Medication Administration

(The "6 Rights" plus 2 Very Important Rights to Decrease Errors)

The nurses' responsibility in safely administering medication is influenced by several major factors. These include guidelines for safe medication administration, pharmacological implications of the medication, and the legal aspects of medication administration. The "5 Rights" to medication administration are what we are going to review here.

As you can see on the next page, these "5 Rights" include:
1. Right client or Who.
2. Right drug or What.
3. Right dosage or Which.
4. Right time or When.
5. Right route of administration or Where.

The 6th Right is the Right for the client to know about the medication and the Right to refuse. Clients must be taught how to safely take the med, the action of the med, and have the opportunity to refuse to take the medication. This is the right of the client!

We have included 2 other Rights that are imperative for safe medication administration. These include:
7. Right rationale/education—Why/Client education.
8. Right documentation—Write.

Nurses must not just implement the top "6 Rights", but must also understand the rationale (reason) for the client receiving the medication. If the client is receiving an antihypertensive medication and just came from dialysis with symptoms of hypovolemia, then would it be appropriate to administer this antihypertensive medication? You are so correct! Of course it would be UNSAFE! Even if you had initiated the "6 Rights", the client may develop more complications from the medication. Always understand the "WHY" prior to administering any medication! Client education is a must! The client needs to understand the reason it is being prescribed, how it should be taken, and what side effects may occur.

The 8th Right is documentation—WRITE. The medication must be accurately documented on the medication record in the chart. Medication errors are a major challenge for clients in hospitals. It is imperative that we initiate these "8 Rights" in order to practice safe medication administration.

THE 8 RIGHTS TO MEDICATION ADMINISTRATION

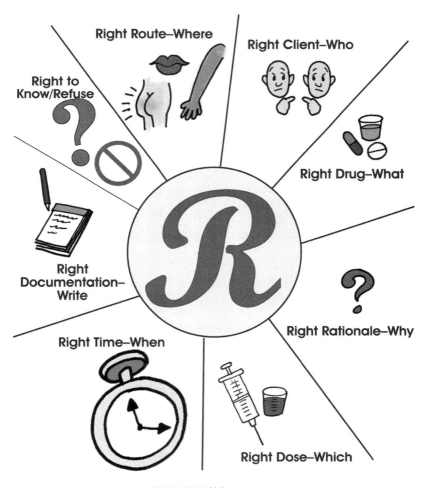

©2008 I CAN Publishing, Inc.

"In all this chaos, we found safety."
UNKNOWN

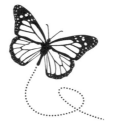

SAFETY & INFECTION CONTROL

Proper Identification

The Joint Commission requirements mandate two identifiers that can include the client's name on the armband, date of birth, or other person-specific identifier. If the client does not have an armband, one identifier may be the client's stated name, and the client's phone number, social security number, or address could serve as a second identifier. In a long-term care facility, behavioral care facility, or home care setting, client's photograph or visual recognition may be used as one identifier. For short-term clients, facilities with unstable staffing, and/or high-risk medications, the two-identifier requirements are necessary. The client does not have to state name as an identifier.

Many institutions are using bar-coded technology to identify clients. The identification band, any client items, and/or specimen will have a bar-code label. Medication administration, nutrition, and/or specimen collection will require client identification through the use of barcode technology if the institution has adapted this technology.

Proper identification should be appropriate to the individuals served and the healthcare setting. Variables that change such as room numbers or bed numbers are NEVER SAFE and/or approved client identifiers. Newborn nurseries will require a different identifier, since many newborns will have the same date of birth.

"**IDENTIFY**" will summarize this information on "PROPER IDENTIFICATION".

- **I** **I**dentifiers (2) are required.
- **D** **D**oes not have to state name as an identifier.
- **E** **E**valuate identification with med administration, specimen collection, and nutrition.
- **N** **N**ewborn nurseries, neonatal units–careful using birth date; many newborns have same.
- **T** **T**he client's photograph or visual recognition–used in long-term care facilities, etc.
- **I** **I**f no armband in place, then the client's stated name, date of birth, social security number, or phone number can provide second identifier.
- **F** **F**or short-term facilities, facilities with staffing challenges, and/or high-risk meds, two identifier requirements are necessary.
- **Y** **Y**es, if armband is on the floor/in the bedside table, this is not reliable. Get a new one!

PROPER IDENTIFICATION

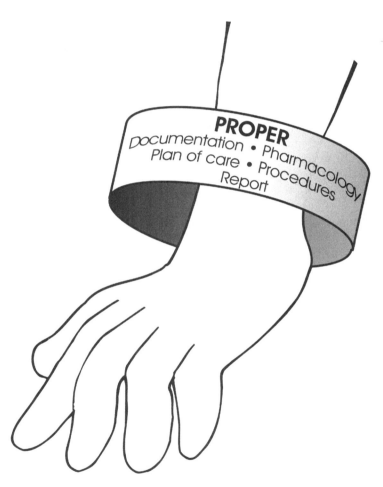

Assignment of Rooms

Nurses are responsible for identifying appropriate room placement for clients when they are being admitted to the hospital. The goal is decrease the **"RISK"** of complications from this process. Nurses and students have requested that we develop a technique to assist in organizing this process. **"RISK"** will assist you in organizing these placements.

If a client has internal **radiation** such as a radium implant, then the client should be placed in isolation to prevent injury to other clients. A client with an **infection** or who is immunocompromised should be placed in appropriate **isolation**. If a client has tuberculosis, varicella, or measles then airborne transmission-based precautions are important to initiate and follow. If a client has neisseria meningitis, mycoplasma pneumonia, streptococcal group A infections, or pertussis then it is important to follow droplet transmission-based precautions. Clients with easily transmitted infections by direct contact such as gastrointestinal, respiratory, skin, or wound should be placed in a private room and have contact transmission-based precautions initiated. If a client is immunocompromised (i.e., from chemotherapy, in preparation for a organ transplant, etc.), then it is important to protect the client from infections. The main point to remember is to consider infection with the selection of roommates for a client.

If a client doesn't have radiation (internal) or is not infected, then perhaps a major concern is with **safety**. Never place a combative or manic client with a depressed client or a client they could injure. If a client is at high risk for seizures due to pregnancy induced hypertension, then the client's room placement is going to be very important so there is not a lot of stimulation in the environment. Another consideration when placing clients in a room is the gender or **sex** of the client.

If none of the above issues are concerns for the client and the client is a child, then **knowing growth and development** is important to consider when placing the child with a roommate. For example, if a 6-year-old child has a fractured femur and there is another 6-year-old with a fracture or a post-op procedure with no infection, then this would be the best room placement due to the growth and developmental needs. If, however, there is another 6 year-old but the child has an infection, this would not be an appropriate roommate for the child due to the risk of transmitting the infection.

In review **"RISK"** will assist you in remembering how to select room assignments for clients.

ASSIGNMENT OF ROOMS

R adiation

I nfection/isolation

S afety, sex

K now growth and development

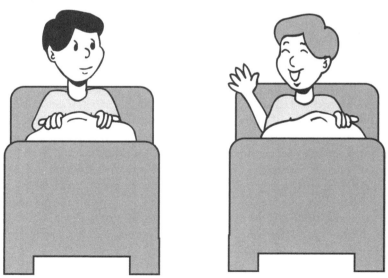

Hand Hygiene

Hand hygiene is the most single effective mechanism for the prevention of transmission of infection in the heathcare setting. **It must be performed prior to and after the use of gloves.** On the right page, "**HANDS**" will assist you in organizing the procedure for hand hygiene with soap and water.

Now that you have reviewed the right page, let's now review the procedure for using antiseptic cleanser. During the procedure of using antiseptic cleanser, the nurse should rub hands together covering all surfaces of the hands and fingers with the cleanser. The hands should be rubbed together until the cleanser is dry. If the hands are visibly soiled, then hand hygiene should be with soap and water

Hand hygiene procedures also include use of alcohol-based hand rubs (containing 60-95% alcohol) and use of antibacterial soap and water using friction for at least 15 seconds. After any contact with blood, body fluids, or excretions or wound dressings, hand hygiene is very important. Prior to performing an aseptic task such as accessing a port or preparing an injection, good hand hygiene is imperative. If hands will be moving from a contaminated-body site to a clean, then hand hygiene is necessary. Always remember, each time gloves are removed, hand hygiene must be performed. Every time a client is touched, hand hygiene is a must even if gloves will be worn. Prior to exiting the client's care area (room) after touching the client or immediate environment, hand hygiene should be performed again.

In addition to hand hygiene, additional prevention will assist in preventing the transmission of infection in the healthcare setting. Always consider all body fluids and blood from every client to be contaminated. When collecting specimens, the nurse should avoid contaminating the outside of the container. Needles and syringes should never be recapped. Household bleach in concentration of 1:100 to 1:10 is an effective germicide in cleansing the work surface areas.

Hand Hygiene must become a habit, so you can practice this without even thinking. This simple nursing action can save your client's life! Once again, this is the single most important and basic action for the prevention of transmission of infection.

Center for Disease Control and Prevention: *2007 Guideline for isolation precautions: preventing transmission of infectious agents in healthcare settings.* Retrieved from http://www.cdc.gov/hicpac/2007ip/2007isolationprecautions.html

HANDS

H andwashing should be done under water flow; wet hands and wrists under running water; hands and forearms lower than elbows

A ntibacterial soap—lather and wash hands using friction for at least 15 seconds

N ote, while rinsing hands under running water, maintain hands lower than elbows

D o NOT allow washed hands to touch inside of sink

S oap and water any time hands are visibly soiled; do not rub when drying; pat thoroughly

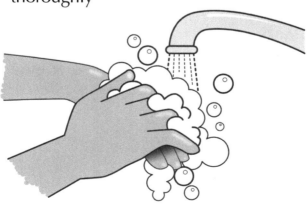

Standard Precautions

Infection control is one very important nursing activity! A major problem in hospitals today is healthcare-associated infections. Something as simple as washing hands (**LATHERING UP**) can significantly decrease infections. Clients, family members, and healthcare providers must understand (**GIVE EXPLANATION**) the importance of infection control. Meticulous attention to aseptic technique when cleaning (**ORIFICES**) is effective in decreasing infections. **VERY SPECIAL HANDLING** of secretions, used equipment, needles, soiled linens, etc. is also important for decreasing infections. Nurses must remember when providing care that **EVERYONE MAY BE INFECTED**. The major concern for the nursing staff is the client who is infected and is unaware. When giving shots, starting IVs, or assisting with invasive procedures, meticulous attention must be paid to **SHARP** needles.

THE KEY TO PRACTICING STANDARD PRECAUTIONS IS TO REMEMBER THE IMPORTANCE OF SAFELY HANDLING BLOOD AND BODY SECRETIONS!

In review, after hand hygiene remember GLOVES when practicing standard precautions.

G GLOVES

L LATHER UP

O ORIFICES

V VERY SPECIAL HANDLING

E EVERYONE MAY BE INFECTED

S SHARPS

Refer to the page 61 for a complete chart on Standard Precautions outlining recommended personal protective equipment based on nursing care.

GLOVES

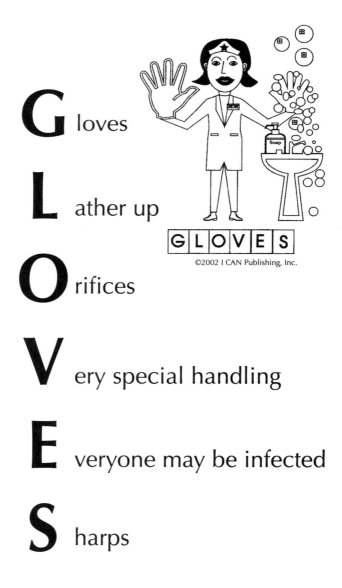

G loves

L ather up

O rifices

V ery special handling

E veryone may be infected

S harps

Standard Precautions

Standard Precautions combine the major features of Universal Precautions (UP) and Body Substance Isolation (BSI), and are based on the principle that all blood, body fluids, secretions, excretions except sweat, nonintact skin, and mucous membranes may contain transmissible infectious agents. Standard Precautions include a group of infection prevention practices that apply to **ALL** clients. These are outlined in the chart on the right.

The client interaction and the extent of anticipated body, blood fluid, or pathogen exposure determines the specific Standard Precaution that is required during caring for the client. For example, if the client is only requiring a venipuncture and is calm and not combative, then only gloves may be needed. If the client requires intubation, then the use of gloves, gown, and face shield or mask and goggles are necessary.

Education and training on the principles and rationale for recommended practices are critical elements of the ongoing success of Standard Precautions because they facilitate appropriate decision-making and promote adherence when healthcare personnel are faced with new circumstances. An example of the importance of the use of Standard Precautions is intubation, especially under emergency circumstances when infectious agents may not be suspected, but later are identified (e.g., SARS-CoV, N. meningitides).

Centers for Disease Control and Prevention (CDC) have included three new elements to the infection control problems that are identified in the course of outbreak investigations. Since these are considered a standard of care and may not be a part of other guidelines, CDC has added these to the Standard Precautions. These include the following: **Hygiene/Cough Etiquette** (*reviewed with Droplet Precautions*), **Safe injection practices**, and **Use of masks for insertion of catheters or injection of material into spinal or epidural spaces via lumbar puncture procedures** (e.g., myelogram, spinal or epidural anesthesia). These new elements of Standard Precautions focus on **protection of clients**. Most elements of Standard Precautions evolved from Universal Precautions that had originally been developed for protection of healthcare personnel.

Refer to chart on the right to assist you in determining the appropriate personal protective equipment (PPE) to apply based on specific aspects of nursing care!

Center for Disease Control and Prevention: *2007 Guideline for isolation precautions: preventing transmission of infectious agents in healthcare settings.* Retrieved from http://www.cdc.gov/hicpac/2007ip/2007isolationprecautions.html

STANDARD PRECAUTIONS: RECOMMENDATIONS FOR THE CARE OF ALL CLIENTS IN ALL HEALTHCARE SETTINGS

COMPONENT OF CARE	RECOMMENDATIONS
Hand hygiene	Between client contacts. Immediately after removing gloves. After touching blood, body fluids, excretions, and contaminated items.
Personal Protective Equipment (PPE) Gloves	Touching blood, body fluids, excretions, contaminated items; mucous membranes, and nonintact skin.
Gown	During client-care activities and procedures when contact of exposed skin/clothing with blood/body fluids, excretions, and secretions are anticipated.
Mask, eye protection (goggles), face shield	Procedures such as suctioning, endotracheal intubation, or any client-care procedures that could generate splashes or fluid sprays of blood and secretions.
Client equipment that is soiled	Safe handling to prevent transfer of microorganisms to the healthcare environment and others; if visibly contaminated, wear gloves; always perform hand hygiene.
Environmental control	Develop protocols and procedures for routing cleaning, care, and disinfection of environmental surfaces, especially areas in the client-care area that are frequently handled and touched.
Needles and other sharps	Do not cap, break, bend, or hand-manipulate used needles. Use a one-handed scoop technique if recapping is necessary. Use puncture-resistant container for all sharps.
Client resuscitation	Prevent contact with mouth and oral secretions by using mouthpiece, resuscitation bag, and other ventilation devices.
Client placement	PRIORITIZE for SINGLE ROOM placement if client is at "**RISK**" for any of these criteria. **R**isk of acquiring/developing adverse outcome from infection. **I**ncrease risk of transmission. **S**ensible hygiene is not followed. **K**(C)ontaminate environment.
Respiratory hygiene/cough etiquette (symptomatic clients present with infectious respiratory secretions at the initial encounter in the system) (i.e., triage, reception areas, doctor's offices, etc.).	Instruct client to cover mouth/nose when sneezing/coughing after using tissues, dispose in a no-touch receptacle; hand hygiene after soiling hands; if can tolerate, wear a surgical mask, and/or maintain separation > 3 feet if possible.
Aerosol-generating procedures on clients with suspected or proven infections transmitted by respiratory aerosols (e.g., SARS).	Wear a fit-tested N95 or higher respirator in addition to gloves, gown, and face/eye protection.

Center for Disease Control and Prevention: *2007 Guideline for isolation precautions: preventing transmission of infectious agents in healthcare settings.* Retrieved from http://www.cdc.gov/hicpac/2007ip/2007isolationprecautions.html

Categories of Transmission-Based Precautions

SPECIFIC PRECAUTIONS

AIRBORNE   DROPLET   CONTACT

ALWAYS USE STANDARD PRECAUTIONS WITH EACH OF THESE SPECIFIED PRECAUTIONS!

=

SAFE CARE!

BASIC FACTS ABOUT PRECAUTIONS

1. When Standard Precautions alone do not interrupt the route(s) of transmission, then **Transmission-Based Precautions** are used.

2. For some diseases that have multiple routes of transmission (e.g., SARS), more than one Transmission-Based Precautions category may be used.

3. When used either singly or in combination, Standard Precautions are **ALWAYS** used with these!

4. Efforts must be made to counteract possible adverse effects on client's (i.e., anxiety, depression and other mood disturbances).

Center for Disease Control and Prevention: *2007 Guideline for isolation precautions: preventing transmission of infectious agents in healthcare settings.* Retrieved from http://www.cdc.gov/hicpac/2007ip/2007isolationprecautions.html

---

I CAN TESTING HINT: On the NCLEX®, you may need to provide client and/or staff education about infection control precautions. This next section in the book will assist you to move the categories of Transmission-Based Precautions into the long-term memory. Prior to teaching, understanding the principles for each of these specific precautions, starting with Standard Precautions, are important for SAFE nursing care!

CATEGORY OF PRECAUTIONS

Infectious Agent	Standard	Airborne	Droplet	Contact	Duration of Precautions
All Clients	S				
Rotavirus	S			Diapers	Extent of illness
Measles (Rubeola Virus)	S	A			Extent of illness
Tuberculosis (TB) Pulmonary	S	A			Three negative sputum smears
Meningococcal disease	S		D		Until therapy for 24 hours
Rubella	S		D	C	7 days after rash onset
AIDS/HIV	S			C	Extent of illness
Clostridium difficile	S			C	Extent of illness
Hepatitis A	S			C	7 days after jaundice onset
Hepatitis B	S			C	Extent of illness
Hepatitis C	S			C	Extent of illness
Herpes Simplex (Recurrent, oral, skin, genital)	S			C	Until lesions crust over
Methicillin–resistant Staphylococcus aureus (MRSA)	S			C	Extent of illness
Salmonella	S			C	Extent of illness
Shigellosis (dysentery)	S			C	Extent of illness
Staphylococcus aureus (infection or colonization)	S			C	Extent of illness
Vancomycin-resistant enterococci (VRE) (infection or colonization)	S			C	Until 3 negative cultures from infectious site (1 week apart)
Varicella Zoster (chickenpox)	S	A		C	Until lesions crust over
Herpes Zoster (shingles) Disseminated or localized if immunocompromised*	S	A*		C	Visible lesions or extent of illness
Respiratory Syncytial Virus (RSV)	S			C	Extent of illness

Airborne Precautions
(Droplets smaller than 5 micrometers) "AIIR"

The sweeper on the right page image is creating negative pressure, so the germs do not go out of the client's room. The organisms that require this Airborne Infection Isolation Room "AIIR" include: **varicella–zoster virus (chickenpox) which also includes a need for contact precautions; Rubeola (measles), Mycobacterium tuberculosis, and smallpox.** The N95 respirator mask which was approved by the National Institute for Occupational Safety and Health (NIOSH) should be worn when entering the room. Limit the times the client is transported out of the room. If transport is required, the client should wear a surgical mask. If the healthcare personnel are not immune to the infection the client has, then they must be restricted from entering the client's room.

In the image on the right page, the client's door is closed and the small germs (droplets smaller than 5 micrometers) are attempting to escape. The negative pressure is preventing this from happening. The N95 mask on the sweeper is to remind you that this type of PPE should be worn upon entering the client's room. Below is a chart to provide you with a simple way to remember that all of these will include both Airborne and Contact Precautions. If there is **only a pulmonary infiltrate** in a client with M. tuberculosis or a client has Rubeola, then the only requirement would be airborne precautions.

Pathogens	Isolation Precautions (always includes Standard Precautions)	
	Airborne	Contact
M. tuberculosis	If pulmonary infiltrate only	If infectious draining fluid present include both.
M. tuberculosis, Respiratory viruses, S. pneumoniae, S. aureus (MSSA or MRSA)–low risk or negative for HIV	X	X
M. tuberculosis, Respiratory viruses, S. pneumoniae, S. aureus (MSSA or MRSA)–High risk for HIV	X	Also use eye/face protection if Aerosol-generating procedure performed or contact with respiratory secretions.
M. tuberculosis. Out of country traveling with active outbreaks of SARS, Avian influenza presenting with M. TB and severe acute respiratory syndrome virus (SARS-CoV), avian influenza	X	Plus eye protection.
Vesicular: Varicella-zoster, Herpes Simplex, Variola (Smallpox)	X	X
Vaccinia virus only if Herpes Simplex, localized zoster in an immunocompetent client	NO	X
Rubeola (measles)	X	NO

References: www.cdc.gov/ncidod/sars); *Center for Disease Control and Prevention: 2007 Guideline for isolation precautions: preventing transmission of infectious agents in healthcare settings.* Retrieved from http://www.cdc.gov/hicpac/2007ip/2007isolationprecautions.html

AIIR

A irborne Infection Isolation Room (AIIR) (Negative pressure)

I nfection examples included in the isolation precaution are TB, smallpox, etc.

I nsist that clients wear a surgical mask if they must be transported (transports should be limited)

R espiratory protection mask should always be worn. (N95) mask recommended, required for (i.e. TB, smallpox)

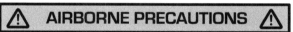

AIRBORNE PRECAUTIONS

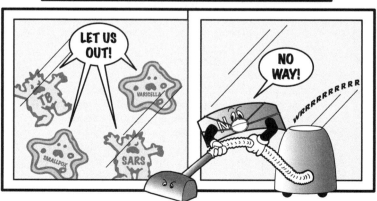

Viral Infections

A major challenge with the Herpes infections is trying to remember which one is a cold sore, shingles, or chickenpox. This has been simplified on the right page, so you can remember this detail. It is so very easy! Just remember Simplex has an "S" for **"SORE"** (*think of a simple "SORE" can be very painful!*); Zoster has an "S" for "SHINGLES". Since they both have an "S", always remember a "SIMPLE SORE" versus zoster for shingles. Varicella a "C" in it for chickenpox and the others do not have a "C" in the word.

The information below will assist you in organizing each of the infections.

- **S** Simplex (Herpes simplex virus type 1) (HSV-1) is a fever blister or cold sore
- **I** Is recurrent; contagious by direct contact; there is no immunity
- **M** Monitor for recurrent episodes that are characterized by appearance of lesions in the same place
- **P** Painful, local reaction consisting of vesicles with an erythematous base; most often around mouth
- **L** Lesions from herpes simplex usually heal without scarring
- **E** Exacerbated by stress, menses, sunlight, trauma, fatigue, or systemic infection
- **X** X out any confusion with HSV-2 which is predominantly associated by occurring below the waist (genital warts)

- **Z** Zoster is the shingles; zoster may cause scarring; Zoster vaccine (Zostavax) is recommended for adults over 60 years old even if they had a prior episode of chickenpox or herpes zoster.
- **O** Often unilateral and may appear on the trunk and may also appear on the face.
- **S** Site may have pain, burning, and neuralgia prior to the outbreak of the vesicles; soothing moist compresses.
- **T** The contact precautions should be followed if hospitalized; the clients who are immunosuppressed or anyone who has not had chickenpox are high risk for developing this infection.
- **E** Erythematous base vesicles that become filled with purulent fluid; vesicles eventually weep and crust.Occur most commonly along a dermatome of thorax, abdomen, forehead and temple, neck and shoulders. These can be in a linear patch and are located along spinal and cranial nerve tracts.
- **R** Related to the chickenpox virus: varicella; Remove pain by administering analgesics; gabapentin (Neurontin) for post-herpetic neuralgia.

Refer to *"PLAN FOR CLIENTS WITH VARICELLA* (Chicken Pox)". The nursing plan is organized around the mnemonic "**ISOLATE**".

SIMPLEX AND ZOSTER

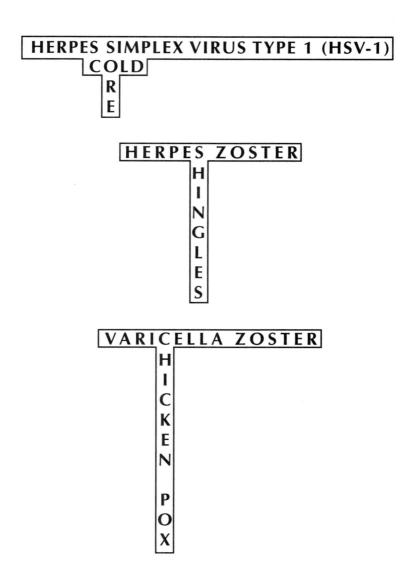

Plan For Clients With Varicella (Chicken Pox)

Herpes virus; varicella zoster is highly contagious and typically occurs in children under 15 years of age. This typically presents with maculopapular rash with vesicular scabs in multiple stages of healing. The incubation period is 14 to 16 days. This pathogen will require **airborne and contact precautions**. The child will be communicable for 1 day prior to when the lesions appear to the time when all lesions have completely formed crusts and will need to remain in isolation.

Assessments

The child will present with a low-grade temperature and with malaise in the prodromal phase. During the acute phase, the child will present with a red maculopapular rash which turns almost immediately to vesicles. These will have an erythematous base with the vesicle oozing and will crust. From 3 to 5 days, new crops of vesicles continue to form, spreading from the trunk to the extremities. The major discomfort to the child during all three stages is pruritus. If these vesicles develop a secondary infection, then this may progress to sepsis, cellulites, or even pneumonia. Prevention of these complications is the priority for nursing interventions. The nurse will "**ISOLATE**" the chicken with chicken pox.

The right page will assist you in organizing the care for prevention of complications with the mnemonic "**ISOLATE**"

- **I** **Isolate** affected child from other children until vesicles have crusted – PRIORITY! Initiate Airborne and Contact Precautions.
- **S** **Skin** care to decrease itching (antihistamines, antipruritics, calamine lotion; a paste of baking soda) may decrease irritation; cool baths may be comforting to the child.
- **O** **Occupy** child with quiet activities to lessen pruritus and prevent scratching.
- **L** **Lessen** duration of symptoms with acyclovir, and it will also decrease number of lesions.
- **A** **Acetaminophen** and/or ibuprofen are effective for fever.
- **T** **The** fingernails should be kept short; apply mittens if necessary.
- **E** **Eliminate** and prevent varicella by administering varicella immunizations. Immunization should not be given to a female who is pregnant or wanting to become pregnant in a few months. Prior to administering to an immune-compromised child, discuss with healthcare provider. Eliminate the use of aspirin for children with varicella.

ISOLATE

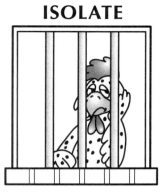

I solate affected child from other children until vesicles have crusted—PRIORITY; Initiate Airborne and Contact precautions; Standard precautions as care necessitates.

S kin care to decrease itching (antihistamines, antipruritics, calamine lotion, paste of baking soda, cool baths)

O ccupy child with quiet activities to lessen pruritus and prevent scratching

L essen duration of symptoms with acyclovir and it will also decrease number of lesions

A cetaminophen and /or ibuprofen for fever

T he fingernails should be kept short; apply mittens if necessary

E liminate use of aspirin

DroPlet Precautions
(Droplets larger than 5 micrometers)

"Patty the Pathogen" on the right page has an infection that is transmitted by respiratory droplets via sneezing, talking, and/ or coughing. Her surgical mask made from the letter "**P**" will assist you in remembering the conditions that require this type of infection control precautions. Note that the majority of these have a "**P**" in the names of the conditions. These include StrePtococcal (group A) **P**hayrngitis, Di**P**theria, Myco-**P**lasma pneumonia, **P**ertussis, **P**neumonic plague, **P**neumonia or scarlet fever in infants & young children. **MumPs (infectious Parotitis)**, Parovirus B 19, **P**arainfluenza virus infection, **P**andemic influenza (human influenza virus), Haemo**P**hilus influenza, type B for infants and children are typically in droplet precautions for 24 hours while antibiotic is being started. Clients with E**P**iglottis due to Haemo**P**hilus influenza, type B will also remain in droplet precautions for first 24 hours, so the antibiotic can be initiated and begin to act on the organism.

There are several diseases that do not fall into the memory technique of The "**P**'s". These include the following: Rubella, and Meningococcal Meningitis, Neisseria Meningitidis.

If possible, place the client in a private room, but if it is necessary due to a decrease in the availability of beds, then two clients may go in the same room if they are infected with the same pathogen requiring the same type of infection control procedures. Whenever the nurse is from 3 to 6 feet from the client, a mask should be worn. There are not any recommendations regarding the use of eye protection. If the client must be transported in the hall, then a mask should be placed on client. Family members and client should be educated regarding "*respiratory hygiene/cough etiquette*" which includes teaching healthcare personnel measures to contain their own respiratory secretions. There should also be signs regarding the importance of covering the mouth and nose with a tissue when sneezing. Tissues should be disposed in non-touch receptacles. Hand hygiene is mandatory for client and all of the healthcare personnel.

Centers for Disease Control and Prevention (CDC) have included three new elements to the infection control problems with one of these being hygiene/Cough Etiquette. The other two new elements will be discussed in the section "*Standard Precautions*" on page 60.

Center for Disease Control and Prevention: *2007 Guideline for isolation precautions: preventing transmission of infectious agents in healthcare settings.* Retrieved from http://www.cdc.gov/hicpac/2007ip/2007isolationprecautions.html

PATTY THE PATHOGEN

Put on your Surgical Facemask— distance 3–6 ft. from client for the P's

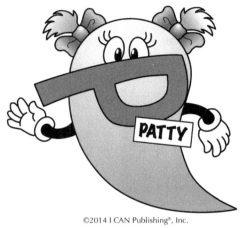

Stre**P**tococcal (group A) **P**hayrngitis

Di**P**theria

Myco**P**lasma pneumonia

Pertussis

Pneumonic plague

Pneumonia or scarlet fever in infants & young children

Priority Nursing Plan For Clients With Clostridium Difficile
"CONTACT PRECAUTIONS"

Private Room: If the client's condition has an uncontrolled drainage, incontinence, etc., then a private room is necessary. Two clients with the same pathogen may be placed in the same room. Personal protective equipment (PPE)–wear a gown when entering the client's room; remove gown prior to leaving. Wear gloves when entering the client's room. Remove gloves prior to leaving the client's room and perform hand hygiene; do not touch anything in client's room as leaving. Wear gloves when touching the intact skin of the client, surfaces, and articles close to the client. **Remove gown, gloves/perform hand hygiene between clients.**

Room Placement: If a private room is not available, then position clients with a > 3 feet spatial separation between beds. This will reduce the opportunities for sharing items between the infected/colonized client and other clients.

Isolation procedures: Use CONTACT PRECAUTIONS for diseases easily transmitted by direct contact such as respiratory tract, skin, gastrointestinal, or wound infections and clients with multidrug-resistant bacteria. Clients with varicella and smallpox also require contact precautions in addition to the airborne precautions. Donning PPE upon room entry and discarding before exiting the room of the client are done to contain pathogens, especially those that have been implicated in transmission through environmental contamination (e.g., C. difficile, VRE, and other intestinal tract pathogens; RSV). **If gloves are visibly soiled from contaminants–change gloves immediately.**

Alcohol is not sporicidal! Do not use for Clostridium difficile. Practice hand hygiene with soap and water. The clients with VRE/MRSA should not be in the room with clostridium difficile and Equipment –Do NOT share! Remember, C. difficile is located on many surfaces including toilet seats, stethoscopes, linens, etc. If common equipment must be used between clients who require contact precautions, then equipment must be disinfected prior to use on another client. Evidence shows that multiple drug-resistant organisms (MDROs), infection or colonization (e.g., MRSA, VRE, VISA/VRSA, resistant S. pneumoniae) can be carried from one person to another via the hands of healthcare personnel.

"**DRAIN**" will summarize a strategy to help you organize what pathogens and clinical findings would require Contact Precautions.

- **D** c**D**iff, **D**rainage from wounds, lesions, Decubitus
- **R** **R**otavirus
- **A** **A**bscess, acute conjunctivitis
- **I** **I**ntestinal tract pathogens, Impetigo
- **N** **N**ote: Hepatitis A, B, and C; Herpes Simplex; Pediculosis (Lice); MDROs, VRE

Center for Disease Control and Prevention: *2007 Guideline for isolation precautions: preventing transmission of infectious agents in healthcare settings.* Retrieved from http://www.cdc.gov/hicpac/2007ip/2007isolationprecautions.html

PRIVATE

P rivate room

R emove gown, gloves/perform hand hygiene between clients

I solation procedures—use CONTACT PRECAUTIONS

V isibly soiled from contaminants—change gloves immediately

A lcohol is not sporicidal!

T he clients with VRE/MRSA—not in room with clostridium difficile

E quipment—Do NOT share! Remember C. diff is located on many surfaces including toilet seats, stethoscopes, linens, etc.

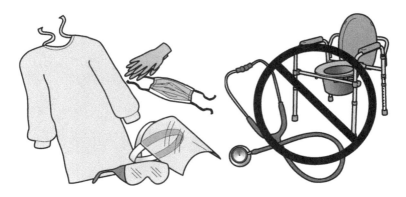

©2014 I CAN Publishing®, Inc.

Clostridium Difficile

C. difficile is an antibiotic associated colitis that is currently the most common hospital acquired infection. The colitis, often caused by the administration of too many antibiotics, resulting in dehydration and client feeling miserable! The word "**BAD**" on the next page will assist you to remember this often death-producing situation.

The "**BAD**" news is that a relapse is common. The good news is this can be prevented by following excellent contact and standard precautions.

CLOSTRIDIUM DIFFICILE

B acterial, hospital acquired

A ntibiotic associated
bdominal cramps

D iarrhea

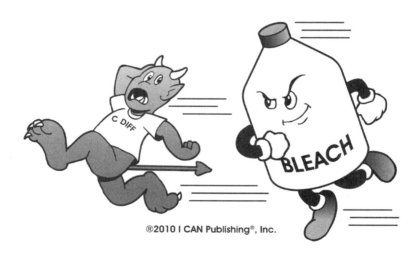

Relapse is common!

Methicillin-Resistant Staphylococcus Aureus (MRSA)

Methicillin-resistant staphylococcus aureus (MRSA) is a common drug-resistant organism found in healthcare facilities. Many different infections may be a result of this pathogen such as respiratory, skin, and urinary infections. As with other organisms, the nurse is not always able to tell that the client is infected. MRSA is spread primarily by direct and indirect contact. Occasionally it is transmitted through the respiratory and urinary tracts. Standard precautions will prevent the spread of MRSA, particularly in the skin and urine infections. If the MRSA is in the wound or urine, contact precautions are used. If the MRSA is in the respiratory tract, such as with TB, then airborne precautions are used.

When incorporating Standard Precautions, **gown**, **gloves**, and **goggles** should be worn. Gloves must be worn when touching body substances, mucous membranes, nonintact skin, and items that are contaminated. They should be changed frequently after contact with infected items and material. If soiling is likely, then gowns should be worn. If body substances are going to be splashed, then a mask/face shield is indicated. Handwashing is always important to consider. Wash hands before and after care.

There should be 3 feet of space between the client/resident and visitors. This can create a feeling of **social isolation** for the client. If it is necessary to transport the client in the hospital, then the client must wear a mask. The linen must be bagged to prevent contamination of self, environment, or outside of bag. Infectious trash must be discarded to prevent contamination of self, environment, or outside of bag. Masks/face shield for staff and visitors must be worn for individuals who are within 3 feet of the client. Noncritical care equipment should be limited to a single client. Hands must always be washed after completion of care and all of the gowns, gloves, etc. have been removed. Standard Precautions are always adapted in addition to the other specific types of isolation.

Since MRSA is such an **active infection**, it is imperative that meticulous attention is paid to isolation techniques. Remember, infection control is one of the top activities on the NCLEX-RN® Test Plan.

MRSA

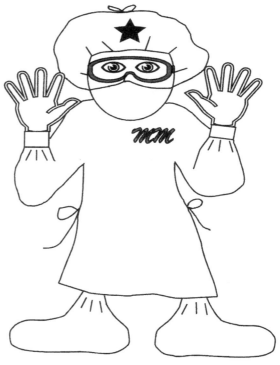

M any cultures

R equires gown, gloves, goggles

S ocial isolation

A ctive infection

Infection Prevention: Positive Pressure

Clients who require neutropenic precautions or are at a high risk for developing an infection from burns, immunocompromised, etc. will need to be protected from any type of organism. The image illustrates this by "Positive Paul" attempting to push any organism out the door by positive pressure. Remember the following to assist you in understanding this concept.

> Positive
> Pressure
> Positively
> Prevents
> Patient infection by
> Pushing air out to
> **PROTECT** client!

P **P**rivate room with a high efficiency particulate air (HEPA) Filtration.

R **R**equires PPE; does not include the use of barrier precautions beyond those indicated for Standard and Transmission-Based Precautions.

O **O**rient client transport and client movement out of the room; to prevent inhalation of fungal spores during periods when construction, renovation, or other dust-generating activities that may be ongoing in and around the health-care facility, it has been advised that severely immunocompromised patients wear a high-efficiency respiratory-protection device (e.g., an N95 respirator) when leaving the Protective Environment.

T **T**hings such as flowers and potted plants with standing water should never be in the room.

E **E**liminate sharing equipment with other clients.

C **C**lose assessments for any subtle signs of infection.

T **T**each client, family, visitors, and staff the importance of following Standard and Transmission-Based Precautions.

Center for Disease Control and Prevention: *2007 Guideline for isolation precautions: preventing transmission of infectious agents in healthcare settings.* Retrieved from http://www.cdc.gov/hicpac/2007ip/2007isolationprecautions.html

POSITIVE PRESSURE: POSITIVE PAUL

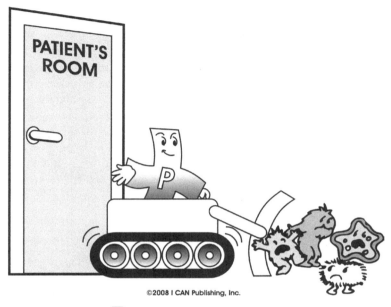

©2008 I CAN Publishing, Inc.

P ositive

P ressure

P ositively

P revents

P atient infection by

P ushing air out

Sequence For Donning PPE

This strategy on the right page was developed to assist you in answering questions regarding organizing the steps for donning personal protective equipment (PPE) in chronological order. In order to simplify this, we have associated this with the numbers 1, 2, 3, 4, to provide you with a visual.

The first step is to put on the gown. Remember the number 1 has the gown wrapped around it. The second step is to put on the mask. The number 2 actually looks like the mask with being able to stretch the 2 out to tie around your head. Also, the mask can rest on the top of the 2 to assist you in remembering this. The third step is the goggles. The number 3 looks like goggles with 2 small areas for the eyes. Also, the goggles sit nicely at the top of the number 3. The last step in donning includes putting on the gloves. Remember, the image has a glove coming out of the top of the 4 and the tail of the 4 on the right. This will help you remember 2 gloves, and we put them on after the other PPE have been applied.

I CAN TESTING HINT: On the NCLEX® you may need to drag and drop these in chronological order to successfully answer the question, *"Put in chronological order the sequence for donning personal protective equipment (PPE)".*

DONNING PPE

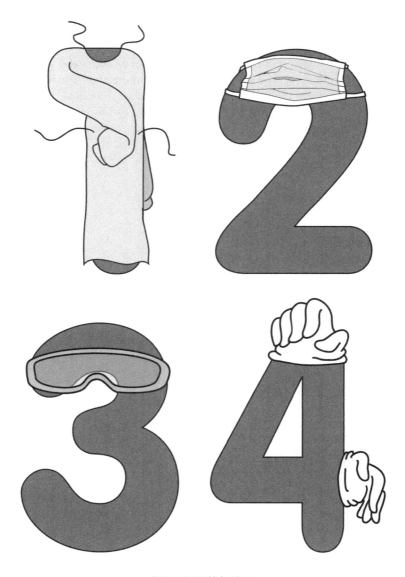

Sequence For Removing PPE

This strategy on the right page was developed to assist you in answering the alternative question on the NCLEX® regarding organizing the steps for removing personal protective equipment (PPE) in chronological order. In order to simplify this, we have associated this with the numbers 1, 2, 3, 4, to provide you with a visual.

The first step is to remove the gloves. This would make sense due to contamination. The second step for removing the PPE would be to remove the goggles. The third step would be to remove the gown followed by the fourth step which is removing the mask. Think about holding your hands over your head and then removing the PPE from head to toe.... First the gloves, then the goggles, then the gown and end by returning to your face by removing the mask.

> **I CAN TESTING HINT:** On the NCLEX®, you may need to drag and drop these in chronological order to successfully answer the question, *"Put in chronological order the sequence for removing personal protective equipment (PPE)".*

REMOVING PPE

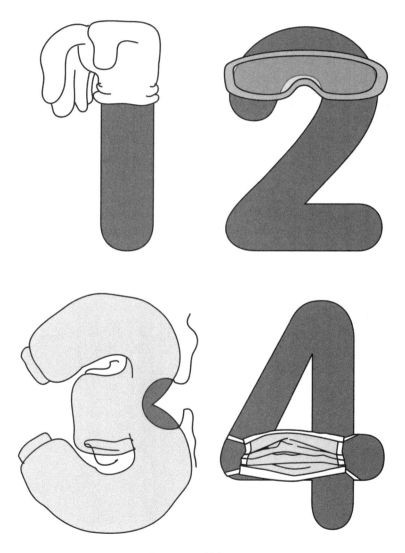

Fever

FEVER is the point where heat production exceeds heat loss. Our little digital thermometer is feeling badly. He has an ice pack on his head. His slippers indicate he is comtemplating a tepid bath. He is taking his acetaminophen or ibuprofen to prevent a rapid rise that may cause seizures. If none of these things work, the 100.4° Fahrehheit that can be tolerated can quickly rise to a dangerous level, especially at peak FEVER time late in the afternoon.

F **FAHRENHEIT** (97 to 100 degrees F) or (36.1 to 37.8 degrees Celsius)

E **ENDOGENOUS PYROGENS** reset the hypothalamic center.

V **VOLUME NEEDS** increase secondary to heat loss (i.e., increased metabolism, shivering, sweating, evaporation, and vasodilation).

E **EVALUATE THE SOURCE VIA LABS:** CBC with differential, urinalysis, blood culture, and chest x-ray. Evaluate trends in Temp. before a major problem with sepsis occurs.

R **RISK FACTOR**S—viral or bacterial illness, environmental factors, tissue damage, biological agents, endocrine disorders

ALERT! GREATER THAN 107° F = DEATH OR IRREVERSIBLE BRAIN DAMAGE!

SAFETY & INFECTION CONTROL | 85

FEVER

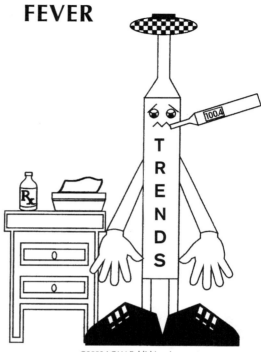

F ahrenheit
(97°-100° F)

E ndogenous pyrogens
Evaluate trends in Temp. before a major problem with sepsis occurs.

V olume needs

E valuate source via labs

R isk factors

Beta Strep

The "3 BEES" help you to remember that with a B STREP infection it is wise to consider getting 3 cultures, administering 3 does of anti-infectives, and if momma BEE is pregnant she should be given her medication at the time of diagnosis as well as 2 more doses during delivery.

B BETA-HEMOLYTIC STREPTOCOCCUS–predominate causative agent in neonatal sepsis

S SCREENING–identify maternal carrier at 35-37 weeks gestation by vaginal swab

T TREATMENT–Currently if the client is found to be positive, the prophylaxis usually starts with labor, rupture of the membranes, or fever over 104° and continues until effective. CBC with differential and blood cultures are useful tests to determine this. If the infant is symptomatic, Penicillin G or other antibiotics are administered. Protocols often change for this treatment.

R RISK FACTORS–maternal GBS during pregnancy, < 37 weeks gestation, sibling with prior GBS infection, rupture of membranes > than 18 hours, intrapartum temp greater than 100.4° Fahrenheit or 38° Celcius

E EVALUATE INFANT for s/s of sepsis usually appearing in first 48 hours–respiratory distress most common (apnea to mild tachypnea, labored breathing, increased oxygen requirements, mechanical ventilation), lethargy, poor feeding, hypoglycemia, temperature instability (hypothermia most common)

P PROPHYLAXIS should be given to mothers at the start of labor or when membranes rupture. If not accomplished due to precipitous delivery, treatment of the neonate should be considered.

BETA STREP

B eta-hemolytic streptococcus

S creening

T reatment

R isk factors

E valuate infant

P rophylaxis

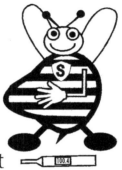
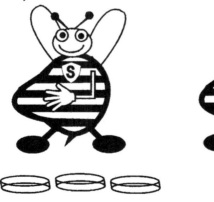
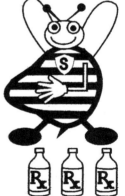

Fall Risk

The frail elder (**A**ge over 85) is a high risk for falls due to the many physiological changes. These problems may be linked to a lack of exercise or to neurological causes, arthritis, or other medical conditions and their treatments. Postural hypotension due to the change in the baroreceptors may also be a contributing factor to falls. Postural hypotension can be a result of dehydration, medications, may be linked to diabetes, Parkinson's disease, or an infection. The physiological changes include:

- Muscle weakness, especially in the legs.
- Poor balance and gait and difficulty in walking.
- Foot problems to include painful feet and wearing unsafe footwear.
- Sensory problems to include declining eye sight, decrease in ability to adjust clearly when moving from darkness and light, poor depth perception, cataracts, glaucoma, poor lighting and wearing multi-focal glasses while walking.
- Peripheral neuropathy with numbness in the feet that may result in the client not knowing where they are stepping.
- Confusion.

A large part of safe care is to educate the staff on fall-reduction protocols. The clients identified as high risk should have an appropriate assessment to implement a plan for fall reduction. For example, keep all personal items within reach of the client and maintain the bed in the low position. Side rails should be used appropriately in addition to advising all the personnel of the clients who are high risk for falling. For these clients, it is imperative to provide appropriate assistance with ambulation. Prior to any ambulation, the environment should provide adequate lighting, and the floor should be cleared of all danger or obstacles such as cords, rugs, etc. that could contribute to falls. All wheelchairs, beds, or stretchers should have the locks secured.

Bones–History of osteoporosis or other bone disorders increase the risk for falls. It is important to attempt to prevent osteoporosis by eating a diet rich in calcium and vitamin D, exercise, and not to drink in excess or smoke. Weight bearing exercises such as walking, hiking, jogging, climbing stairs, and dancing, etc. should be included in a prevention program.

Coagulation–There is an increased risk of a subdural hematoma and other bleeding complications if the client falls.

Drugs such as anticholinergics, diuretics, anti-hypertensives may contribute to falls. The more medications a client takes, the greater the risk for falling. Clients who take four or more prescription drugs have a greater risk of falling than clients who take fewer drugs.

Surgery–Risk for injury from a fall could cause wound dehiscence or damage to their surgical site.

ABCS

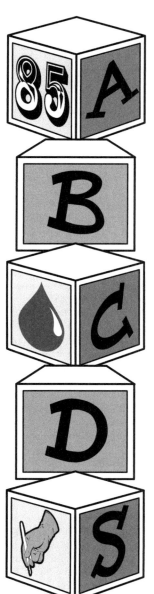

AGE OVER 85—Frail elders are high risk for falls

BONES—History of osteoporosis or other bone disorders are more likely to be high risk for falls

COAGULATION—Increased risk of subdural hematoma and other bleeding complications

DRUGS—Use of specific drugs such as diuretics, anti-hypertensives, anticholinergics, etc.

SURGERY—Risk for injury from a fall such as wound dehiscence, damage to their surgical site

©2014 I CAN Publishing®, Inc.

I CAN TESTING HINT: When you are given an age, disease, and/or medication, pay attention! *"Protect client from injury related to falls"* is in the top ten NCLEX® standards. It is important to understand the risks in order to understand how to prioritize nursing care with a focus on fall prevention.

Anaphylactic Reactions: Priority Nursing Care That "Limits Dyspnea"

Anaphylactic reactions may occur in clients who are highly sensitized to a specific allergen. If the nursing care "**LIMITS**" these allergens, then the risk factors will be decreased. Physiologically, the antigen-antibody response results in the release of histamine that causes vasodilation and increases the permeability of the capillaries. The quicker the onset of clinical findings after the exposure, the more severe the reaction will be. "**LIMITS**" on the right page will assist you in organizing many of these allergens and "**DYSPNEA**" outlines the clinical manifestations that may occur as a result of the physiological changes from the histamine release. These clinical findings depend on the degree of hypersensitivity and the amount of allergen exposure the client experiences.

Mild to moderate symptoms may include the following: itching (pruritus, urticaria), peripheral tingling, nasal congestion, lips and tongue edema, flushing, and anxiety. These may rapidly progress to "**DYSPNEA**" (laryngeal edema, bronchospsam), GI cramping, tachycardia, cyanosis, and hypotension. These clinical findings can be fatal without immediate intervention.

With the focus of the NCLEX® being clinical decision making, this concept is a great way to evaluate your ability to prioritize nursing care. In order to assist you in organizing this information, we have organized it around the "**5 A's**".

Assess for allergies–Always try to prevent this from occurring by identifying potential risks, "**LIMITS**".

Antihistamines–MILD to MODERATE reactions–antihistamines and/or epinephrine **0.2 to 0.5 mL (1:1000 solution)**, administered **subcutaneously or intramuscularly.** When administering epinephrine, the CORRECT concentrate is crucial. **Subcutaneous or IM–concentrations of 0.1% to 1:1000**; Intracardiac or Intravenous solutions–concentrations of 0.01% or 1:10,000. Due to potential fatal reactions, intravenous solutions are more dilute. **SEVERE** reactions–Epinephrine **0.5 mL (concentration of 1:10,000)**, administered intravenously at 5 to 10 minute intervals which provides client with 1 mg over at least 1 minute. Remember: **SAFETY IS A PRIORITY! IV is MORE DILUTE!**

Airway–Keep client from going to "**POT**"! This is a medical emergency. Anaphylaxis requires an immediate response!

    P Patent airway–intubation or tracheostomy may be necessary
    O Oxygen in high concentrations
    T The meds include: albuterol, corticosteroid, epinephrine

Adequate circulation–Due to the loss of fluid to third–space shifts and vasodilation, IV fluids (Lactated Ringer's or 0.9% saline), vasopressor agents, and volume expanders are used to maintain circulation. Vital signs are used to evaluate the titration of fluid replacement. SAFETY is a priority on the NCLEX®! REMEMBER, it is the responsibility of the nurse to monitor the fluid status carefully because once the fluid starts to shift back into the vascular compartment, it is easy to cause fluid overload!

Alert–Wear identification tag or medic-alert bracelet to identity any allergies. Once an allergic reaction occurs, the next exposure could progress to an emergency from an anaphylaxis reaction. Prevention is important!

LIMITS & DYSPNEA

L atex (high risk if allergic to Kiwi, avocados, chestnuts, bananas, paypaya)

I nfluenza, Insect stings (i.e., bee, wasp, ant)

M easles (eggs); Meds (i.e., penicillins may be allergic to cephalosporins) (hypersensitivity to trimethoprim may be allergic to sulfonamides)

I nfusion (blood)

T ape

S hellfish (allergic to Iodine); other food allergies may include peanuts or eggs

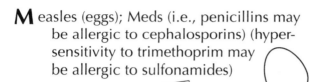

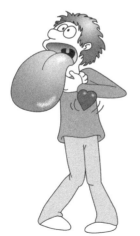

D yspnea, tight throat, bronchospasm, laryngeal edema

Y es, onset is rapid

S welling and tingling in mouth, face, throat, and tongue

P ruritus

N ote BP ↓

E levated HR

A loss of consciousness

©2014 I CAN Publishing®, Inc.

I CAN TESTING HINT: Anaphylaxis is a medical emergency and requires immediate intervention. Bronchospasms and edema of the airway are typically the cause of death from an anaphylactic reaction.

Safe Use of Equipment

Due to the number of injuries that have occurred with clients from malfunctioning equipment, it is imperative that nurses understand the importance of "**SAFE**" use.

The **System** must be without problems in order to maintain client safety.

Accident prevention can be achieved 100% of the time when the nurse evaluates **the proper functioning of the equipment PRIOR to use**. There would never be ANY client deaths from a medication due to an inappropriate bolus from the PCA pump if the nurse developed the habit of ALWAYS checking the equipment first. Equipment must also be operated appropriately. Nursing personnel should have appropriate education related to operating, managing, and troubleshooting equipment. It is unsafe practice to operate any piece of equipment without appropriate knowledge. The education files for staff will have forms for documentation indicating there was a teaching session, and a return demonstration was performed evaluating appropriate understanding of how to operate equipment safely. **Evaluating effectiveness** of the equipment is of paramount importance in providing safe care!

SAFE USE OF EQUIPMENT

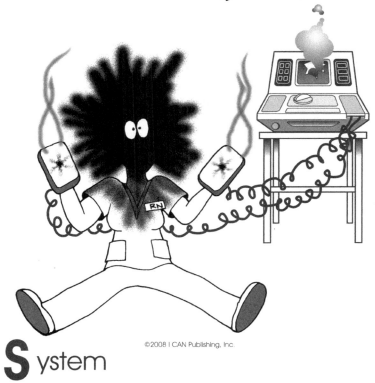

S ystem

A ccident prevention

F unctions properly prior to using

E valuate effectiveness

Priority Plan Regarding Restraints

Client safety is always the priority care for any nursing intervention. The use of restraints may be to protect the client and/or others. The order for restraints should include the type and location of the restraint, and the time frame the order covers. The behavior type for which the restraint is to be used should also be included in the order.

"**RESTRAINT**" on the right page will assist you in providing safe nursing practice for the client in restraints.

In addition to safety for the client, the family should be informed regarding the rationale for and the purpose of the restraints. It is very important to explore all the alternatives to restraints prior to using these.

When answering questions regarding restraints on the NCLEX®, always remember the importance of applying and maintaining the prescribed restraints/bed alarms/safety devices according to facility policy. The client's response to the restraints should be monitored and documented in addition to evaluating the appropriateness of the type of restraints being used. Our goal as nurses is to always be a client advocate.

RESTRAINT

R estraints require an order from the healthcare provider per protocol (q 24 hours).

E mergency—physical restraints may be used for a brief period of time, but must get order.

S afety for the client and others are the goals and purpose for the procedure.

T he restraints and the client's physiological needs should be assessed on a regular basis per hospital protocol.

R emove restraints and provide range of motion every 2 hours.

A ssess and document neruovascular status of client's extremities at the time of each check.

I nvolve family.

N o securing restraints to the side rails; secure to the bed frame.

T he alternatives to restraints should be investigated prior to use (i.e, family involvement, orientation, etc.).

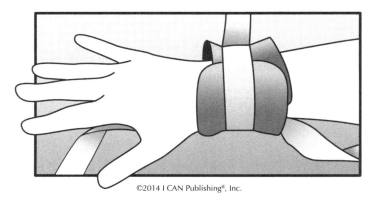

©2014 I CAN Publishing®, Inc.

Applications of Heat and Cold

Warm compresses (heat application) are used for vasodilation and to decrease pain. These compresses will also assist with healing and to soften exudates. Types of heat application include: heat lamp, sitz bath, moist heat pack, and/or pad that circulates warmed water to distribute dry heat to body parts. The heat sources should be covered to protect the skin. The compresses are typically used for 20 to 30 minutes. When using hot baths, it is important to instruct client to be cautious because of the vasodilation effects that may result in postural hypotension. When providing safe care, it is also important to understand when NOT to use the compresses. "**BURN**" will assist you in remembering when **NOT** to use warm compresses.

Cold compresses are used to promote vasoconstriction, stop bleeding, stop pain by decreasing sensitivity to pain receptors through numbing them, and decrease temperature or edema. If the cold compress is applied immediately after an injury, the edema will be reduced. Types of cold applications include ice bag, cold compress or cold pack, ice collar, and/or hypothermia blanket. Safety is always a priority, so always use a towel or cloth to cover the source to protect the skin. "**COLD**" will assist you in remembering when **NOT** to use cold compresses.

I CAN TESTING HINT: A nursing priority is to **NOT** use hot or cold compresses with conditions of **alteration in circulation** such as diabetes or peripheral vascular disease. **Heat is used for vasodilation** and decreases pain. **Cold is used for vasoconstriction**, and stops bleeding, pain and reduces edema.

BURN / COLD

NO WARM COMPRESSES
B leeding site
U cannot feel (Decrease sensation)
R adiation
N ot to injury in last 24 hours

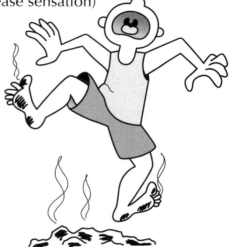

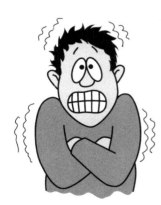

NO COLD COMPRESSES
C irculation decreased
O pen wound
c **L** oth use over compress; do not put on bare skin
D o not use cold with radiation or Raynaud's phenomenon

©2014 I CAN Publishing®, Inc.

Disaster Plan

A disaster plan needs to be activated when there is a life threatening risk and a large number of clients must be evacuated from the hospital, assisted living units, etc. "MERRY" needs a way to remember which clients to remove first from the rooms. **ABC** will assist in organizing this information!

- **A AMBULATORY**–The priority is to evacuate the largest volume of clients initially.

- **B BEDRIDDEN**–The bedridden clients will be the next group to be evacuated from the rooms. Actually, the ambulatory group may be able to assist in getting this group evacuated more quickly.

- **C CRITICAL CARE**–The last group of clients to be evacuated will be the critically ill.

The ultimate objective in a disaster plan is to evacuate volumes of clients. If the clients with numerous tubes and IVs are evacuated initially, this will slow the process down. Fewer clients will be safely rescued from the disaster.

DISASTER PLAN

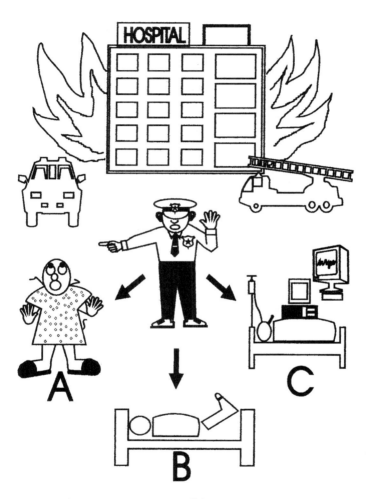

Triage

Triage is a standardized system of sorting clients according to medical needs when there are minimal or no resources available for every person to receive treatment. The goals for triaging clients are to determine whether a client is appropriate for a specific level of care and to optimize the use of hospital resources. Triage scoring (color) levels that are used during a mass casualty include the following: immediate care (red), delayed (yellow), minor (green), and expectant or morgue (black). A TRIAGE scoring (color) levels during a mass casualty incident (MCI) is to help the staff provide the greatest good for the greatest number.

An easy way to remember this is that if the stop light is **red** and the client goes through this light, then it will result in an accident requiring **immediate assistance**. If the care does not occur within one hour of the accident, then the client will most likely not survive. Any compromise to the casualty's cardiovascular system, respirations, hemorrhage or shock control could be fatal. Other clients that may fall into this category include individuals who are paralyzed, have an obstructed airway, acute myocardial infarction, and/or are unconscious.

If a client was to go through a **yellow** light, there may or may not be an accident. If an accident does occur, it will most likely not be as serious as it would have been going through a red light, and may allow for a **delay** in treatment. The casualty does require treatment, but can wait until the red clients have been evaluated and had an intervention. These may include complications such as (e.g., open thoracic wound and/or abdominal wound that is penetrating).

If the client was to go through a **green** light and there was an accident, the injury most likely would be **minimal**. A delay in treatment would present no threat to the client. These clients typically do not require monitoring and stabilization. These injuries may include a broken arm and/or cuts on extremities requiring stitches.

The color **black** is what people many times will wear to a funeral, so remember that black indicates the client is most likely not going to survive due to the level of care required to intervene with the injury. Although the client may not survive, it is important to provide palliative care and pain relief. These types of clients may include conditions such as chest or head trauma, massive burns, cardiac arrest, etc. These clients will most likely go to the **morgue**.

I CAN TESTING HINT: This image on the right page will assist you in answering NCLEX® questions regarding triaging clients. If a question requires you to place in chronological order which client you would provide care for, the stoplight will assist in remembering this concept. Remember, red requires immediate care; yellow can be delayed up to 6 hours; green requires minimal care; and black indicates client will most likely not survive.

STOP LIGHT

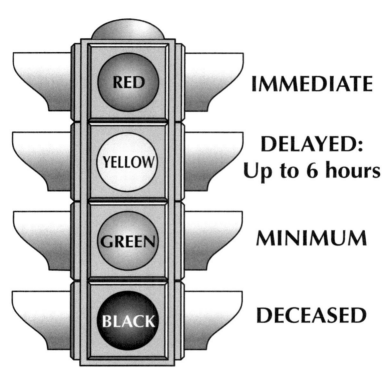

"Your actions show what your heart is made of."
UNKNOWN

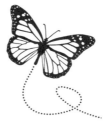

CARDIAC SYSTEM

Tools of Physical Assessment

The tools of Physical Assessment are the most important in assessing, evaluating and monitoring the client's care. The appropriate tools include inspection, auscultation, percussion and palpation. Inspection is the use of the eyes to gather data. Careful observation can reveal clues about the client's respiratory system, musculoskeletal and neurological system, skin integrity, and the emotional and mental status.

Auscultation is the process of listening to sounds produced by the organs and tissues of the body. It is a clinical tool used most frequently to assess the heart, lungs, neck and abdomen. These sounds are characterized according to pitch, intensity, quality and duration.

Percussion is used for assessing the size, position and density of underlying structures. This technique consists of a sharp tapping that produces vibrations and subsequent sound waves. These sound waves are interpreted by the experienced percussor as air, fluid or solid material in an underlying structure.

Palpation is the use of hands and fingers to gather data through touch. The characteristics of body texture, temperature, size, shape and movement may be distinguished by different parts of the hands and fingers. The palm and ulnar surfaces are used to distinguish vibrations and the dorsal surface is best for estimating temperature. A bimanual technique uses both hands to entrap an organ or mass between the fingertips to better assess its size and shape.

Practice, practice and practice improve this skill.

TOOLS OF PHYSICAL ASSESSMENT

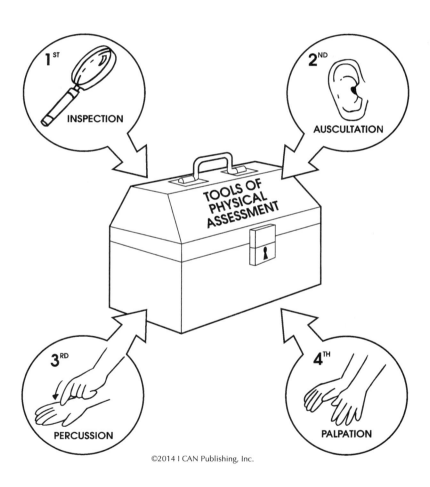

Stethoscope

The stethoscope is indispensable for determining the sounds inside the body. The image on the next page will assist you in determining when to use the diaphragm or the bell of the stethoscope to hear the best sounds.

The diaphragm is used to hear high pitched heart sounds such as S_1 and S_2, murmurs of aortic and mitral valve regurgitation, pericardial, and abdominal friction rub sounds.

The bell is used to hear lower pitched heart sounds such as S_3, S_4 and a murmur of mitral stenosis.

STETHOSCOPE

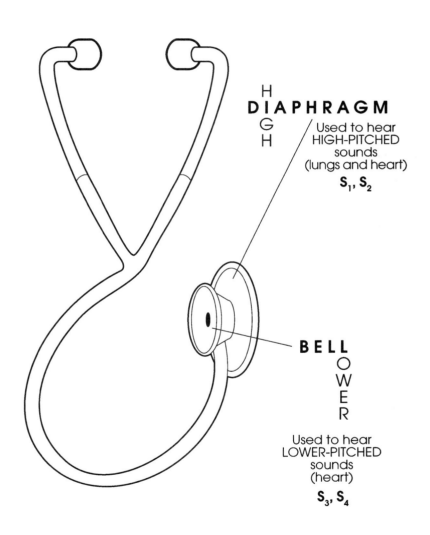

Vital Signs

Vital signs are just that. **VITAL to LIFE**. If we have no BP, inspiration, temperature or pulse, we are dead. That makes these the most important assessments that a nurse can make. A flow sheet on a history of vital signs will give the nurse valuable information on which to make life-saving decisions.

The ordinary definition of a normal blood pressure varies with the client, but can range around 120/80. If the client has hypertension, the nurse may hear the BP over 200/100. This high a BP is a priority for the nurse to take action as it is "stroke territory." Clients on BP medication must be taught to monitor their own BP to make sure it stays within a normal range (usually below 120/80).

Cuff size is important in determining an accurate BP. For example, do not use a neonatal cuff (2" wide) on a 250-pound man. It may cut his arm, and the reading will be inaccurate. "Hard cuffs" commonly found on automatic BP readers, often leave big bruises on little old ladies that are taking coumadin. Be cautious when taking the BP of the client on blood thinners.

LOC (level of consciousness) is essential as all vital signs may be within normal limits, but the client may be unresponsive and unconscious.

Breathing is a must. *"Assessment of the breath includes the number of times that we breathe per minute = respiratory rate).* An adult's respiratory rate is approximately 20 times per minute. *(Refer to the chart on page 110-111 for respiratory rate change at different ages.)* If an adult has a high respiratory rate, there may be an alteration in air exchange. High or low rate (under 12) is a high priority for nursing action. We also want to determine if the client is having difficulty breathing by assessing for dyspnea or shortness of breath (SOB). Is there a scared look on their face? Are they using chest and neck muscles to breathe? Does it hurt for them to breathe? These are vital assessments!

Skin assessment provides us with a lot of information. We can determine if they are hot, dry, cold or clammy. Assessing the body temperature is confirmation of what we feel. We can also determine if they are shivering by touching them. Maybe one of the most important things that we are doing is touching them to let them know that we care and to calm them.

Evaluating the pulse involves the heart rate *(around 70-80 for an adult, check chart for changes in other age groups)*. While we are feeling the pulse, we can tell if it is regular, irregular, bounding, thready, strong or weak. An abnormal pulse is a high priority for nursing action.

Evaluating for pain is also a priority because it may result in vital sign changes. When people are hurting, their pulse and respiratory rate elevates. In fact, the pulse is a good indication for evaluating the effectiveness of pain medication.

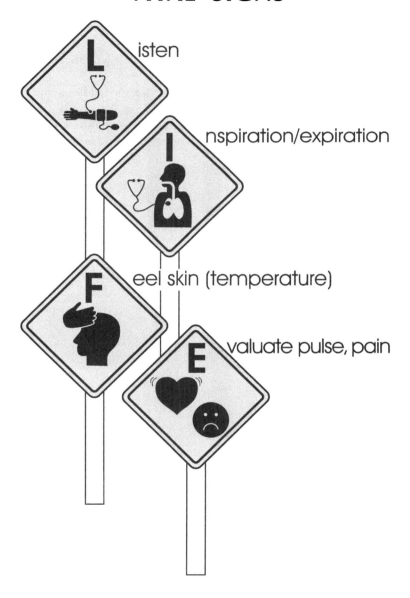

The vital signs on this page will assist you in remembering what assessments are vital to "LIFE"!

Vital Sign Values

Many learners indicate they have a hard time remembering the respiratory rate and the heart rate for the various stages of development. It in reality is quite simple! All you do is start with the neonate for your guidelines.

In order to determine the respiratory rate for the toddler, subtract 10 from the neonate, and the heart rate for the toddler can be determined by subtracting 20 from the neonate. Continue in this fashion for each of the stages. The next page outlines the averages to validate your figures.

Now, was that so hard?

VITAL SIGN VALUES

Neonate

    Respiratory   40

    Heart Rate   140

Toddler (age 2–4)

    Respiratory   30

    Heart Rate   120

Child (6–10)

    Respiratory   20

    Heart Rate   100

Adult

    Respiratory   12–18

    Heart Rate   60–100

©1994 I CAN Publishing, Inc.

Cardiac Sounds

Cardiac sounds are one effective assessment for identifying alterations in the cardiaovascular system. S_1 is ordinarily auscultated over the tricuspid/mitral sites. It is heard in the beginning of the cardiac cycle (systole) and is described as the sound "Lubb".

S_2 is auscultated over the pulmonic/aortic site. It is heard at the end of the cardiac cycle (diastole). This sound is described as "Dubb".

S_3 is usually ascultated over the apex in the left side-lying position. It is heard in early diastole. The sound is described as "Ken-tuck-y." Hearing the S_3 may indicate heart failure, which also has 3 syllables (heart fail-ure).

S_4 can be auscultated over the apex in the left side-lying position. It is heard in late diastole and is described as "Tenn-e-see." Hearing the S_4 may indicate hypertension, which also has 4 syllables (hy-per-ten-sion). The PMI or Point of Maximal Intensity is usually located near the left midclavicular line at the 5th intercostal space.

CARDIAC SOUNDS

NORMAL

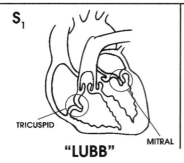

"LUBB"
Closure of
mitral and tricuspid valves

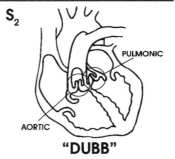

"DUBB"
Closure of
aortic and pulmonic valves

ABNORMAL

S_3

**Heart Fail-ure
(3 syllables)**
Physiologic
(usually in children and young adults)

S_4

**Hy-per-ten-sion
(4 syllables)**

©2002 I CAN Publishing, Inc.

Diagnostic Procedures

As you review diagnostic procedures throughout the different systems of nursing, there are specific areas to focus on to assist in maintaining safety for your clients before, during and after any procedure. We want to "**ACT NOW**" to prevent any complications with these information-gathering procedures. While DIAGNOSTICS will be in each system throughout the book, "**ACT NOW**" will assist you in organizing some general plans that will apply to the majority of the procedures across the systems.

A   **ALLERGIES** are an issue because many diagnostic tests use dyes. Assess for allergies, especially with iodine and shellfish which have iodine in them, prior to any procedure that uses dye. After these procedures, fluids will be encouraged to flush the dye out of the body. Some examples of procedures requiring dyes include myelograms, cardiac catheterizations, computerized axial tomography (CAT Scans), IVP's etc. (Refer to PRIORITY OF CARE PRIOR TO A "GRAM" in this Cardiac chapter.) We have developed several tools to assist in making your life so much easier. These strategies will apply to many similar procedures. After you review these several times, they will remain in your long-term memory. *Remember, the geriatric client excretes dyes slowly. Use with caution.*

C   **CONSENT FORMS** must be signed. The client should be well informed of the risks and benefits of the procedures.

T   **TEACH** the client regarding his participation and the data that the test will provide.

N   **NPO** is required for many tests. Clients and ancillary staff must be aware of this.

PO   **POSITION** is important during and after many procedures. This information should be part of the pretest education.

W   **WHAT ARE THE VITAL SIGNS?** VS's are an excellent way to determine the client's reaction to a procedure, especially if dye has been used. VS's can assist in evaluating if too much fluid has been removed such as with a paracentesis, or if there is a complication with hemorrhaging following the procedure.

Note, on the bottom right page there are several questions. These will be consistently reviewed throughout the chapters where the procedures are reviewed. The reference for the "DIAGNOSTICS" that will be outlined on each right page when reviewing the procedures throughout the book is, The National Council of State Boards of Nursing, Inc. (NCSBN) 2012. NCSBN Research Brief, Volume 53/ January 2012, *2011 RN Practice Analysis: Linking the NCLEX-RN® Examination to Practice.*

ACT NOW

A llergies

C onsent

T each

N P O

p**O** sition

W hat are the vital signs?

Three questions a safe nurse will be able to answer regarding diagnostic tests.

- What is the priority of care prior to the test? (e.g., teaching, consent, allergies, holding meds or food, etc.)

- What is the priority of care during the procedure? (e.g., positioning, anesthesia, invasive/noninvasive, etc.)

- What is the priority of care after the procedure? (e.g., reporting, monitoring, teaching, positioning, etc.)

Diagnostics For The Cardiac System

ECG: (Initiate, maintain, monitor, interpret, and intervene)

Holter Monitor: A small portable ECG unit with a recorder to record client's heart activity for a 24 to 48 hour period. Client documents any pain, activities, and/or palpitations. Client should not remove leads, but can continue with normal activity. No baths or showers should be taken while monitor is in place. The log and record of cardiac activity will be analyzed by HCP.

Echocardiogram: (Noninvasive) Ultrasound of the heart. Diagnose valve disorders and cardiomyopathy. Explain test is pain free, may take up to 1 hour; lie on left side and remain still during the procedure; no specific post-procedure instructions need to be followed.

Angiography: Also referred to as a cardiac catheterization and is an invasive diagnostic procedure. Determines the presence and degree of coronary artery blockage. *Refer to "Priority Care Prior to a GRAM" for specifics; Cardiac Chapter.* Administer premedication as prescribed. Client will be awake and sedated during procedure. *Refer to "Priority Care After a GRAM" for specifics; Cardiac Chapter.* Maintain bed rest per protocol; avoid flexion of the extremity keeping it straight for 3 to 6 hours or as prescribed by HCP or protocol

Stress Test: (Noninvasive) Client walks on a treadmill providing information about the workload of the heart. When client's heart rate reaches a certain rate, the test is discontinued. Advise to wear comfortable shoes and clothes. Instruct to be NPO 2 to 4 hours prior to the procedure based on hospital protocol and avoid alcohol, tobacco, and caffeine. Client will be monitored by ECG and blood pressure checked frequently until the assessments return to baseline and are stable.

Hemodynamic Monitoring: *Refer to "Hemodynamics: A New Approach to Values!"*

Serum Laboratory Studies: Cardiac Markers–In the bloodstream, the content of cells that were injured.

Creatinine kinase (CK): CK isoenzyme MB (CK-MB) is specific to heart muscle. Normal range is 0% of total CK (30 to 170 units/L); an increase of greater than 5% of total CK is highly suggestive of an MI. Levels will be elevated following an MI within 4 to 6 hours, peaking in 12 to 24 hours.

Cardiac troponin T: A myocardial muscle protein with a normal value less than 0.2 ng/mL with an elevation within 3 to 5 hours following myocardial injury and peaks within 12 to 24 hours.

Cardiac troponin I: A myocardial muscle protein with a normal value less than 0.03 ng/mL with an elevation and peaks as the same as troponin T.

Nursing Care: Time is important! On admission, evaluate enzymes and then assess in a serial manner following initial lab test. Troponin levels being elevated are the most significant of heart damage.

Serum Electrolytes: *Refer to Fluid and Electrolyte chapter for an easy way to remember Hyperkalemia and Hypokalemia.*

B-Type Natriuretic Peptide (BNP): A whole blood marker for assessing and treating heart failure. Left ventricular function may be evaluated through a series of BNP labs. The normal value is less than 100 pg/mL.

DIAGNOSTICS FOR THE CARDIAC SYSTEM

"DIAGNOSTIC" exams can be hazardous to the health of our clients.

It is our mission to keep them safe!

The designated NCLEX® standards are outlined below to assist you in organizing the assessments, nursing interventions, and evaluation that must be incorporated into our critical thinking and clinical reasoning for clients experiencing a diagnostic procedure, treatment, or laboratory procedure.

D iagnostic test results—monitor; intervene for complications.

I njury and/or complications from procedure should be prevented.

A ssist with invasive procedures (e.g., thoracentesis, bronchoscopy).

G lucose monitoring, ECG, O_2 saturation, etc. may be performed.

N ote client's response to procedures and treatments.

O btain specimens other than blood (e.g., wound, stool, etc.).

S igns and symptoms of trends and/or changes-monitor, and intervene.

T each client and family about procedures and treatments.

I dentify vital signs and monitor for changes and intervene.

C omplications should be noted and followed immediately with an action.

This image is to remind you that "Sure Look" Holmes is looking into the hippo's mouth to assure he is safe! Just as "Sure Look" Holmes, the nurse is not responsible for ordering these tests, but to maintain client SAFETY prior to, during, and after these diagnostics have been completed.

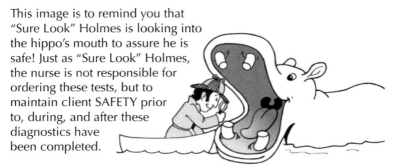

©2014 I CAN Publishing®, Inc.

Priority Care Prior to a "Gram"

There are numerous diagnostics that end in "**GRAM**" such as myelo**gram**, intravenous retrograde pyelo**gram** (IVP), renal arterio**gram** (angio**gram**). One exception to the "**GRAM**" rule is a cardiac catheterization also requires dye to be used as a contrast for providing data regarding the status of the coronary arteries; however, this is also called a coronary angio**gram**. Another example of a test requiring dye that does not end in "**GRAM**" would be a computerized axial tomography (CAT Scan) with contrast.

While each of these diagnostic tests visualize a different part of the body, they require similar nursing care prior to the procedure. These are outlined on the right page with the mnemonic "**DYES**". Remember your job as a nurse is not to order the procedure; however, it is to provide SAFE care.

Prior to the procedure, it is always important to **determine** if the client has any allergies to shellfish/iodine. If they do, there is a risk of experiencing an allergic reaction from the dyes used for the contrast media. It is important to evaluate the age of the client, their renal function, specific medical diagnosis, and medications client is taking. If the client is elderly, there will be a normal physiological decline in the renal function. If they have diabetes mellitus in addition to their advanced age, this could also contribute to additional risks from a diagnostic test requiring dye.

If the client is taking glucophage (Metformin), the healthcare provider needs to be informed due to the risk of the development of lactic acidosis. Glucophage (Metformin) should be discontinued prior to any procedure with a dye due to the risk involved. Once the dye has been excreted, then the medication can be restarted.

Advise client to **drink** and be well hydrated prior to procedure, and **yes, NPO** for 6-8 hrs prior to the procedure. When the dye is being injected, the nurse needs to explain that client may **experience a feeling of warmth**. There may even be an oral **metallic taste**. Prior to the procedure, another important aspect of care is to **evaluate and record quality of distal pulses** for comparison after the test. This will provide a baseline for the neurovascular evaluation following the procedure to determine if there is adequate arterial perfusion. Due to the dyes needing to be excreted via the kidneys, it is imperative for the nurse to know what the **renal function** is prior to the procedure. It is important for the client to be taught prior to the procedure the importance to remain very **still during the procedure** to prevent injury.

> **I CAN TESTING HINT:** When answering questions regarding prior to procedures requiring dyes, remember to "**ARM**" yourself with the priority nursing care! Does the client have **allergies** to shellfish/iodine? What is the **age** of the client? What is the renal function for the client (BUN, creatinine)? Does the client have any diseases such as diabetes mellitus that would compromise the **renal function**? Does the client take **metformin** (Glucophage) or any other medications that could contribute to renal toxicity? In some situations on the NCLEX®, there may be an example of a question that asks about the priority of care for a client with an order for an arteriogram who is 86 years old, has diabetes mellitus, and has a creatinine level of 2.2 mg/dL. The SAFE practice would be to recognize the risk involved with the dyes and "*Question the appropriateness of the order*". If you select an answer about asking if client is allergic to dyes, this would not address the concerns with the age of the client, the creatinine level, and/or the fact the client has diabetes mellitus. The key to success is to read the question carefully, and use your clinical knowledge to make the best decision with the information you have.

DYES

D etermine if any allergies to shell fish/iodine; Drink and be well hydrated prior to procedure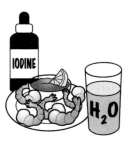

Y es, NPO for 6–8 hrs prior to procedure; void before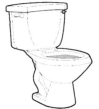

E xperience a feeling of warmth; metallic taste—oral; if taking glucophage (Metformin) advise HCP to hold; evaluate renal function; evaluate pulse distal to injection site and compare to unaffected extremity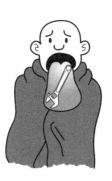

S till during the procedure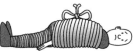

Priority Care After a "Gram"

The goal following a procedure ending in "**GRAM**", in addition to a cardiac catheterization, is to prevent the client's post procedure from being "**HARD**" and without complications.

Due to the dyes injected, it is important to **hydrate** client well to flush out the dye.

Encourage oral intake of fluids. IV access may be obtained if client is unable to drink enough oral fluids. The venipuncture site should be **assessed** q 15-30 min. for bleeding, hematoma, or signs of an infection. Symptoms of infection will be typically assessed later than the bleeding and/or hematoma; however, the evaluation will be an ongoing. With this process, the nurse should monitor the trends with the changes in the client's clinical presentation. If the client does begin bleeding, the vital signs will also show a trend with the HR slowly increasing. The BP will not decrease until later. It is the nurse's responsibility to intervene prior to the client experiencing later changes with bleeding. Another priority for the client during the post procedure period is to **review** for hypersensitivity from dyes in case client was not aware of allergies prior to the procedures. The client should be assessed for urticaria, pruritus, wheezing, or stridor indicating an anaphylactic reaction from the dye. The pulses and neurovascular status (site, color, sensation of the extremity) **distal** to the injection site should be assessed for peripheral perfusion, and compare pre and post procedure neurovascular assessments. Notify the healthcare provider for any alteration in circulation (perfusion) or neurovascular changes in extremity. Assess for any dysrhythmias.

HARD

Hydrate well to flush out the dye

Assess venipuncture site q 15–30 min. for bleeding, hematoma, infection

Review symptoms of hypersensitivity in case client not aware of allergies

Distal pulses to the injection site—assess for occluded blood flow

Cyanotic Heart Defects

Some folks have a hard time remembering which of those congenital heart defects are cyanotic versus which are acyanotic.

NO PROBLEM, just remember all congenital heart defects that begin with the letter "T" are cyanotic defects. Color the "T" on the next page blue to help you remember this easy concept.

FOUR T'S

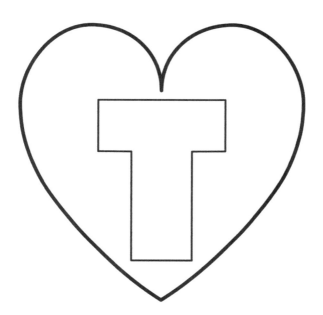

T etralogy

T runcus

T ransposition

T ricuspid

©1992 Sylvia Rayfield & Associates

Tetralogy of Fallot

Tetralogy of Fallot is often referred to as that complicated congenital heart defect that causes children to "squat" or "**DROP**" to the floor. When they get tired or out of breath, this position will decrease the amount of venous return to the heart. **DROP** will assist you in reviewing the four physiological defects with the heart in Tetralogy of Fallot.

D **DISPLACED AORTA** which allows unoxygenated blood into the oxygenated system causing cyanosis (overriding aorta).

R **RIGHT VENTRICLE HYPERTROPHIES** due to working so hard pumping against pressure. The more the heart muscle works the bigger it gets.

O **OPENING IN THE SEPTUM** is a "hole" that allows shunting of unoxygenated blood to mix with oxygenated blood (ventricular septal defect).

P **PULMONARY VALVE** partially closes making the right ventricle work, thus causing the right ventricle to hypertrophy.

These children are often small, tired, delicate and need surgery before leading a better quality of life. Teach parents to pace the child's activities, provide good nutrition to build strength and to renew themselves. Due to the challenges of these children, the parents need emotional support!

TETRALOGY OF FALLOT

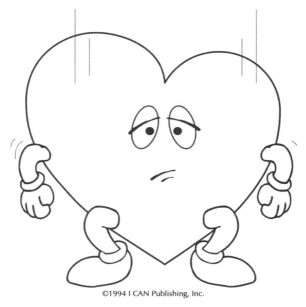

Displaced aorta

Right ventricle hypertrophy

Opening in septum

Pulmonary valve stenosis

Assessments for Congenital Heart Disease

This is to assist with remembering the nursing evaluation for an infant who has a serious defect requiring home care prior to corrective surgery. Think of a **HEART** since this is the location of surgery.

H   **HEART MURMUR**–A murmur will be assessed especially with ventricular septal defects (VSD), atrial septal defects (ASD), and patent ductus arteriosus (PDA).

E   **EVALUATE WEIGHT GAIN**–Due to their intolerance to suck well, they will have a slow weight gain. Some of these infants will be fed via a feeding tube because of their weakness.

A   **ACTIVITY INTOLERANCE**–The infant fatigues easily. Conserve oxygen by anticipating their needs, so they won't cry.

R   **RESPIRATORY INFECTIONS**–Due to pooling of blood in the pulmonary region, these infants have an increased frequency in respiratory infections.

T   **TACHYCARDIA**–An elevation in the resting heart and respiratory rate are signs of hypoxia. Assess these changes carefully! They will give you a lot of information.

S   **SUPPORT**–Allow family to grieve over loss of perfect infant. Foster early parent-infant attachment; encourage touching, holding and loving.

HEARTS

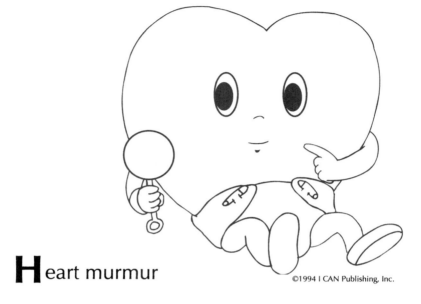

Heart murmur

Evaluate weight

Activity intolerance

Respiratory infections

Tachycardia & Tachypnea

Support

Symptoms of Hypoxia In An Infant

The normal vital signs for a neonate through infancy is 30-60 breaths/min with an average of 40/min. The pulse is 120-160 bpm. Remember at rest the number to remember is 4! If the pulse is approximately 140 bpm and the RR is approximately 40/min, then this is within the normal range. The key here is at REST. **Tachycardia and tachypnea** at rest are indicative of hypoxia and require further assessment and intervention. Periods of apnea lasting for longer than 10-15 seconds need to be further evaluated.

It is imperative when answering test questions or caring for infants in the hospital, that the nurse assesses for clinical trends in the infant that may indicate hypoxia. It is easy when you organize these findings around the word "**GRUNTS**", since this is how the infant will present if hypoxia is present. Crackles and wheezing are symptoms of fluid or infection in the lungs. **Grunting and nasal flaring** are signs of respiratory distress. An infant who is **restless** may also be presenting with hypoxia. **Retracting** is a symptom of respiratory distress. This indicates the infant is working hard to oxygenate the lungs. The infant who is **uninterested in feeding** is typically hypoxic and needs further assessment and intervention. If an infant is presenting with **stridor**, there may be upper airway swelling.

The strategy for answering questions regarding prioritizing which client to see first may be to recognize which infant is presenting with normal clinical findings versus signs of hypoxia. If you have an infant who "**GRUNTS**" while resting, this infant is a priority to assess or intervene with immediately. Remember, the NCLEX® is all about SAFE care! Part of safe care is also to recognize trends in the vital signs and clinical findings prior to the infant being in major distress.

I CAN TESTING HINT: Another way to organizes these symptoms is to remember "**GFRRTT**", grunting, flaring, restless, retracting, tachypnea, tachycardia. This infant would be the priority to evaluate due to hypoxia! Of course, whenever any client is experiencing hypoxia the color can quickly progress from being pale to cyanotic. As nurses, our responsibility is to recognize symptoms of hypoxia and intervene to prevent the progression to cyanosis.

GRUNTS

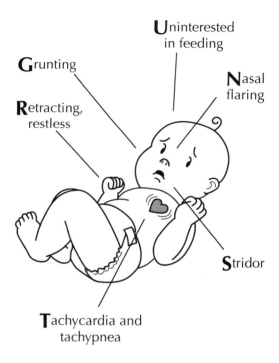

©2014 I CAN Publishing®, Inc.

G runting

R etracting, restless

U ninterested in feeding

N asal flaring

T achycardia and tachypnea

S tridor

Kawasaki Disease

Kawasaki Disease is a **systemic vasculitis** with unknown etiology. F**RED** on the right page is very RED! This is an easy way to remember some of the signs and symptoms that may occur with this medical condition. "**STRAWBERRY**" will assist you in organizing the assessment findings for FRED who is very RED. Clients with Kawasaki Disease will present with a **RED polymorphous rash over the trunk** and perineal area and will present with a temperature >102.2° F. **RED (and peeling) soles and palms** will also be a presenting sign of Kawasaki Disease. **REDNESS in the eyes** (conjunctivitis) may also be a presenting symptom in addition to a strawberry **RED tongue. Bright RED cracked lips** will contribute to the discomfort of this child. This is the reason we named the child FRED, since "RED" is part of the name, and this will assist you in recalling the major presenting signs for this client.

Aneurysms (coronary artery) are the worst that can happen in addition to myocardial infarction. This condition is a **major cause of heart disease for young children**. Due to the many discomforts involved with Kawasaki Disease, the nurse needs to **watch for irritability** and/or lethargy. The child may become RED due to crying from being uncomfortable. Due to the increased need for oxygenation, excessive crying is not good for a child with cardiac disease. Complications may also include **edema** (peripheral) and **reduced urine output**.

Kawasaki Disease typically occurs in children less than five years-old. The strategy for answering questions on the exam would be to remember FRED is **RED** with a "**STRAWBERRY**" tongue. He has a high fever with most of the presenting signs representing the color RED. This disease is usually treated with very high dose IV globulin for 7-10 days and aspirin. Due to the risk of Reye's Syndrome, aspirin is typically not administered; however, this would be an exception to this rule. Due to the high dose of globulin that is administered, safe client care would contraindicate the administration of a live vaccine for one year.

STRAWBERRY

S ystemic vaculitis with unknown etiology

T runk—RED rash over trunk and perineal area; temperature > 102.2° F

R EDNESS in the eyes (conjunctivitis); strawberry red tongue

A neurysms (coronary artery) worse that can happen and myocardial infarction

W atch for irritability and/or lethargy

B right RED cracked lips

E dema (peripheral)

R ED (and peeling) soles and palms

R educed urine output

Y oung children—a major cause of heart disease

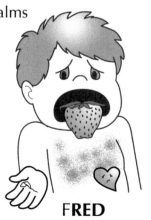

FRED

System-Specific Assessments For Heart Failure

Heart failure (previously referred to as congestive heart failure {CHF}) involves cardiac decompensation, cardiac insufficiency, ventricular failure, and results in the lack of ability of the heart to meet the tissue metabolic demands due to the inability of the heart to pump adequate amounts of blood.

Physiology of Ventricular Failure: The left ventricular (LV) is unable to generate the necessary pressure to eject blood effectively through the aorta resulting in a decrease in the adequate cardiac output (CO). As a result **left ventricular hypertrophy (LVH) develops**, and there is an increased pulmonary capillary bed pressure causing **lungs to become congested**. This will result in an impaired gas exchange. A decrease in the left ventricular (LV) ejection fraction (EF) is the hallmark of ventricular failure.

Diastolic failure is the inability of the ventricles to relax during diastole (filling). Cardiac output and stroke volume are decreased. Both **systemic** and pulmonary systems may have venus engorgement.

Risk Factors:
- Congenital heart disease
- Hypertension
- Fluid overload–myocardial disease, valvular disease

Assessment Findings of Heart Failure:

Left-Sided (Pulmonary Symptoms = **LUNGS**); *refer to image on right page*

Right-Sided (Systemic Symptoms = **EDEMA**); *refer to image on right page*

Chronic Heart Failure = **LACES**; *Remember, if clients have CHF, they may have limited energy to "LACE" their shoes.*

    Lethargy (fatigue)
    Activity limitations
    Cough/chest congestion
    Edema
    Shortness of breath

HEART FAILURE

Left sided Heart failure = **Lungs**

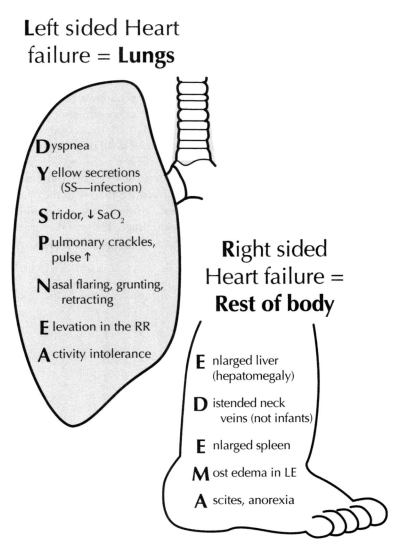

D yspnea
Y ellow secretions (SS—infection)
S tridor, ↓ SaO$_2$
P ulmonary crackles, pulse ↑
N asal flaring, grunting, retracting
E levation in the RR
A ctivity intolerance

Right sided Heart failure = **Rest of body**

E nlarged liver (hepatomegaly)
D istended neck veins (not infants)
E nlarged spleen
M ost edema in LE
A scites, anorexia

Reduce Cardiac Workload

The car on the next page is carrying a **SPARE** "heart tire." The goal for nursing care is to decrease the stress and strain on the heart after a myocardial infarction. *(It is the same as our goal when we drive our automobile; we do not want our tire to be damaged. The spare tire never quite replaces the original.)* After a myocardial infarction, modification in diet and lifestyle are important nursing implications. Lifestyle and diet changes should include **restriction of sodium and saturated fat** and a reduction or avoidance of alcohol consumption. It is important to **provide a calm**, quiet environment and comfort measures to ensure effectiveness of pain medications. Immediately after a MI the nurse should allow the client time to rest between treatments, and limit visitors and extra activity. Cardiac **after load** can be decreased by medications such as vasodilators. These medications will relax the vascular smooth muscle, producing vasodilation of the arterioles which reduces the cardiac after load. Anxiety can increase the oxygen requirements significantly; therefore, it is important to **reduce anxiety** in the client's life and encourage **daily renewal and rest**. This is an important time in a client's life to learn new relaxation techniques. The ultimate goal is for the client to return to his/her activities of daily living and to live a happy, healthy, productive life!

REDUCE CARDIAC WORKLOAD

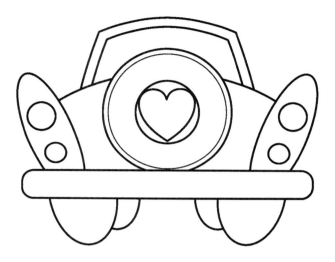

S odium and saturated fat intake

P rovide a calm environment

A fter load reduced

R educe anxiety

E motional rest

Cardiac Management

OANM will assist you in remembering medications to administer to clients with chest pain.

O **OXYGEN** Oxygen will reduce complications from ischemia.

A **ASPIRIN** Aspirin is administered for its blood-thinning properties.

N **NITROGLYCERIN** Nitroglycerin will increase the blood supply to the heart by dilating the coronary arteries. The cardiac workload is reduced due to decrease in venous return as a result of the peripheral vasodilation.

M **MORPHINE** This analgesic will reduce the pain, which subsequently will decrease the ischemia.

Remember: If you need to prioritize, OANM will do it. Oxygen first, Aspirin second, Nitro, and then Morphine.

CARDIAC MANAGEMENT

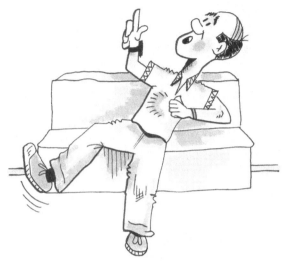

Oxygen

Aspirin

Nitroglycerin

Morphine

Ace Inhibitors

What is an ACE Inhibitor?

It lowers blood pressure by stopping the angiotensin converting enzyme (ACE) in the lung, which reduces the vasoconstrictor, angiotensin II. This indeed will lower your blood pressure.

How do I remember all of these medications?

It's actually insanely easy!!! Let us introduce you to the "**Pril**" sisters who are taking a "**strol**" through the park to prevent cardiac problems. Strol will assist you to remember the actions of the ACE inhibitors. "**CHF**" will help you in remembering some undesirable effects from these drugs. CHF is used as a mnemonic to assist you in remembering that a client can receive these medications if they have hypertension and have experienced congestive heart failure. Since these drugs work directly at blocking the angiotensin converting enzyme (ACE), and it does not work directly on the heart, then these drugs are appropriate for clients with CHF.

What are some examples of these drugs?

    Capto**pril**
    Enala**pril**
    Lisino**pril**
    Fosino**pril**
    Rami**pril**
    Benzae**pril**

What do I need to evaluate?

1. Blood pressure—Since these medications reduce vasoconstriction, the pressure may go down too low. Observe for dizziness and/or tachycardia.

2. Some undesirable effects include an annoying dry cough, angioedema of the face, lips, tongue, and pharynx. Uncommon side effects include rash and taste disturbances.

3. Monitor for hypotension and hyperkalemia.

4. With Captopril, agranulocytosis or neutropenia may occur (ask about sore throats).

PRIL SISTERS

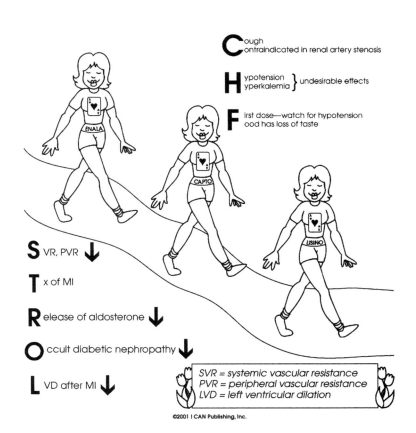

C ough
  ontraindicated in renal artery stenosis

H ypotension } undesirable effects
  yperkalemia

F irst dose—watch for hypotension
  ood has loss of taste

S VR, PVR ↓

T x of MI

R elease of aldosterone ↓

O ccult diabetic nephropathy ↓

L VD after MI ↓

SVR = systemic vascular resistance
PVR = peripheral vascular resistance
LVD = left ventricular dilation

©2001 I CAN Publishing, Inc.

Beta Blockers

Beta Blockers are a group of drugs that can be remembered using the acronym BETA. People taking these drugs may need TLC (tender loving care) because they may become drowsy or fatigued.

B **BROCHOSPASM** (so we don't want to give them to people with asthma or brochoconstrictive disease!)

E **ELICITS A DECREASE IN CARDIAC OUTPUT AND CONTRACTILITY.**

T **TREATS HYPERTENSION /ANGINA/MIGRAINES/ PANIC ATTACKS.**

A **AV CONDUCTION DECREASES** (short for treats arrhythmias, especially fast ones by decreasing the heart rate and cardiac output!)

REMEMBER–STOP BETA BLOCKERS WITH BRONCHOCONSTRICTIVE DISEASE

T **TENORMIN** (atenolol) used for hypertension and angina (watch for renal impairment as this drug is renally excreted).

L **LOPRESSOR** (metoptolol) used for hypertension and angina (contraindicated in sinus bradycardia, 2nd or 3rd degree block, metabolized in liver and NOT renally excreted).

C **CORGARD** (nadolol) used for hypertension and angina (renally excreted, contraindicated in bronchial asthma, sinus bradycardia or 2nd or 3rd degree heart block).

NOTICE ALL THE GENERIC NAMES END IN "LOL"!

ROAD BLOCKS TO BETA BLOCKERS

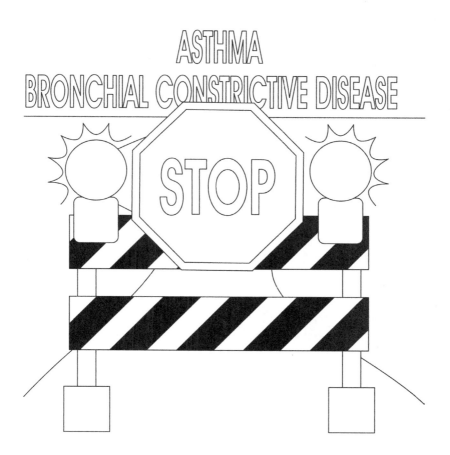

Calcium Channel Blockers

Calcium Channel Blockers are used to treat hypertension, angina, and migraine headaches. This group of medications are often called "Don't Give a Flip Pills" by the clients who take them because that's exactly how they feel. Their blood pressure is lowered (calcium influx blocked), pulse is decreased, and if they move too quickly they get dizzy. They are much happier being a couch potato and taking life easy. A few examples of the calcium channel blockers include **Cardi**zem, **Ca**rdene, Pro**ca**rdia, and **Ca**lan. Each of these common Calcium Channel Blockers have a "**Ca**" in them which makes it easy to remember! These medications should be administered with meals and milk. Some general undesirable effects of these medications include **constipation, bradycardia, peripheral edema, hypotension, dizziness, heart blocks, and worsening of CHF.**

Remember—Calcium Channel blockers should not be given in clients who are in **congestive heart failure** *or* **cardiogenic shock** *because they can decrease the heart rate too much.*

CALCIUM CHANNEL BLOCKERS

"DON'T GIVE A FLIP PILLS"

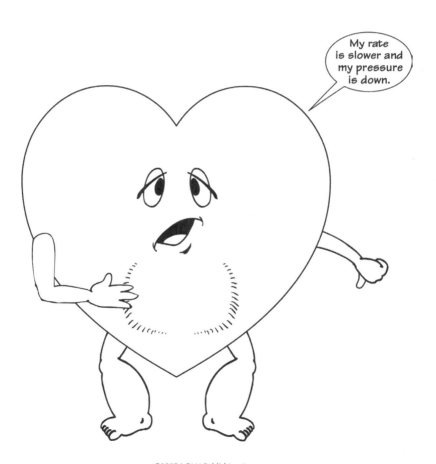

Loop Diuretics

"Lou La Bell" has been given a loop diuretic such as Lasix or Ethacrynate Sodium and is very **dizzy**. Her blood pressure has decreased too much after her excessive peeing. You would also feel as if you were spinning in a tube over the falls if you lost this much urine (volume). It may be very useful to teach her to get up slowly so she won't fall.

The life guard must blow his whistle in order to get her some assistance. She feels that the **ringing** in her ears just won't go away. **Dizziness** and **ringing** in the ears are major adverse reactions from loop diuretics.

A few other adverse reactions include: **hypokalemia, hypocalcemia (tetany), hyperglycemia**, and **hyperuricemia**. While aplastic anemia and agranulocytosis may occur, they are RARE!

Remember—Keep a close watch on blood pressure, potassium and calcium levels. Teach foods high in potassium and calcium. See ABC Fruit and Veggie Plate. Potassium supplements may be necessary.

LOU LA BELL

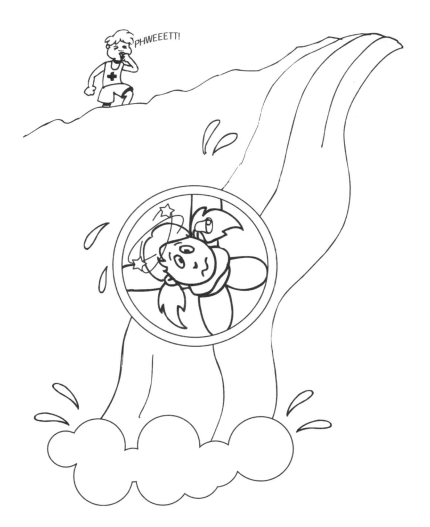

Atrial Dysrhythmias

If atrial fibrillation or atrial flutter occur greater than 48 hours in a client with normal cardiac function, diltiazem (Cardizem) is one agent that may be effective in controlling the **heart rate**. If the duration of the dysrhythmia is < 48 hours, consider the use of only one of the following agents for **converting the rhythm**: Amiodarone, Ibutilide, Flecainide, Propafenone, or Pocainamide. DC cardioversion. If the duration is > 48 hours or unknown, use antiarrhythmic agents with extreme caution. Avoid nonemergent cardioversion unless anticoagulation or clot precautions are taken. For specific management refer to *Handbook of Emergency Cardiovascular Care for Healthcare Providers* by American Heart Association. The management of delayed cardioversion and anticoagulation therapy are beyond the scope of this book.

In a client with an impaired heart (EF < 40% or CHF) and the AF > 48 hours duration, one of the following agents are recommended for controlling the **heart rate**: Digoxin, Diltiazem, Amiodarone. For this same client converting the AF in < 48 hours may be accomplished with Amiodarone. DC cardioversion. If the AF has persisted > 48 hours, manage the anticoagulation and DC cardioversion. (*American Heart Association*)

Cardioversion may be indicated for heart rates >150 bpm with serious signs and symptoms related to tachycardia. Place the defibrillator/monitor in synchronized (sync) mode. The cardioversion may be painful due to the electric current going through the chest, therefore premedicate whenever possible.

Be prepared for the cardioversion to convert the rhythm to ventricular fibrillation. As our mothers always told us, too much of a good thing can be bad for us. Sometimes "stuff just happens!"

ATRIAL ACTIONS

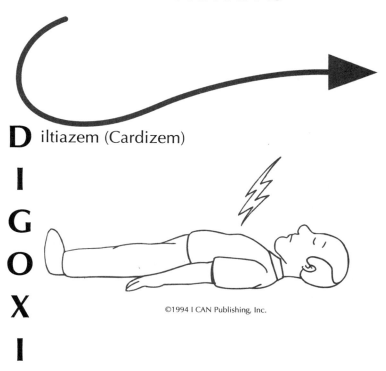

D iltiazem (Cardizem)

I

G

O

X

I

N ow lie 'em down for cardioversion

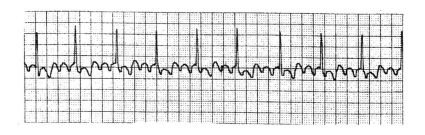

Defibrillate or Cardiovert?
That is the Question!

When you are first learning about cardiac dysrhythmias, it can be very confusing about the appropriate interventions particularly when it comes to defibrillation versus cardioversion.

Here are some basic facts that can help you become a cardiac whiz!

Elect to Cardiovert–Get in Sync!!! "CARDIOVERT"

- **C** **Conscious** client with sedation
- **A** Anticoagulation prior to cardioversion
- **R** Requires shock be synchronized, use low joules; synchronize on the "R" wave!
- **D** **Done only by HCP**
- **I** IV will be needed
- **O** Oxygen before & after, NOT during
- **V** Vital signs & ECG rhythm-evaluate throughout
- **E** **Elective Procedure, need consent**
- **R** Rhythms to cardioversion include atrial fibrillation
- **T** Tell everyone to clear prior to shock; use conduction medium to prevent burns

Defibrillate–Do or DIE!!! "DEFIBRILLATE"

- **D** Defibrillate only on an **unconscious** client
- **E** **Emergency**–Call a Code
- **F** **Fibrillation ventricular or pulseless ventricular tachycardia**
- **I** IV needed for drugs according to ACLS protocol
- **B** Begin CPR & continue in between defibrillations
- **R** Respiratory, need to support
- **I** Increase joules as needed (defib x 3 only at max joules)
- **L** Locate crash cart
- **L** Learn to correctly place paddles
- **A** Always use conduction medium to prevent burns
- **T** Tell everyone to clear prior to shock
- **E** Evaluate vital signs, rhythm & response to meds

Be SAFE for Both Cardioversion and Defibrillation
- **S** Skin protect from burns with conduction medium
- **A** Always place paddles correctly
- **F** Find crash cart to have at bedside
- **E** Everyone clear prior to shock

DEFIBRILLATE OR CARDIOVERT?

CARDIOVERSION

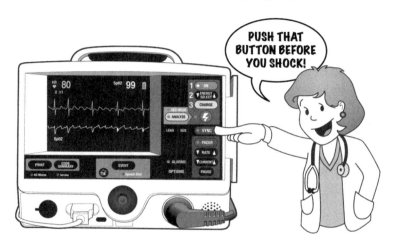

VERSUS DEFRIBILLATION

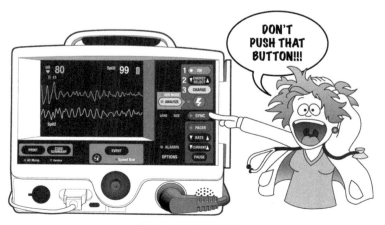

Heart Blocks

Heart Blocks are caused by a delay or interruption in electrical conduction between the atria and ventricles. This delay may be caused by cardiac disease process, Beta Blockers, and Calcium Channel Blockers. An electronic **Pacemaker** (transcutaneous pacing, TCP) is usually the preferred treatment for the more severe heart blocks. Drugs are often tried to correct this rhythm and **Atropine** is frequently the choice. Atropine blocks the vagus nerve impulses on the SA node causing an increased heart rate. **Ephinephrine** will also cause an increased heart rate.

According to current American Heart Association guidelines, if the client is exhibiting serious signs and symptoms due to the bradycardia, then the intervention sequence would be as outlined below.

Atropine–First Degree
Transcutaneous pacing if available–Second/Third Degree
Dopamine
Epinephrine

(For specific dosage, refer to *Handbook of Emergency Cardiovascular Care for Healthcare Providers* by the American Heart Association.)

If the client begins experiencing a Type II second-degree AV block or Third-degree AV block, prepare for transvenous pacer. If the symptoms develop, use the transcutaneous pacemaker until the transvenous pacer is placed.

*If a pacemaker is inserted, teach client how to monitor their pulse which is an indicator of pacemaker function. Teach symptoms of pacemaker dysfunction and pertinent detail regarding "power" failure in permanent pacemakers. Provide a safe environment by eliminating all possible electrical hazards. Instruct these clients to wear medical identification.

For additional specific algorithms refer to www.ACLS.net.
A special thank you to ACLS for outlining algorithms which are easy to remember!

HEART BLOCKS

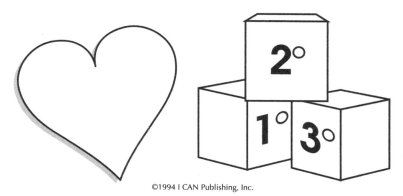

©1994 I CAN Publishing, Inc.

PACEMAKER
ATROPINE
PI

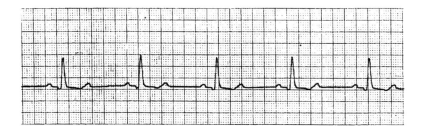

Hemodynamics: A New Approach to Values! (The 6s)

Do you ever have a hard time remembering the values for key hemodynamic readings? Do you ever get stressed out because you are concerned with SAFETY for the client due to hemodynamic monitoring? Those concerns can end now because this can be as easy as the end of hemodynamics, "**MICS**" rhymes with **SIX**, and the key values are **6** or 6 x 2 = **12**. Another way to remember this is there are **12 letters in hemodynamics**!

The information on this page will include the specific hemodynamic values for the CVP and CO with a brief description. There will also be a brief review of potential complications from the CVP line. On pages 154-155, **MPAP** and **PAWP** are reviewed.

Let's begin with CVP! **Central venous pressure (CVP)** is a measurement of the pressure in the right atrium or within the large veins in the thoracic cavity. An intravenous catheter is placed in the superior vena cava or in the right atrium or jugular vein. The CVP reading may also be assessed from the proximal lumen of the pulmonary artery catheter. The normal range for the value is from **2-6** mm Hg. The "**6 hearts**" on the right page will help you visualize the value for this measurement. The key is to note the **trends** with this value. If the reading was 4 and in 1 hour the value increased to 12, then the client needs to be further evaluated.

There are several reasons that the value may increase or decrease. Remember "**VEIN**" since the value evaluates venous pressure. This will assist you with clinical decision making with your hospitalized client, on exams in school, and / or on the NCLEX®.

- **V** **V**enous return to the heart (↑ CVP may indicate hypervolemia; ↓ may indicate hypovolemia).
- **E** **E**valuates function of the left side of the heart (↑ CVP may indicate poor contractility; ↓ may indicate vasodilation).
- **I** **I**ntrathoracic pressure (an increase in this pressure can result with a ↑ CVP).
- **N** **N**ote that coughing or straining may result in a ↑ CVP.

Infection and/or air emboli are two potential complications that could occur with the hemodynamic lines. Safe nursing practice is always focusing on prevention first, and then ongoing assessment of the signs and symptoms for potential complications.

Use surgical aseptic technique with all dressing changes (mask, sterile gloves, maintain sterile field). Monitor for evidence of an infection such as a trend in the temperature increasing, subtle redness at the site, and/or elevated WBC count. The catheter should be stabilized on the skin at the insertion site. An occlusive sterile dressing should be applied. Always remember the importance of excellent hand hygiene for any procedure, before and after. Excellent nursing care is the key to the prevention of complications.

Plaque or a clot may become dislodged during the procedure. Patency of the CVP line is maintained via IV infusion drip to prevent thromboembolism. The nurse must avoid introduction of air into flushing system to prevent air embolism.

Complications that may occur during the insertion of the line include the risk of a pneumothorax and/or dysrhythmias. This would require immediate medical intervention.

The **cardiac output (CO)** is the measurement of the amount of blood pumped in 1 minute (60 seconds). The normal range is **4-6** L/min.

THE 6s

CVP = Central venous pressure (2–6 mm Hg)   **6**
CO   = Cardiac output (4–6 L/min)   **6**

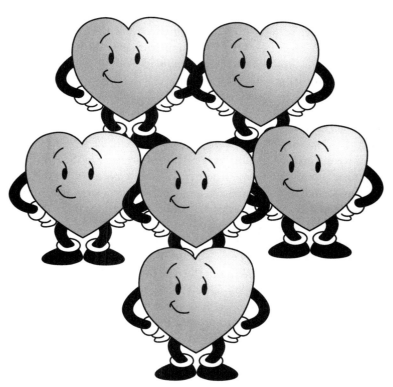

Hemodynamics: A New Approach to Values! (The 12s)

The pulmonary artery pressure monitoring (Swan-Gantz Catheter) is a multilumen catheter that is inserted and advanced through the right atrium and right ventricle into the pulmonary artery. The patency of this line is maintained by an heparainized saline solution.

The "**12 hearts**" on the right page will assist you in remembering the approximate value for the MPAP and the PAWP. The pulmonary artery pressure value is 15-26 mm Hg systolic, with the **mean pulmonary arterial pressure (MPAP)** at approximately **12** to 15 mm Hg. The MPAP is typically increased in clients with chronic pulmonary diseases and clients with heart failure.

The pulmonary capillary wedge pressure (PAWP or PCWP) has a normal range from 4–**12** mm Hg. It is determined as a mean pressure. To evaluate this value, a small balloon on the catheter tip that is in the distal branch of the pulmonary artery is inflated or wedged. This wedge pressure is a direct reflection of pressure in the left cardiac chambers and reflects ventricular end diastolic pressure. If the trend increases, then this may indicate an increase in pressures and/or fluid. If the trend decreases, then this may indicate a need for fluid, dehydration, or severe dilation.

Just as with the CVP line, there are risks with sepsis, air emboli, ventricular dysrhythmias typically during insertion (*refer to previous page on CVP for description*), but the risk that is unique to the pulmonary artery pressure (Swan-Ganz Catheter) is pulmonary infarction. When the PCWP is evaluated, it is imperative that the balloon or the wedge be deflated in order to prevent the complication of pulmonary infarction.

I CAN TESTING HINT: First, when the CVP and PAWP readings are high, this most likely indicates too much fluid. When they are low, the client may be experiencing hypovolemia.

Second, CVP evaluates the right side of the heart (venous) and the Pulmonary Artery Pressure evaluates the left side of the heart (arterial).

THE 12s

MPAP = Mean Pulmonary Artery Pressure (12–15 mm Hg) **12**

PAWP = Pulmonary Artery Wedge Pressure (4–12 mmHg) **12**

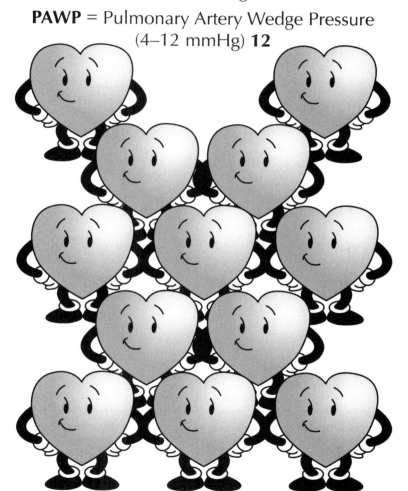

Peripherally Inserted Central Catheter Care

The mnemonic on the right page provides you with a strategy to organize the care for an alternative question evaluating your understanding on how to provide nursing care of a PICC line in chronological order.

> **I CAN TESTING HINT:** Remember to use a 10 mL syringe or larger to avoid excess pressure per square inch (PSI) that could cause catheter fracture/rupture.

PERIPHERAL

P eripheral site assessed per protocol; note redness, swelling, etc.

E xchange tubing and positive pressure cap with new ones per facility protocol (typically a minimum of 3 days for the hospitalized client).

R emember to use **10 mL or larger** syringe to flush line.

I nsertion port should be cleaned with alcohol for 3 seconds; dry prior to accessing it.

P erform flushing for intermittent medication administration per protocol, usually with **10 mL** of 0.9% sodium chloride before, between, and after medications.

H ave 3 **10 mL** syringes available for blood samples; withdraw 10 mL of blood and discard; take a second syringe and withdraw 10 mL of blood for sample; take the a third syringe and flush with 10 mL of 0.9% sodium chloride *(follow specific facility/hospital flushing guidelines)*.

E valuate dressing for wetness, looseness, or soiled and change; use a transparent dressing and follow facility protocol for dressing changes, usually every 7 days with the exception of a problem of being loose, soiled or wet.

R emind client not to immerse arm in water.

A void water exposure by covering dressing to shower.

L imb (arm) with PICC line should not have blood pressure taken.

Peripheral Vascular Disease: Arterial Versus Venous

Peripheral arterial disease (PAD) is a narrowing and obstruction of the arteries, especially in the lower extremities. This obstruction may result in a decreased oxygen supply to the tissues. Due to the obstruction, there is a delay in the capillary refill making it greater than 3 seconds. The description of the ulcers that may result from this are described on the right page. The pulses may be decreased or even absent with this complication resulting in a cool extremity.

Keep the blood flowing by: (*So Art can flow down the slide easily!*)
Avoiding remaining in one position for too long.
Avoiding pressure in the popliteal area.
Avoiding crossing legs at the knees.
Avoiding positions, bandages, or clothing that restrict circulation to the lower extremities such as girdles, hose, elastic bandages, etc.

Notice *Art* is having a hard time getting down the slide into the extremity which is exactly the issue with the blood not getting down to the extremity. Remember **arterial** blood flows **away** from the heart. This is the reason the color may progress from pale to being gray, eventually presenting with no pulse. Refer to **"PAIN"** for the nursing care with inadequate peripheral artery perfusion on page 161.

Peripheral venous disorders (PVD) are problems with the veins that interfere with adequate return of the blood flow from the extremities. Three peripheral venous disorders that are the most familiar to nurses include: varicose veins, venous insufficiency, venous thromboembolism (VTE).

The bottom line here is that Vik is unable to climb back up to the heart! Due to lack of blood return, then the extremities get edematous where the blood is pooling. Sequential compression stockings can assist with the prevention of the blood pooling for the immobilized client. The image on the right page will assist you in remembering the symptoms of this disorder. Notice that these symptoms from venous insufficiency are all about stasis of the blood and inability for it to return to the heart.

"EDEMA" will assist you in organizing the nursing care for PVD.

E Encourage mobility; elastic support stockings: Hospitalized clients should wear all the time. Clients at home should wear the support stockings during the day. Put on before getting out of bed and remove when going to bed. Do not hang feet dependently when putting on stockings; elevate the legs or put them parallel on the bed.

D Do not cross legs when sitting or lying in bed. Do not wear restrictive clothing.

E Educate client to elevate legs for about 20 minutes every 4 or 5 hours.

M Maintain adequate hydration; avoid dehydration. Monitor safe use of sequential compression stockings.

A Avoid prolonged sitting; every 1 to 2 hours client should walk around.

ARTERIAL VERSUS VENOUS

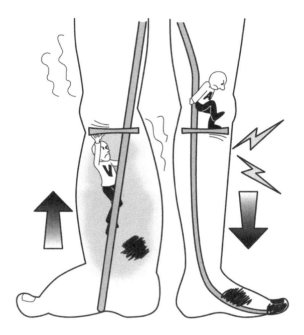

Venous
Apperance—irregular shape

Pain—when leg is dependent, dull, heavy and achy

Color—beefy red/granulation; ruddy skin

Drainage—exudative wounds

Location of sores—ankles

Arterial
Appearance—regular borders, round

Pain—burning and throbbing (intermittent claudication pain)

Color—pale or gray; may progress to black eschar

Drainage—No drainage

Location of sores—toes and feet

Circulation
Lower leg edema

Pulse present

Circulation
No edema

No pulse or weak pulse

Priority Plan For Clients With Inadequate Peripheral Artery Perfusion

Alteration in peripheral artery perfusion results from atherosclerosis that typically occurs in the arteries of the lower extremities and is characterized by inadequate blood flow. Atherosclerosis occurs as a result of a gradual thickening of the intima and media of the arteries, resulting in the progressive narrowing of the vessel lumen. The arteries may become rough and fragile from the formation of the plaques on the arterial walls. Peripheral artery disease may be classified as inflow (distal aorta and iliac arteries) or outflow (femoral, popliteal, and tibial artery). This tissue damage occurs distal to the arterial obstruction. Examples of PAD may include: Buerger's disease, Raynaud's disease or Raynaud's phenomenon, etc.

The assessments have been outlined on previous pages. This strategy is to assist you with a SAFE nursing plan of care. We have chosen the mnemonic "**PAIN**" since this is the result of inadequate peripheral artery perfusion. In order to promote vasodilation and to avoid vasoconstriction, **provide with a warm environment**; promote walking (30-60 min/day, 3-5 days a week). **Avoid exposure to cold**, stress, caffeine, smoking, nicotine (all of which result in vasoconstriction); avoid standing in one position for prolonged periods of time. Complete abstinence from smoking or chewing tobacco is the most effective way to prevent vasoconstriction (vasoconstrictive effects last up to 1 hour after each cigarette is smoked). Instruct client to **avoid crossing legs at the knees or ankles**. Avoid pressure in the posterior popliteal area. Advise client not to wear restrictive garments. Recommend client to elevate legs to reduce swelling; however, not to elevate legs above the level of the heart. This extreme elevation slows arterial blood flow to the feet. Due to the alteration in perfusion, the client may have a tendency to have cool extremities.

Insulate socks to keep feet warm. Inspect feet and extremities for discolored areas. **Never apply direct heat** to affected extremity since sensitivity is decreased and may result in a risk for burning.

The client should initially exercise gradually and slowly increase. Advise the client to walk to the point of pain, stop and rest, and then resume walking a little further.

Notice some trends in care! Nothing that will result in constriction, no crossing of legs, no restrictive clothes, do not get cold (keep warm), no chewing tobacco (cigarettes)! **The Cs** may also help you in recalling this information! Pathophysiology will help you understand the nursing care, so you will always be able to remember this concept. The goal is to prevent the problem from ever occurring; however, once peripheral artery perfusion is altered then your plan is to support the "**PAIN**" and provide SAFE care.

PAIN

P rovide with a warm environment to prevent vasoconstriction; promote walking (30–60 min/day, 3–5 days a week)

A void exposure to cold, stress, caffeine, smoking, nicotine (all of which result in vasoconstriciton); avoid standing in one position for prolonged periods of time. Avoid crossing legs at the knees or ankles while in bed. Avoid pressure in the posterior popliteal area.

I nsulate socks to keep feet warm; inspect feet and extremities for discolored areas

N ever apply direct heat to affected extremity since sensitivity is decreased; risk for burning

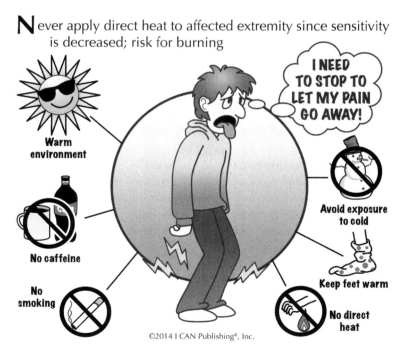

Raynaud's Phenomenon: Prevention of Vasospasms

Raynaud's phenomenon consists of intermittent episodic spasms of the arterioles, most frequently in the fingers, toes, ears, and tip of the nose. The spasms may not be correlated with other peripheral vascular problems.

The risk factors for Raynaud's Phenomenon include occupation related, females 20-40 years of age, and/or an autoimmune response. Clinical assessment findings may be precipitated by exposure to a cold object (environment), caffeine, cigarettes (nicotine), and chaos in the client's life (emotional upset).

Decreased perfusion results in "**PAIN**".

P **P**allor; pulses usually remain adequate
A **A**ppearance of waxy tissue in the vasoconstrictive phase
I **I**ncrease in aching, tingling, and throbbing in the hyperemic phase
N **N**umbness and tingling

Complications may progress to ulceration to gangrene. There is no cure. The treatment is based on the symptoms. Medications that may be used include calcium channel blockers, vasodilators.

The right page is a strategy to assist you in organizing the nursing care necessary to prevent vasospasms. "**STRESS**" will help you remember the priority care for clients with Raynaud's phenomenon. A great place to begin is with **stress management**. This could include music, reading, meditating, or any activity that assists the client to decrease stress (*palm trees and the beach will do it for me!*). **The hands, feet, nose, and ears need to be protected when exposed to cold weather.** This will prevent constriction that may assist in decreasing episodic attacks. **Refrigerated** or freezer objects are also a concern for this client. Client should be advised to wear gloves/socks with any exposure to cold. If possible, maintain a **warm environment. Stress the importance of avoiding caffeine and tobacco products.**

Do you notice the similarity with this phenomenon and nursing care for alteration in peripheral artery perfusion on the previous page? The link here is that we need to keep client warm and free of nicotine and caffeine. This will be the same for any medical condition that may result in arterial insufficiency or spasms. It is always a great idea to incorporate stress management with all of our clients. See how EASY it can be when we focus on the priority care and associate it with other concepts that require similar nursing care! You CAN do this!!

STRESS

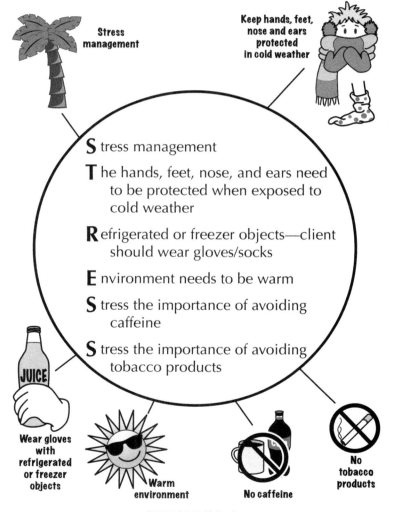

S tress management

T he hands, feet, nose, and ears need to be protected when exposed to cold weather

R efrigerated or freezer objects—client should wear gloves/socks

E nvironment needs to be warm

S tress the importance of avoiding caffeine

S tress the importance of avoiding tobacco products

©2014 I CAN Publishing®, Inc.

"To know even one life has breathed
easier because you have lived.
This is to have succeeded."

RALPH WALDO EMERSON

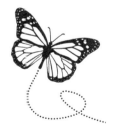

RESPIRATORY / ACID BASE

Breath Sounds

Normal breath sounds have been organized into three categories based upon the intensity, pitch, and duration of the inspiratory and expiratory phases.

The bronchial sounds are heard over the manubrium (if heard at all). The expiration sounds are longer than inspiration sounds. They are louder and higher in pitch. If these are auscultated anywhere other than the manubrium, they are considered to be abnormal and may indicate a complication with a lobar pneumonia.

The bronchovesicular sounds are heard often in the 1st and 2nd interspaces anteriorly and between the scapulae. The inspiratory and expiratory sounds are about equal in length. These sounds are intermediate. Differences in pitch and intensity are often more easily assessed during expiration. If bronchovesicular sounds are heard in other locations distant from what is listed above, then the air-filled lung may have been replaced by fluid or solid lung tissue.

The vesicular breath sounds may be auscultated over most of both lungs. Inspiratory sounds last longer than expiratory ones. Vesicular breath sounds are soft and low-pitched.

BREATH SOUNDS

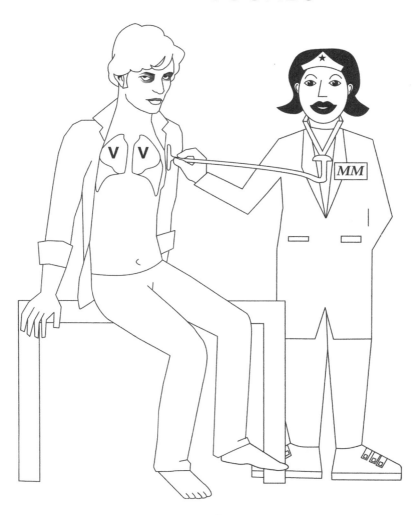

Transmitted Voice Sounds

When the lung is normal and filled with air, spoken words are indistinct and muffled. The spoken "ee" is heard as "ee." Whispered words are faint and indistinct if heard at all. They are normally accompanied by vesicular breath sounds and normal tactile fremitus.

When these sounds go through an airless lung such as in lobar pneumonia or toward the top of a large pleural effusion, these spoken sounds (99, ee, 1, 2, 3) are louder and clearer (bronchophony). The spoken "ee" is heard as "ay" and whispered words are louder and clearer (whispered pectoriloquy). These transmitted voice sounds are usually accompanied by bronchial or bronchovesicular breath sounds and increased tactile fremitus.

Note: Remember to end in "phony" (phonics) to understand clarity. Increase in clarity = consolidation!!

TRANSMITTED VOICE SOUNDS

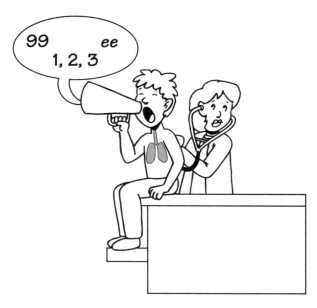

Ego**phony** "ee"   =   "ay" sound
Broncho**phony** "99"   =   clarity of sounds
Whispered Pectoriloquy   =   clarity of sounds
"whisper 99 or 1,2,3"

↓
Clarity of Sounds
↓
CONSOLIDATION

©2002 I CAN Publishing, Inc.

Diagnostics For The Respiratory System

Chest X-Ray: An x-ray of the chest and lungs. No special care prior/afterwards.

Bronchoscopy: Invasive; a test to visualize the airway (larynx, trachea, and bronchi). **Before procedure:** Typically NPO 6-12 hours (per protocol) prior to procedure. Preop med and upper airway is anesthetized. *Refer to "Assessments After Any Test That Ends in SCCPY" for specific care after procedure.*

Thoracentesis: A test that withdraws fluid from pleural cavity. Performed under local anesthesia. *Refer to "Priority Care for a CENTESIS" for specific care.*

Pulmonary Angiography: The pulmonary arteries have contrast media injected into them to visualize the pulmonary system. Pulmonary emboli are diagnosed with this procedure. *Refer to "Priority Care Prior to a GRAM" for specific care.*

Magnetic Resonance Imaging (MRI): Refer to Diagnostics for the Neurological System.

Computerized Axial Tomography (CAT Scan): Refer to Diagnostics for the Neurological System.

Pulmonary Function Test: Measures lung volume and does not require medication. Client must be alert and cooperative. Client breathes into a cylinder and the process is recorded in a computer. Prior to treatment, client should not smoke for 12 hours or use bronchodilator for 6 hours.

Lung Scan (V/Q Scan): Ventilation perfusion measures how well air reaches the lungs, requires consent and utilizes a radioisotope for imaging. Determine possible allergy to radioisotope used in the exam. Client not sedated or on dietary restrictions for exam.

PPD: An intradermal skin test for tuberculosis. Safe nurses must know how to determine positive/negative. PPD is injected intradermally in forearm.

Pulse Oximetry: Noninvasive measurement of the oxygen saturation of the blood. A sensor probe is placed on the finger or earlobe with a wave of infrared light passing through the tissue to measure the oxygen-saturated hemoglobin. Normal range is 95% or higher. Acceptable ranges for SaO_2 may be 91% to 100%. The nurse should confirm the oxygen delivery system is functioning and client is receiving what is prescribed. Position in semi-Fowler's or Fowler's position to optimize ventilation. Encourage deep breathing. Of course, the nursing responsibility is also to prevent false readings to assure safe and accurate interpretation. "**COLDS**" will assist you with this process. A cold extremity will result in an inaccurate reading.

- **C** Circulation (peripheral) inadequate
- **O** Oximeter fell off or client is wearing nail polish
- **L** Low temperature (hypothermia)
- **D** Decreased hemoglobin
- **S** Swelling (edema)

Remember normal values for a geriatric client may be lower than for a younger adult.

ABGs: Used to measure the pH and partial pressure of the dissolved gases (O_2 and CO_2) of the arterial blood.

DIAGNOSTICS FOR THE RESPIRATORY SYSTEM

"DIAGNOSTIC" exams can be hazardous to the health of our clients.

It is our mission to keep them safe!

The designated NCLEX® standards are outlined below to assist you in organizing the assessments, nursing interventions, and evaluation that must be incorporated into our critical thinking and clinical reasoning for clients experiencing a diagnostic procedure, treatment, or laboratory procedure.

D iagnostic test results—monitor; intervene for complications.

I njury and/or complications from procedure should be prevented.

A ssist with invasive procedures (e.g., thoracentesis, bronchoscopy).

G lucose monitoring, ECG, O_2 saturation, etc. may be performed.

N ote client's response to procedures and treatments.

O btain specimens other than blood (e.g., wound, stool, etc.).

S igns and symptoms of trends and/or changes-monitor, and intervene.

T each client and family about procedures and treatments.

I dentify vital signs and monitor for changes and intervene.

C omplications should be noted and followed immediately with an action.

This image is to remind you that "Sure Look" Holmes is looking into the hippo's mouth to assure he is safe! Just as "Sure Look" Holmes, the nurse is not responsible for ordering these tests, but to maintain client SAFETY prior to, during, and after these diagnostics have been completed.

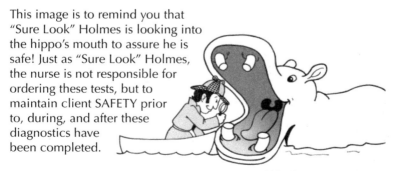

©2014 I CAN Publishing®, Inc.

Priority Care For a "Centesis"

The definition of "CENTESIS" is the act of puncturing a body cavity or organ with a hollow needle in order to draw out fluid. Several diagnostic tests that include this procedure of a "CENTESIS" include a thora**centesis**, para**centesis**, or an am nio**centesis**. "CENTESIS" on the right page will review nursing care. The fun fact is that there are many similarities among these procedures.

A thora**CENTESIS** is the withdrawal of fluid from the pleural cavity to diagnose.

A para**CENTESIS** involves a catheter being inserted into the peritoneal cavity, most often just below the umbilicus. This is done to assess for presence of ascites and/or to identify the cause of acute abdominal problems such as perforation or hemorrhage. Bloody fluids, presence of fecal or bacterial material, an elevated red or white blood cell count occur with a positive test result; immediate surgery may be required.

Arthro**CENTESIS**: Samples of synovial fluid are obtained from an incision of a joint capsule. Local anesthesia is induced. Prior to aspiration of the fluid, aseptic preparation is completed. Synovial fluid is examined for infection and bleeding into the joint and diagnose arthritis.

Amnio**CENTESIS** is an invasive procedure performed on the mother at 14 to 16 weeks of pregnancy to obtain amniotic fluid for evaluation of the risk of delivering a fetus with a chromosomal abnormality. The procedure can also be performed at approximately 35 weeks' gestation to evaluate for fetal lung maturity. The placenta is located by ultrasound examination and the needle is inserted through the abdomen (puncture site has been anesthetized). After the amniotic fluid is aspirated, it is sent to lab for testing.

Due to the risks involved with these procedures, it is imperative to obtain client identity and the **consent** prior to the client having one of these procedures. There must be an **explanation** and review the importance of being absolutely still during procedure. Positions will vary based on location.

Note, ideally client would be positioned on the side of the bed upright with the arms and head over the bedside table is experiencing a thora**CENTESIS**. If client is unable to be positioned ideally then place on **affected side with the head of the bed slightly elevated**. Area containing the fluid should be dependent. After a thora**CENTESIS**, client should be positioned on the unaffected side. Needle insertion by the provider of care is determined by x-ray for thora**CENTESIS**. Clients experiencing a para**CENTESIS** should be placed in the semi-Fowler's position.

The **vital signs** should be assessed for any trends prior to, during, and after procedures (bleeding, breathing). Respirations and **breath sounds** should be assessed for possible pneumothorax. Talking and coughing are out during the thora**CENTESIS**. If too much fluid is removed during a para**CENTESIS**, then the client will present with hypotension and hypovolemia. The client should be evaluated for perforation of the bowel which would present as peritonitis: board like abdomen, decrease in bowel sounds, abdominal distention, and/or rigid abdomen. With the para**CENTESIS**, the client may present with a complication of the introduction of air into the abdominal cavity. The client may present with right referred shoulder pain (caused by the air under the diaphragm). For a para**CENTESIS**, have client void prior to the procedure if client has a full bladder to prevent bladder perforation. With the pregnant mother who had an amniocentesis, complications although unlikely (less than 1% of the cases) may include some mild discomfort at the needle site, or rarely abdominal wall hematoma. There is a risk for miscarriage.

Following a thora**CENTESIS**, **infuse cytotoxic** drugs into the pleural space if client has a malignancy.

CENTESIS

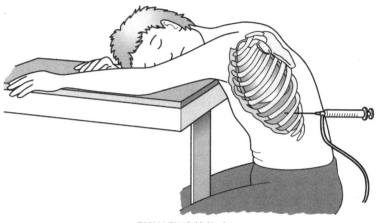

C onsent

E xplain

N ote what to expect

T he vital signs

E levate HOB

S o, area can be aspirated place on affected side

I nfusion cytotoxic drugs

S ide up with puncture; Sounds (breath), Support

Assessments After Any Test That Ends in "Scopy"

The definition of "**SCOPE**" is to look over, examine, or check out. If the procedure is a broncho**scopy**, then it provides direct visualization of the larynx, trachea, and bronchi. If the exam is an endo**scopy**, then these procedures would visualize the designated regions of the gastrointestinal tract via a flexible, fiber optic, lighted scope.

It is important that you are able to provide SAFE care following the procedures, so we have organized the nursing assessments on the right page to assist you in answering questions and providing nursing care. The key to success is to recognize expected versus unexpected outcomes and intervene appropriately.

Following these procedures, it is expected for the client to experience a **sore throat**. The nurse may provide the client with throat lozengers or warm saline solution gargles for the relief of the sore throat. Assessments such as stridor, shortness of breath, and hoarseness are not expected, and should be reported immediately to the healthcare provider. It is also expected for the client to **cough** up small amount of blood-tinged sputum. Hemoptysis would be indicative of bleeding and would not be expected. This would also need to be reported immediately to the healthcare provider. Due to the **presentation** of **the expected depression of the gag reflex**, all po intake should be **omitted** until the gag reflex, swallowing, and level of consciousness (LOC) return. **Evaluation** is a must!

Evaluate the upper airway following procedure (broncho**scopy**), since it is anesthetized topically during procedure; evaluate for pneumothorax or frank bleeding if bronchoscope is done for cytologic exam. Evaluate vital signs: HR, RR, BP; O_2 saturation; level of conscious. Following an endo**scopy**, observe for signs of perforation: upper GI bleeding-dysphagia, substernal or epigastric pain; lower GI bleeding-rectal bleeding, increasing abdominal distention. Assist client to upright position: assess for orthostatic hypotension.

A cysto**scopy** is a direct method to visualize the urethra and bladder by using a tubular lighted scope (cysto**scope**). This scope may be inserted via the urethra or percutaneously. "**SCOPE**" is different for this procedure.

- **S** Systolic blood pressure monitor for hypotension and orthostatic hypotension.
- **C** Conscious sedation or anesthesia may be used.
- **O** Oral fluids should be forced or administer fluids intravenously.
- **P** Position—Lithotomy may be used; preoperative med is given.
- **E** Evaluate urine output after procedure; check for frequency, dysuria, pink-tinged color (**these are expected and will decrease with time**). **Bright red blood in urine is NOT normal** and must be reported to healthcare provider.

I CAN TESTING HINT: The keys to NCLEX® and clinical success are to know what outcomes are expected versus unexpected in order to provide SAFE care.

SCOPE

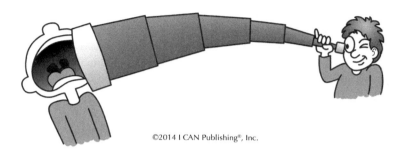

S ore throat—expected; stridor, shortness of breath, and hoarseness—notify health care provider (unexpected)

C oughs up small amount of blood tinged sputum—expected

O mit any po intake until gag reflex, swallowing, and LOC return

P resents with a depressed gag reflex following procedure—expected

E valuation is a must! Evaluate the upper airway following procedure (bronchoscopy) since it is anesthetized topically during procedure; evaluate for pneumothorax or frank bleeding if bronchoscope is done for cytologic exam. Evaluate vital signs: HR, RR, BP; O_2 saturation; level of conscious. Following an endoscopy, observe for signs of perforation.

Pulmonary Edema

This condition is a result of too much fluid in the lungs, both in the interstitial and in the alveolar spaces. Pulmonary edema results from severe impairment of the left heart function. "**DOG MAD**" COMES TO THE RESCUE!

D **DIURETICS** that are rapid-acting, such as furosemide (Lasix) and bumetanide (Bumex), dump the fluid over-load through the kidneys. Monitor potassium level. Hypokalemia precipitates digitalis toxicity. (Therapeutic level of potassium is 3.5-5.0 mEq/L.) Daily weight will help evaluate the fluid loss along with an accurate intake and output record.

O **OXYGEN** is given to saturate red blood cells and provide more oxygen to the tissues. Oxygen is usually given via nasal cannula. **CARDIAC OUTPUT** improved with dobutamine (Dobutrex).

G **GASES** are evaluated to maintain pH, PO_2 and PCO_2 within appropriate limits. (Refer to ACID-BASE.)

M **MORPHINE** will decrease preload, allowing blood to pool in the extremities. As a result, the heart will not work as hard. A major problem is anxiety, due to feeling they are drowning in their secretions. Although morphine will decrease the anxiety, monitor for potential respiratory depression.

A **AFTERLOAD DECREASED:** Ace Inhibitors, Beta Blockers, Nitroprusside (can also decrease preload)

D **DECREASED PRELOAD:** Nitroglycerin, Morphine, furosemide (Lasix)

DOG MAD

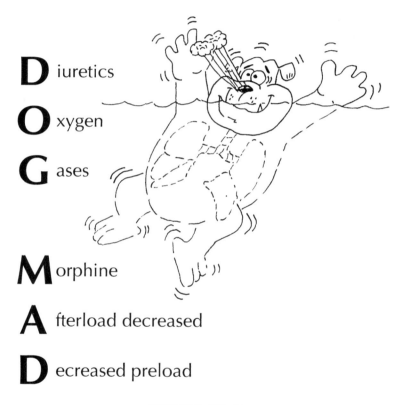

D iuretics

O xygen

G ases

M orphine

A fterload decreased

D ecreased preload

©2014 I CAN Publishing®, Inc.

Acid-Base

Draw a line down the middle of the right page. At the top of the left column put the numbers 7.35. At the top of the right column put 7.45. The normal blood pH should stay between these numbers. A pH below 7.35 indicates acidosis. A pH above 7.45 indicates alkalosis. Under 7.35 write CO_2 (body turns carbon dioxide to carbonic acid). Under 7.45 write HCO_3. Under HCO_3 write HCO_3 again and again. If we had enough paper we would write HCO_3 20 times because normal ratio of HCO_3 to pCO_2 is 20:1. The objective is to keep the pH between 7.35 and 7.45 which is done with buffer systems.

COLOR the van red. The red van represents the blood buffer system. Imagine the van driving through the arteries and veins of your body. When the pH gets below 7.35 (acidosis) the back van door opens, out jumps 20 little bicarbs, neutralizes the acid and gets back in the van to drive off! If the ph gets above 7.45 (alkalosis) the front van door opens, big powerful CO_2 jumps out, neutralizes and gets back in to drive off. This blood buffer is the first buffer system to respond to pH variations. The lungs follow by adjusting the respirations to regulate the CO_2. The third buffer system that helps maintain the pH are the kidneys.

ACID-BASE

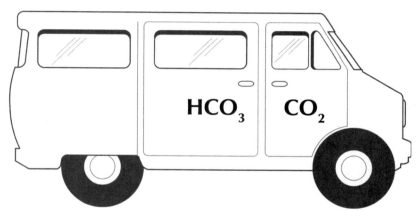

Acid-Base Status

To determine acid-base status (respiratory or metabolic), picture yourself in Rome. You are on a playground with Phonetia (pH), Carbo (HCO_3), and Paco (pCO_2).

Phonetia and Paco hop on the see-saw and begin to play. Up and down, up and down. When the pH and pCO_2 are in opposite directions from "normal," the status is respiratory (respiratory = opposite).

Phonetia tires of playing with Paco and runs off to join Carbo who is on a swing. Both go up and both go down, always together. When pH and HCO_3 are either both up or both down, the status is metabolic (metabolic = equal).

pH > 7.45 = alkalosis
pH < 7.35 = acidosis

(Turn page for COMPENSATORY MECHANISMS).

Reprinted with permission from Creative Educators, Jefferson, LA

ACID-BASE STATUS

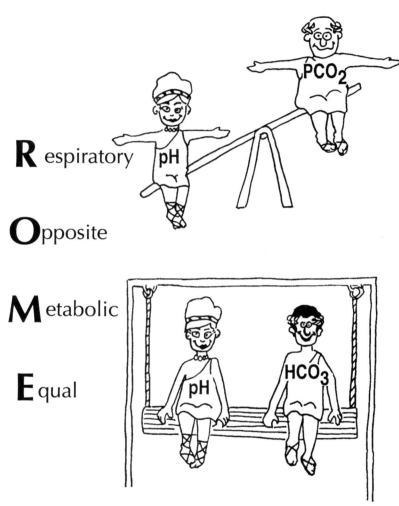

Respiratory

Opposite

Metabolic

Equal

Reprinted with permission ©1994 Creative Educators

Compensatory Mechanisms

(This will make more sense to you if you first refer to Acid-Base Status on page 180.)

Compensation occurs in respiratory situations when Carbo gets mad at Phonetia for playing with Paco and hops on Paco's side of the see-saw! Imagine all three on the same see-saw.

Compensation occurs in metabolic situations when Paco decides to crash the swinging twosome and hops on with Phonetia and Carbo. Now all go up or all go down.

Reprinted with permission from Creative Educators, Jefferson, LA

COMPENSATORY MECHANISMS

Respiratory

Metabolic

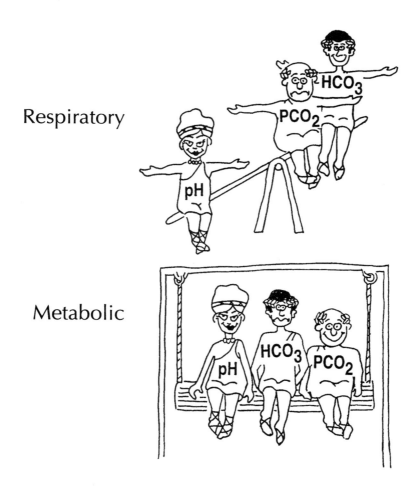

Reprinted with permission ©1994 Creative Educators

Acid-Base

This referee is calling the shots in Acid-Base. He will help you remember if **ACID** or **BASE** is lost. Think, **A**bove the waist **A**cid is lost. **B**elow the waist **B**ase is lost. The stomach, above the waist, contains HCl (H^+ is an acid). HCl acid is lost during vomiting or when the client has a nasogastric tube. As a result, the client may develop a problem with alkalosis. When a client is hyperventilating, he increases the loss of carbon dioxide which also results in alkalosis.

The bowel below the waist contains alkaline substances which are lost during diarrhea. If alkali are lost, then the client may become acidotic.

There's a BIG exception here! Deep, prolonged vomiting will reach below the waist and lose alkaline intestinal juices resulting in a ketoacidotic state.

CALLING THE SHOTS IN ACID VS. BASE

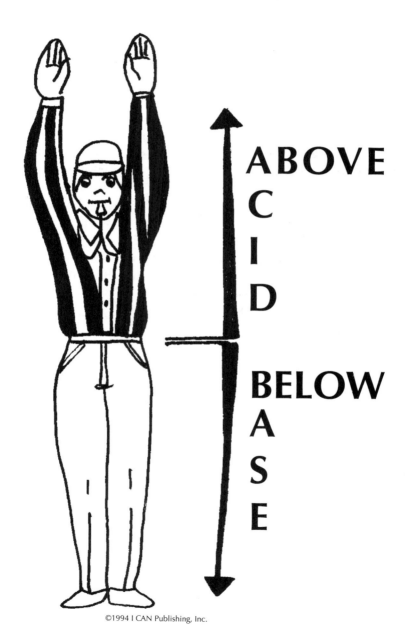

Shock

When you think about the pathophysiology of shock, the classifications (except cardiogenic) have the common bond of decreased venous return (DVR).

HYPOVOLEMIC SHOCK (Hemorrhagic)–If an arm is cut off, that blood is certainly not returning to the heart. DVR! Another example of hypovolemic shock is the guy decides to roof his house on the 4th of July, and sweats out his volume, resulting in dehydration. Less blood to pump = DVR!

NEUROGENIC SHOCK–A severed spinal cord from a gunshot wound or fall allows blood to pool. Nerves have been cut; there is less venous constriction due to absent nerve stimulation. Spinal anesthesia and barbiturate overdose will cause the same response.

SEPTIC SHOCK (toxic)–An overwhelming infection; generally gram negative organisms will cause a dilation of the blood vessels resulting in a DVR.

VASOGENIC SHOCK (anaphylactic)–A DVR results from an antigen-antibody reaction with release of histamine. Blood that pools causes DVR! Less blood to pump = DVR!

(Refer to **Shock Interventions.**)

In contrast, CARDIOGENIC SHOCK is volume overload NOT volume deficit.

SHOCK

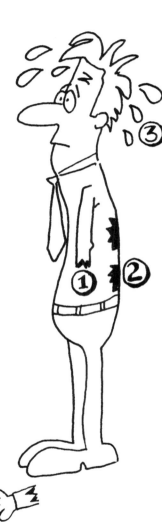

Shock is Decreased Venous Return

except Cardiogenic

Help Stamp Out Shock

S   **SOLUTIONS** add volume and will increase venous return. Increase the rate. A combination of fluids, blood and plasma expanders (dextran, plasma and albumin) are commonly used. Watch for I.V.s with meds in them. We wouldn't want to turn up the I.V. rate of Pitocin!

H   **HEMODYNAMICS** are a way to measure potential shock and evaluate interventions. CVP–(normal is a lucky 6) low CVP means DVR, (decreased venous return) or fluid deficit. Elevated CVP means fluid overload as seen in cardiogenic shock. Low BP reading is one parameter that spells trouble.

Monitor it every few minutes. As meds are given to increase the BP, it may come up quickly.

EARLY CHANGES	LATE CHANGES
Anxious	Coma
Heart rate elevated	Heart rate elevated and weak
Respirations elevated and deep	Respirations elevated and shallow
Skin cool, moist	Skin cold, clammy
Blood pressure no change	Blood pressure decreased
Normal skin color	Pale skin color

O   **OXYGEN** will saturate those red blood cells and decrease tissue starvation.

C   **CHECK** the skin which is often cold and clammy.

K   **KICK** up those feet and legs! There's a lot of blood volume in those legs. Elevate them and let gravity help increase venous return. Don't put the head down. Trendelenburg position may increase cranial pressure, ocular pressure and pressure on the diaphragm.

HELP STAMP OUT SHOCK

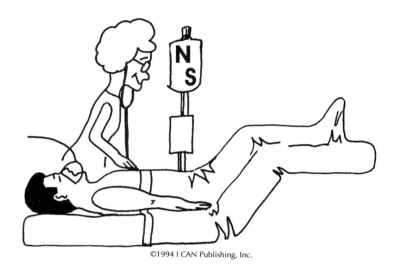

Solutions

Hemodynamic changes

Oxygen

Checking

Kick 'em up

Lung Sounds

Just breathing in and out makes a normal lung sound that can be heard with a stethoscope. Listen to both sides of the chest because the right side can have clear lung sounds while the left side can have "rales," "wheezes" or some adventitious breath sounds. Listen to the anterior (front) and posterior (back) sounds. How do we know if we hear rales? Rales, sounding like Rice Krispies doing "snap, crackle and pop," are most commonly heard around alveolar sacs more distal to the bronchial tubes. Rales have also been compared to the fizzling of a carbonated drink and are usually heard midway through the inspiratory phase. Wheezes are most often found over the midline or bronchi indicating constriction. Wheezes are continuous sounds, although they are heard more on expiration. Imagine hearing a whistle blow! This is similar to a wheeze.

The bottom line is that breath sounds should be clear and air should be heard moving on both inspiration and expiration. The key is to know what the normal is, so you can detect a difference.

ABNORMAL LUNG SOUNDS

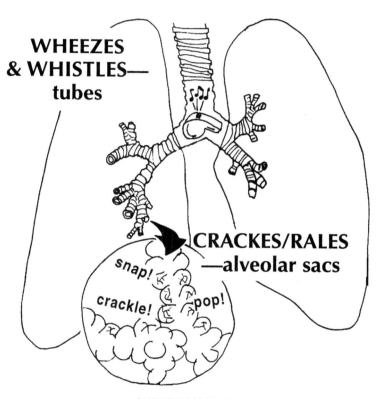

COPD

Chronic Obstructive Pulmonary Disease is referred to as emphysema. A major risk factor is cigarette smoking.

C   **COUGH** is chronic and nonproductive making it hard to breathe or rest well. A chest x-ray is often ordered to confirm the diagnosis and to look for pneumonia. Nope, one does not have to be NPO for a chest x-ray.

O   **OXYGEN** starvation demands oxygen. A good rule of thumb for the O_2 flow is 2-4 liters. High concentrations of oxygen depress the drive to breathe and cause respiratory distress. ABG's (arterial blood gases) are an excellent way to measure what's happening.

P   **PULMONARY FUNCTION TEST** shows a decrease in lung function possibly calling for postural drainage to reduce secretions and increase oxygen exchange.

D   **DON'T SMOKE** is probably excellent advice. Emotional support usually helps; nagging doesn't. Drugs and other stuff often given for COPD are included on page 194.

CHRONIC OBSTRUCTIVE PULMONARY DISEASE

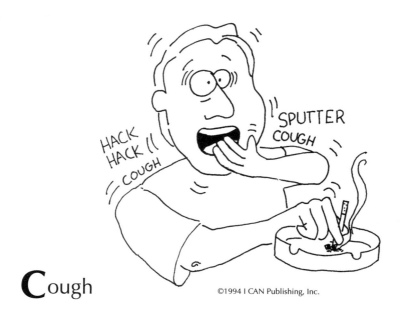

Cough

Oxygen and ABG's

Pulmonary function and postural drainage

Don't smoke

Interventions For COPD (Chronic Obstructive Pulmonary Disease)

Since our primary objective for these clients is to enhance oxygen exchange, it makes sense to look at these medicines around the ABCs.

A   **ANTI-INFLAMMATORY (CORTICOSTEROIDS)** May be used to decrease inflammation. Example: Betamethasone *(Remember: Excellent oral hygiene to prevent candida infections from corticosteroids).*

B   **BRONCHODILATORS**–Epinephrine (adrenalin) is also used to relax smooth muscle of bronchials. Do not use if client has hypertension or cardiac arrhythmias. Example: Albuterol.

C   **CHEST PHYSIOTHERAPY**–Help remove secretions from the lungs. (Refer to Postural Drainage.)

D   **DELIVER OXYGEN AT 2 LITERS**–High concentrations of oxygen would eliminate the client's hypoxic drive and cause respiratory distress.

E   **EXPECTORANTS**–These will assist in decreasing the viscosity of the mucous.

F   **FORCE FLUIDS**–Fluids will facilitate the removal of secretions.

INTERVENTIONS FOR COPD
(A B Cs)

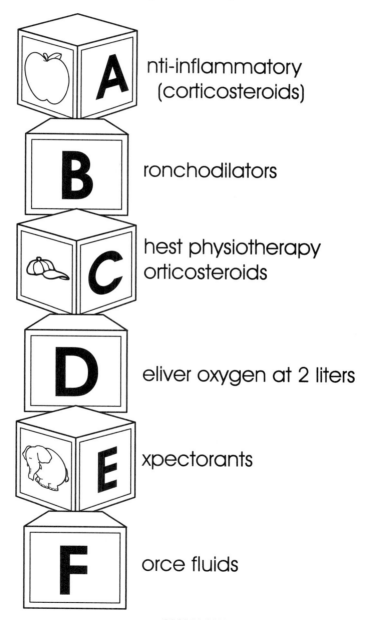

A - nti-inflammatory (corticosteroids)

B - ronchodilators

C - hest physiotherapy orticosteroids

D - eliver oxygen at 2 liters

E - xpectorants

F - orce fluids

©1994 I CAN

Asthma

INFL A MMATION–Asthma is a chronic inflammatory process that produces mucosal edema, mucus secretion, and airway inflammation.

S SYMPTOMS–Wheezing, chest tightness, shortness of breath, cough. Use of accessory muscles in breathing. Symptoms of hypoxia and cyanosis occur late. Increased anxiety, restlessness, and exercise intolerance. Excessive sputum production.

T TREATMENT–includes beta$_2$ adrenergic medications by nebulizer or metered dose inhalers. Epinephrine, antibiotics (if an infection is present), bronchodilators, expectorants. Inhalation of steroids to prevent edema. Supplemental oxygen for hypoxemia.

IN H ALERS–Inhalation of steroids to prevent edema. Beta$_2$-Adrenergic Agonists stimulate beta receptors in the lung, relax bronchial smooth muscle, increase vital capacity, and decrease airway resistance.

M MECHANISMS–Intermittent narrowing of the airway is caused by constriction of the smooth muscles of the bronchi and bronchioles. Excessive mucus production and mucosal edema of the respiratory tract are other mechanisms that contribute to asthma. Constriction of smooth muscle results in a significant increased airway resistance, resulting in trapped air in the lung. Emotional factors are also known to play an important role in precipitating an asthmatic attack for the child.

A AVOID ALLERGENS–Educate client regarding the importance of avoiding allergens that have been identified as precipitating factors resulting in an asthmatic attack.

ASTHMA

infl **A**mmation

Symptoms

Treatment

in**H**alers

Mechanisms

Avoidance

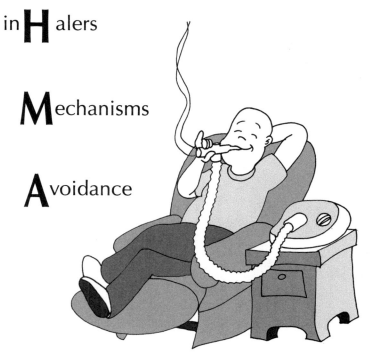

Beta$_2$-Adrenergic Agonists

"**MAX AIR**," our friend on the next page, is holding several balloons to assist you in remembering some key points with these medications. Notice the balloons on the left are the clinical outcomes we expect from "**MAX AIR**." Beta$_2$-Adrenergic Agonists stimulate the beta receptors in the lung, resulting in the relaxation of bronchial smooth muscles. This action results in an increased vital capacity which allows clients to breathe easier, resulting in the ability to blow up balloons.

Unfortunately, there are some undesirable effects that may occur while taking these medications. The balloons on the right will help you remember some key points. Tachycardia, irregular heart beat, hypertension, or cardiac dysrhythmias may occur. In addition to cardiac irregularities, other undesirable effects that may occur include nervousness, tremors, restlessness, insomnia, headache; nausea, or vomiting.

NOTE: For specific details about these drugs refer to *Pharmacology Made Insanely Easy* by Loretta Manning and Sylvia Rayfield.

BETA$_2$-ADRENERGIC AGONISTS

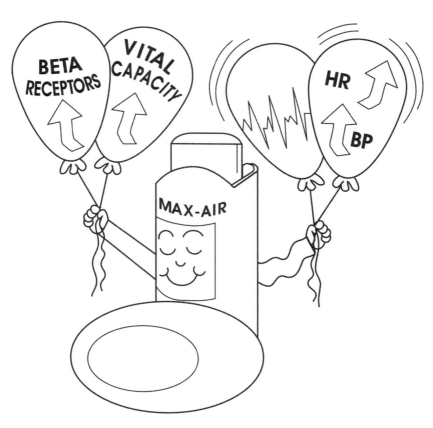

Cystic Fibrosis

This little guy is a "**SICKER KID**." His disease is inherited from an autosomal recessive trait. The exocrine glands that normally produce the enzymes lipase (digests fats), trypsin (digests protein) and amylase (digests starches) are not functioning normally. He's doing without a good part of his nutrition (about 40% of his food gets ingested). The other issue is that cystic fibrosis causes these enzymes to become so tenacious that they cause other problems. Organs affected by this disease include the lungs, pancreas, GI tract, and liver. "**Sicker Kid**" will assist you in remembering the major concepts in cystic fibrosis.

S **STEATORRHEA** (fat in stool) smelly stools with increased amount.

SWEAT TEST indicating high salt content may be diagnostic. Adequate salt intake is important.

I **ILEUS-MECONIUM** may be present in newborns. The small intestine is blocked with thick mucous causing symptoms of intestinal obstruction.

C **CONSTANT HUNGER** because of poor food absorption.

K **VITAMINS K, A, D, E** (fat soluble) may be supplemented.

E **ENZYME (pancreatic) REPLACEMENT** is mandatory. Administer prior to meals and snacks.

R **REDUCTION OF DIETARY FAT** is at a minimum. Increase intake of pancreatic enzymes with increased fat intake.

K **KEEP CALORIES UP.** Use **simple sugars** as a source of energy.

I **INFECTION** may be a way of life, especially respiratory infections due to pulmonary congestion. Administer oxygen and IV fluids to keep secretions thin.

D **DRINK PLENTY OF FLUIDS** to prevent dehydration and to keep mucous thin. DIET high in calorie, high protein, fats as tolerated or increased, and increase salt intake.

CYSTIC FIBROSIS

S teatorrhea
   weat test

I leus-meconium

C onstant hunger

K vitamins

E nzyme replacement

R eduction of fat is out!

K eep calories up

I nfection

D rink plenty of fluids

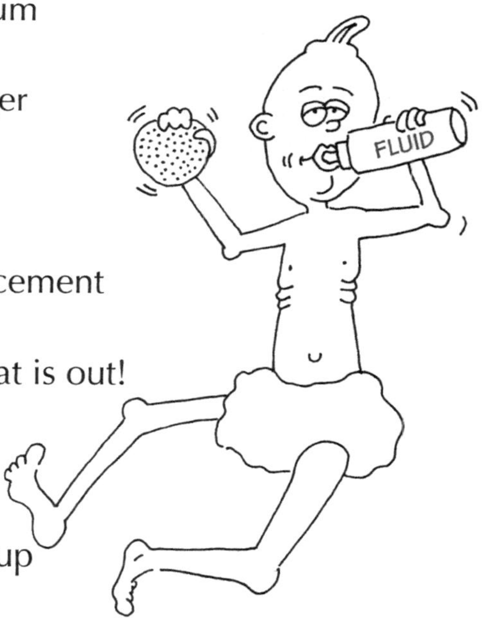

Water-Sealed Chest Drainage

The water seal (or dry seal on some equipment) operates as a one-way valve. It prevents air, under atmospheric pressure, from reentering the pleural cavity. When the client inspires, the air and fluid exit the pleural cavity via the chest tube. The dry seal or water prevent the air and fluid from reentering.

Equipment

A three-chamber disposable chest drainage system: This is a molded plastic system that provides a collection chamber, a water-sealed chamber, and a suction-control chamber. There should be a continuous gentle bubbling in the water in the suction control chamber when suction is applied.

Purposes

Chest Tubes inserted in pleural space to drain fluid, blood, or air
Helps lung expansion
Establishes normal intrapleural pressure
Sitting or lying position during insertion
The negative pressure is restored

Proper Functioning

The water level in the water-seal chamber and in the tubing from client should fluctuate (tidal) : rise on inspiration and fall on expiration.

Initial bubbling may occur in the water-sealed chamber with coughing as air is moved out of the plural cavity and intermittent bubbling with respirations until the lung is re-expanded.

Deep respiration may also result in initial bubbling in the water- sealed chamber.

Assess for continuous bubbling in the fluid where the water seal is maintained; this should NOT occur! This indicates a LEAK!

Look only for continuous bubbling in the third chamber for suction control!

Maintenance of Water-Sealed System

Equipment for drainage should all be kept below the chest-tube insertion site.

Evaluate for dependent loops in the tubing; this increases resistance to drainage.

Extra tubing should be coiled in the bed and flow in a straight line to the system.

Evaluate all connections to make certain they are taped.

Evaluate and note characteristics and amount of the drainage; mark level on the collection chamber per protocol.

Eliminate vigorous "milking" or stripping of the chest tubes, since it ↑ pleural pressure.

Evaluate when the collection chamber is half full and change the system.

Eliminate clamping chest tubes during transport.

PLEUR-EVAC

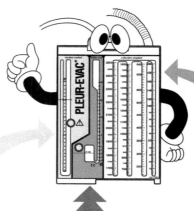

Water seals—adding sterile fluid to chamber 2 cm.
Air leak assessed by fast and continuous bubbling in this chamber!
Tidaling is expected in water seal chamber.
Elimination of tidaling water seal—lung re-expanded
Remember not to strip or milk tubing routinely

Suction control—The suction needs to have an order regarding the amount.

Drainage characteristics
Review hourly and mark level on the collection chamber
Assess output in comparison to previous hour
Identify if there has been a trend with an increase or decrease in output
Note when the chamber is half full

Ventilator Care

This poor guy has found himself on a ventilator. To accurately evaluate the effectiveness of the vent, closely **VIEW** the client's **ARTERIAL BLOOD GASES**. Pressure should be maintained at the puncture site for a minimum of 5 minutes. After changing any ventilatory settings or suctioning the client, wait for 30 minutes to draw the ABG's. After procedures, carefully evaluate client's vital signs, pulse oximetry, color, etc., and check that **VENT** alarms are on. To determine the adequacy of air exchange (**AIRWAY**), **EVALUATE** the **BREATH SOUNDS**. Look for equal chest movement, client's color and respirations. Calmly explain **EQUIPMENT** and alarms to both the client and family. Keep **EQUIPMENT** at the bedside such as a bag and valve mask resuscitator, suction equipment, oxygen, etc. Ventilators are such a scary proposition that people become stressed. **NOTICE GI COMPLICATIONS** from potential **STRESS ULCERS**. The majority of clients will require a H_2 Histamine Antagonist.

Adequate **NUTRITION** is mandatory and will facilitate weaning. The gastrointestinal (GI) tract is preferred if it is functioning well. The nutritional support provided via the GI tract improves the blood flow to the intestine, the mucosal integrity is preserved, and the incidence of sepsis is decreased. If there is a need to administer either bolus or continuous feedings, then the use of a small-bore transpyloric tube emptying in the duodenum is the recommended route. During the feeding the **head of the bed should be elevated 30 degrees.**

The nurse must **TAKE NOTICE OF PRESSURE ALARMS** on the ventilator. An easy way to remember this information is that if the low alarm goes off, the priority of care is to check for a leak. This sounds when tidal volume cannot be delivered due to a leak or break in the system. The connections on the ventilator need to be checked for any break in the system. The tracheostomy or endotracheal (ET) tube cuff may be leaking, so check for air escaping around cuff. If cuff is ruptured, then the tracheostomy tube may need to be replaced. To assist you in remembering this, *note there is a l in low and in leak.*

If the high pressure alarm goes off, *remember* **high** *rhymes with* **dry**. This occurs when the tidal volume cannot be delivered at the set pressure limit. The client may need **suctioning to clear out the secretions**; may be biting on the tube; coughing and/or experiencing an increase in level of anxiety (*may need a sedative*), or there may be water in the ventilator tubes. Never allow the condensation in the tubing to flow back into fluid reservoir. The tubes or client needs to dry out.

VENTILATOR CARE

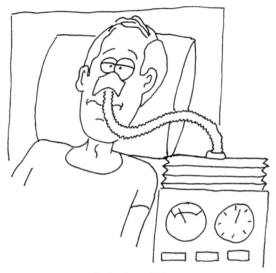

V iew ABGs, Airway, Respiratory status (breath sounds, RR, O_2 saturation, etc.)

E levate HOB 30–45 degrees, Equipment (ambu bag, oxygen, suction)

N otice G.I. complications (stress ulcer), nutrition

T ake notice of settings and alarms

S uction to maintain endotracheal (tracheostomy tube patent)

Tuberculosis

INA has the typical signs and symptoms of tuberculosis including fatigue, weight loss, anorexia, chronic productive cough, night sweats, and hemoptysis (advanced stage). In order to help the *mycobacterium tuberculosis* rise out of her, there are several medications which may be prescribed. "**RISE**" will assist in remembering these medications.

R   **RIFAMPIN**–This medication is most often prescribed with isoniazid (INH). The secretions (sweat, urine) may turn orange. Hepatitis may be a complication, especially in alcoholics. Rifampin should be administered once daily on an empty stomach.

I   **ISONIAZID (INH)**–This is the primary medication used in prophylactic treatment of tuberculosis. Adverse reactions include hepatitis, and/or hepatotoxicity. Peripheral neuropathies can be prevented by pretreating with pyridoxine (vitamin B6). INH should be administered once daily on an empty stomach.

S   **STREPTOMYCIN**–Two major adverse effects from this medication are ototoxicity and nephrotoxicity. Due to the susceptibility to cranial nerve VIII, this medication is generally avoided in the elderly. Use it with caution if clients have renal disease. Hearing must be evaluated frequently. Streptomycin may not be given po.

E   **ETHAMBUTOL**–This medication is frequently administered with rifampin and INH. Assess vision prior to therapy to identify side effects of optic neuritis which may result in loss of central vision from this medication. Ethambutol should be administered once daily with food or meals to decrease gastric irritation.

INA TUBERCULOSIS

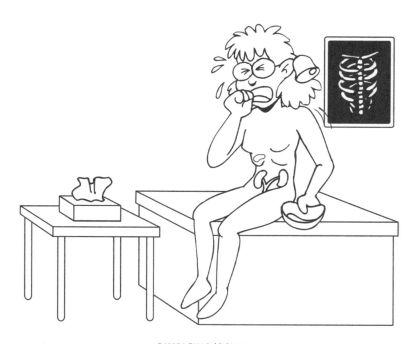

"Whatever you do, do it well. Do it so well that when people see you do it, they will want to come back and see you do it again and they will want to bring others and show them how well you do what you do."

WALT DISNEY

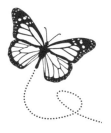

FLUID VOLUME / RENAL SYSTEM

Fluid Volume Status

The arrow indicates that fluid (plasma) volume decreases during dehydration. This will cause an increase in the sodium blood level above the normal range of 135-145 mEq/L. The hematocrit will also rise (above 45%) due to the same principle.

The opposite occurs during pregnancy. Due to increased fluid (plasma) levels, the hematocrit and the serum sodium levels decrease. This dilution of the red blood cells is referred to as pseudoanemia. Evaluation of the serum sodium and hematocrit levels are excellent indicators of the fluid volume status. Several important nursing interventions for these clients include: daily weights, intake and output records, specific gravity evaluation of the urine, assessing the skin turgor, and lips and mucous membranes. An important assessment for infants regarding their fluid status is to observe if the fontanels are depressed or bulging.

This is an excellent tool to assist you in remembering the concept of the fluid volume status.

Assessment for fluid volume may be determined by blood work.
Normal Sodium blood level 135-145 mEq/L
Normal Potassium level 3.5-5 mEq/L
Normal Hemoglobin ranges with age-adults 12-14 g/dL
Normal Red Cell Count adult women 4.2-5.4, men 4.7-6.1 million/uL
Or
Skin Turgor, lips, mucous membranes, daily weights

FLUID VOLUME STATUS

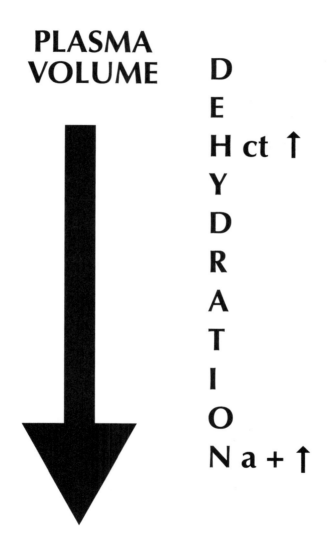

Fluid Shifts

Fluid shifts are easier to figure out if you remember this nursery rhyme:

"Mary had a little lamb and everywhere Mary went, the lamb was sure to go." Mary is salt (NaCl), and the lamb is water. Everywhere salt goes, water follows.

You may be asking yourself, how does this fit in with my nursing care? Frequently, we need to do health teaching for clients who are taking certain medications. The group that comes to our mind are the thiazides. Would we want these individuals eating a high sodium diet? Of course not! That would defeat the purpose for these diuretics.

Diuretics are given to remove fluid from the body. If we increase the sodium intake for these clients, they will continue to retain fluid. Everywhere salt (NaCl) goes water follows.

FLUID SHIFTS

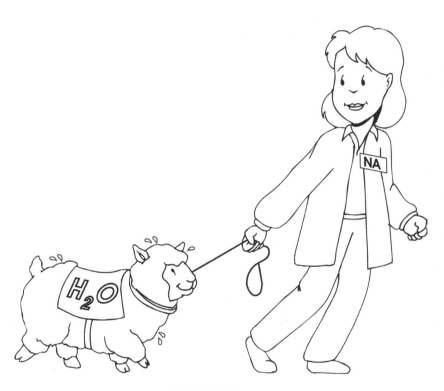

"Mary had a little lamb and everywhere Mary went the lamb was sure to go."

Hypernatremia
Serum Na⁺ > 145 mEq/L

Nursing students and graduates consistently struggle with this concept! In order to simplify this for you, we have provided you with several images to review on the right page that are discussed throughout this book (in addition to a couple new ones) to help you link these medical conditions to the potential complication with hypernatremia. The medical condition will be reviewed in the designated chapters.

The bottom line is that with each of these medical conditions, the result is the same, HYPERNATREMIA!

The next step is for you to review the clinical assessment findings that the client with hypernatremia may experience. The two mnemonics below will assist you in reviewing these findings for hypernatremia. The first one reviews fluid deficit (hemoconcentration of Na⁺, water loss) from complications with decreased fluid intake, excessive water loss from diarrhea, or being febrile. Refer to the cactus on the right page. The skin of the cactus is very rough and "DRIED" out just as the lips and mucous membranes of a client would be very dry.

D	Dry mucous membranes; decrease in urine output; Deep muscle reflexes increased
R	Red, flushed skin; restless (irritable), progressing to confusion
I	Increased temperature; increase in urine concentration
E	Elevated HR
D	Decreased weight; decreased CVP

Fluid Excess from Na⁺ retention can occur from excessive salt intake, increased renal retention, or Cushing's syndrome

- E Edema (pitting)
- D Decrease in the hematocrit
- E Elevated weight; elevated BP
- M Mentation decreased (lethargic)
- A A flushing of the skin

The **bottom line** is that whether hypernatremia is from **fluid deficit** or **fluid excess from sodium retention** the priority is for the nursing care to focus on returning the level of sodium to the normal range, so the nurse will "**RESTRICT**" extra sodium and support the client's symptoms during this process. The last thing the nurse would want to do is to provide extra sodium to these clients with hypernatremia. While the cause of the hypernatremia may be different, the nursing care is similar! (**Review both causes of hypernatremia.*)

R	Restrict fluid intake if experiencing fluid retention
E	Evaluate for cerebral changes such as headache, nausea; evaluate for seizures**
S	Strict intake and output; seizure precautions**
T	The blood pressure is elevated (fluid excess); the VS need to be monitored**; the oral hygiene**
R	Review origin of hypernatremia**
I	If there is a fluid deficit, administer Hypotonic IV fluids
C	Check daily weight**; neurological assessments
T	The excess fluid may be removed by diuretics

HYPERNATREMIA

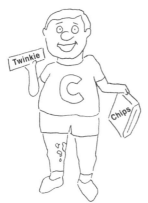

Cushing's Syndrome
"Cushy Carl": ↑ amounts of adrenal adrenocortical hormones ↑ Na⁺. Result, **HYPERNATREMIA!**

Diabetes Insipidus
↓ antidiuretic hormone from the brain resulting in extreme urinary losses; cannot drink enough fluids to match losses causing severe dehydration and ↑ Na⁺. Result, **HYPERNATREMIA!**

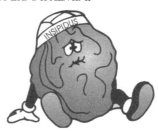

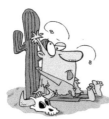

Fluid deficit (hemoconcentration of Na⁺, water loss) from complications with decreased fluid intake, excessive water loss from heat (*i.e., excessive water loss from diarrhea, vomiting, or being febrile*). Result, **HYPERNATREMIA!**

Variations in body fluid and tend to lose more fluid. Result, **HYPERNATREMIA!**

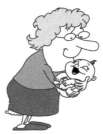

High sodium foods, salt tablets, etc. Result, **HYPERNATREMIA!**

Hyponatremia
Serum Na⁺ < 135 mEq/L

Just as we did for hypernatremia, we have provided you with several images to review on the right page that are discussed throughout this book (in addition to a couple of new ones) to help link these medical conditions to the potential complication with hyponatremia. The medical condition will be reviewed in the designated chapters.

Some other examples of hyponatremia may include a client who has become dehydrated from overheating, resulting in a loss of sodium. Massive tissue injury such as burns and/or trauma may also result in complications with hyponatremia. Another cause of hyponatremia may be the increased renal excretion from specific medications such as thiazide or loop diuretics. High amounts of excess fluid may result in another complication with hyponatremia from dilutional hyponatremia. The bottom line is that with each of these medical conditions, the result is the same, HYPONATREMIA!

The two mnemonics below will assist you in reviewing the clinical assessment findings for hyponatremia from sodium loss and for hyponatremia from too much fluid retention. Note, that with each of these categories of sodium deficit, the risk for seizures is a safety priority! A little hint to make your life easier is that the risk for seizures can also result from hypernatremia

---

Clinical Assessment Findings: Solution deficit (Na⁺ loss)
- **C** Cold and clammy skin; Cramps in abdomen
- **O** Oliguria
- **L** LOC changes, confusion, seizures**
- **D** Decreased blood pressure; decreased muscle strength (weak)

Dilutional Hyponatremia (Water excess) "High Fluid Retention"
- **H** Hypertension
- **I** Increase in muscle twitching** and cramping; increase in urine
- **G** Gain in weight
- **H** Headaches, confusion, seizures**

The **bottom line is that whether hyponatremia is from Na⁺ loss or water excess, the neurological changes will be consistent. This is screaming SEIZURE PRECAUTIONS!** Remember SAFETY is the priority for any client. The nursing care must focus on returning the level of "SODIUM" to the normal range and support the client's symptoms during this process.

- **S** **Seizure precautions!** May administer IV hypertonic solution containing 3% NaCl.
- **O** Occurs in Addison disease; diabeteics acidosis, and renal disease; clients NPO; SIADH; perspiring, vomiting, diarrhea; burns or excessive administration of D₅W
- **D** Deficit of sodium: 0.9% NaCl (normal saline) or 0.45% NaCl
- **I** If retaining fluids, restrict fluids; Irrigate NG tube with normal saline solution
- **U** Understand the cause of the hyponatremia
- **M** Monitor blood pressure, I&O, weight (best indicator of fluid status), skin turgor; Neurological assessments (pupils, etc.); maintain fall precautions

HYPONATREMIA

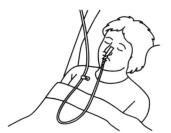

NG Tube to Low Suction
Na⁺ and water levels ↓ in the extracellular area, but sodium **LOSS** is greater.

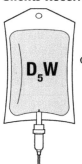

Clients Receiving Only D_5W
Expands extracellular fluid; water ↑ ; dilutes Na⁺; Na⁺ not replaced with this IV fluid results in **HYPONATREMIA!**

Cystic Fibrosis
Sweat glands: excretion of excess amounts of Na⁺; result, **HYPONATREMIA!**

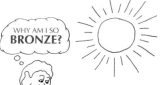

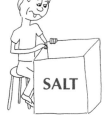

Anemic Adam
"Anemic Adam" is experiencing a ↓ in aldosterone secretion which leads to ↓ Na⁺ absorption.

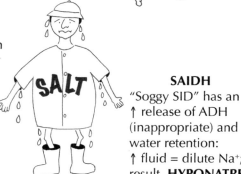

SAIDH
"Soggy SID" has an ↑ release of ADH (inappropriate) and ↑ water retention:
↑ fluid = dilute Na⁺; result, **HYPONATREMIA!**

Hyperkalemia
Serum K⁺ > 5.0 mEq/L; Critical Level >6.5 mEq/L

The s**K**⁺ier is at the top of "**Mount T**" (**spiked T or tall T waves**)! The s**K**⁺ier is a risk taker and has no fear of "**DEATH**"; however, he is a new s**K**⁺ier, and did not understand that he should have gradually worked up to a Black Diamond Slope. Once he realized this, he became **HYPER**, with tremors, diarrhea, and an irregular heart rhythm with a slow beat! If he does not start coming down from the top of "**Mount T**", "**DEATH**" could be imminent!

D	**Dysrhythmias**–Irregular Rhythm, Bradycardia
E	**ECG Changes**–Tall Peaked T Waves
A	**Abdominal cramping**; diarrhea
T	**The muscles twitch**
H	**Hypotension**; has irritability/restlessness

The s**K**⁺ier's decision to start at the top of "**Mount T**" has caused his hyperkalemia. Clients, however, can develop hyperkalemia from a result of many causes. These may include renal failure; massive tissue injury from burns, trauma; fever, sepsis; the use of potassium sparing diuretics; excessive administration of IV potassium; salt substitutes; ACE Inhibitors; acidosis.

The s**K**⁺ier needs to successfully start down the mountain as he "**DROPS**" his skis in the snow to begin the journey of skiing down to the bottom. This will assist you in organizing the nursing care for this electrolyte imbalance.

D	**Dysrhythmia**, spiked or tall T wave (peaked), widened QRS, prolonged PR interval -monitor
R	**Review** and monitor K⁺ levels ongoing
O	**Orders**: Kayexalate or dextrose with regular insulin
P	**Provide potassium**-restricted foods, Potassium-losing diuretics (Lasix)
S	**Stop** infusion of IV potassium; Salt substitutes are not allowed

Unfortunately, he was not successful on his journey down, and wrecks at the bottom of the mountain resulting in massive tissue injury! Turn to the next page to see what happens to the s**K**⁺ier's T waves and the clinical assessments after the fall!

Concept developed by Dr. Melissa Geist

HYPERKALEMIA

D ysrythmias—Irregular rhythm, bradycardia

E CG Changes—Tall peaked T waves

A bdominal cramping, diarrhea

T he muscles twitch, cramp

H ypotension; has irritability/restlessness

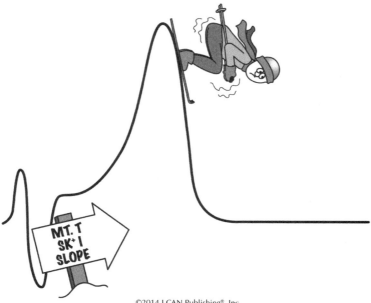

Hypokalemia
Serum K⁺ <3.5 mEq/L; Critical Level < 2.5 mEq/L

The sK⁺ier from the previous page who was on the top of "Mount T" fell on his way down the slope! When he flattened out with the fall, his **T wave also becomes flat**. He got wobbly (lethargic), could not hold on to his poles (hyporeflexia); after the fall he got more confused! He developed bradycardia with a weak irregular pulse and ECG changes were S-T depression, U waves, PVCs. From the trauma of falling, he developed decreased bowel sounds, nausea, and vomiting. This sK⁺ier is so very "**WEAK**" after the fall! This will assist you in remembering some of the signs and symptoms:

> **W** **Weak** and irregular pulse; waves–U (ECG changes); weakness of muscles; weakness of skeletal muscles
> **E** **Evaluate** for hyporeflexia; irritability, anxiety followed by confusion and eventually a coma; decreased RR; I & O
> **A** **Arrhythmias**–Flat T waves (no K⁺ for repolarization); abdominal distention; alkalosis
> **K** **K⁺** (serum) < 3.5 mEq/L; Constipation, ↓ bowel sounds

Clients who are experiencing hypokalemia may be presenting with a decreased intake of foods high in potassium; excessive GI loss from vomiting, diarrhea, and fistulas; nasogastric suction without replacement; skin loss: diaphoresis; excessive renal excretion; alkalosis; loop diuretics, steroid therapy; increasing aldosterone; diabetics: Insulin and glucose move K⁺ into cell.

The nursing care for the sK⁺ier is to help increase his potassium level. "**POTASSIUM**" will assist in decreasing the problem with hypokalemia.

> **P** **Potatoes**, Avocados, broccoli, etc. (↑ K⁺)
> **O** **Oral** potassium supplements
> **T** **T waves** depressed (flattened)–monitor
> **A** **Arrhythmias**–monitor
> **S** **Shallow** ineffective respirations–monitor
> **S** **Sounds** of breathing diminished–monitor
> **I** **IV** supplement is NEVER an IV push!!! Never IM or Sub Q
> **U** **Urine** output monitor–monitor
> **M** **Muscle** weakness–fall precautions; monitor K⁺ & digitalis level (low serum K⁺ can potentiate digitalis toxicity)

HYPOKALEMIA

W eak and irregular pulse; muscle weakness

E valuate for hyporeflexia; decreased RR; I & O

A rrhythmias—Flat T wave (no K^+ for repolarization)

K (serum) < 3.5 mEq/L

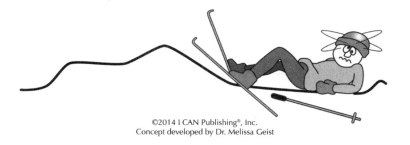

Hypercalcemia
Serum CA^{++} level > 10.5 mg/dL (4.5 mg/dL)

"**FAT CA^{++}T**" on the right page will help you remember the signs and symptoms of hypercalcemia, ($\uparrow$ Ca^{++}) forever! Look at his **tummy**, perhaps full of milk (calcium); he looks like we do after having a big meal. He is **slowing down** and ready for a siesta! He is **D**rowsy with a **D**ecrease in the muscle tone, and as we would expect there is CNS **D**epression in addition to a (**D**ecreased) or shortened QT interval and (**D**ecreased) or shortened ST segment in the cardiac conduction system. I think you have the point that everything has slowed **D**own! If you need some additional assessment findings, here are a few more. These may include **D**ecrease in the LOC (confusion), **D**epression; anorexia, nausea, and **D**ecrease in bowel movements (constipation). The bottom line is that many of the signs and symptoms come from the effects of excess calcium in the cells, which causes a **DECREASE in cell membrane excitability**, especially in the tissues of skeletal muscle, heart muscle, and the nervous system.

Let's take a minute and summarize these clinical assessment findings, so you can see just how easy this is! The key to remember is "**FAT CA^{++}T**" is **Drowsy** from all of the milk (**Ca^{++}**)!

The Ds
Drowsy
Decrease in muscle tone
Depressed CNS
Decrease in bowel movements (constipation)
Decreased or shortened QT interval
Decreased or shortened ST segment

The two major causes of hypercalcemia are **hyperparathyroidism and cancer**. Other causes may include a false high resulting from prolonged blood draws with an excessively tight tourniquet; prolonged bed rest; chronic renal failure associated with hyperparathyroidism; hypophosphatemia; uses of lithium, thiazide diuretics, and vitamin D overdose.

The nursing plan of care for clients with hypercalcemia would include fluids (0.9%NS IV) to promote excretion; increase fluid intake; furosemide (Lasix) to facilitate removal of Ca^{++}; foods low in calcium; increase fiber in diet; focus on cardiac monitoring; dialysis; neurological assessment; seizure precautions; encourage mobility, and initiate fall prevention protocol.

"**FAT CA^{++}T**" needs some of the calcium removed. Until that happens, assess and provide safety by preventing complications.

I CAN TESTING HINT: The 6 Fs will assist you in remembering the priority nursing care for these clients.
- $\uparrow$ Fluids
- $\uparrow$ Fiber
- Fluids (IV) that are ordered
- Furosemide (Lasix)
- Fall precautions
- Focus on seizure precautions

HYPERCALCEMIA

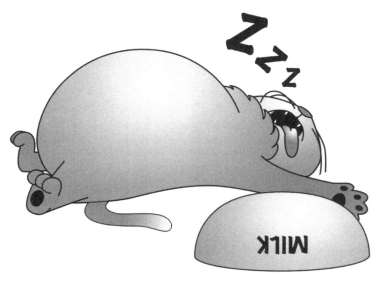

D rowsy

D ecrease in muscle tone

D epressed CNS

D ecreased QT interval

D ecreased ST segment

D ecrease in bowel movement (constipation)

Hypocalcemia
Serum Ca^{++} < 9 mg/dL (4.5 mg/dL)

"**SKINNY CA⁺⁺T**" is on the edge, and "Wow!" he is so irritable that he has a "**TWITCH**"! He may be very hungry from not having much milk (Ca^{++}). It must be that the stepbrother, "FAT CA^{++} T" got all of the milk in the bowl! The "**TWITCH**" of the "**SKINNY CA⁺⁺T**" will help you review and visualize the nursing assessments that can occur with this calcium deficiency.

A great learning strategy is that if you learn the hyper, then the hypo will be opposite. For example, "FAT CA^{++}T" was slow, CNS depression, constipated, etc. Notice, now with hypocalcemia (tummy with no milk!), the cat is now twitching, may have hyperactive reflexes, and diarrhea!

T	**Trousseau's** Sign (hand finger spasms)
W	**Watch** for dysrhythmias (↓ pulse, ↑ ST–ECG)
I	**Increase** in bowel sounds; diarrhea
T	**Tetany**, twitching, seizures
C	**Chvostek's** sign (facial twitching)
H	**Hypotension**, Hyperactive DTR

"**SKINNY CA⁺⁺T**" can occur from several diagnoses. These may include, but not be limited to hypoparathyroidism, parathyroid removed with a thyroidectomy, hyperphosphatemia, multiple blood transfusions, acute pancreatitis, malnutrition, acute renal failure, and alkalosis.

The priority care for this client is to provide a "**SAFE**" environment!

S	**Seizure** precautions; environmental stimuli ↓
A	**Administer** calcium supplements
F	**Foods** high in calcium (i.e., dairy, green); educate client
E	**Emergency** equipment on standby

> **I CAN TESTING HINT:** If you are making the decision about priority setting, and there is no indication in the question about a dysrhythmia or indication of seizure activity; start with something as basic as giving the "**SKINNY CA⁺⁺T**" some milk (*diet high in calcium*)! Maslow's Hierarchy of Needs starts with basic needs! Let's not make this difficult! Of course, you MUST READ the question carefully because the concept being tested may also be about safety with the risk of seizures or the clinical assessment findings for a client presenting with hypocalcemia, etc.

HYPOCALCEMIA

T rousseau's Sign (hand finger spasms)

W atch for dysrhythmias (↓ pulse, ↑ ST- ECG)

I ncrease in bowel sounds; diarrhea

T etany, twitching, seizures

C hvostek's sign (facial twitching)

H ypotension, Hyperactive DTR

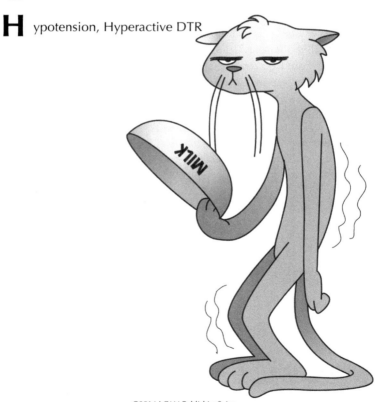

Renal Pathology

This system can be quite simple when you compare it to a water faucet and pitcher as we have on the image page. In the normal (healthy) faucet, the flow is great. There is no obstruction, and the filter is fine.

Notice in the **PRERENAL** diagram, there is decrease in the flow of water (urine). There is faucet (renal) ischemia—a decrease in the water pressure. Have you ever tried getting hot water out of the faucet while the dish washer is on? This can occur in the renal system from hemorrhage, shock, burns or decreased cardiac output.

In the **INTRARENAL** diagram, there is decreased output and some WBCs and protein which do not normally belong in the urine. This is due to kidney tissue pathology. In the faucet, it is as if someone came along and cut an opening in the filter on the spicket. This may be from glomerulonephritis, pyelonephritis, severe crushing injury, chemicals or medications.

In the **POSTRENAL** diagram, there is an obstruction in the water flow. This could be from the lime build up in the system which is causing a decrease in the free fluid. This is exactly what happens in the renal system. Some examples are: urinary calculi, benign prostatic hypertrophy (BPH) and cancer.

Remember to check renal function tests, BUN 10–20 mg/dL, creatinine 0.6–1.2 mg/dL. As the renal function decreases, these values will increase.

RENAL PATHOLOGY

Normal — 50–60mL

Prerenal — <30mL

Intrarenal

Postrenal

©2014 I CAN Publishing®, Inc.

Drugs That Can Cause Nephrotoxicity

The right page outlines several of the nephrotoxic drugs that should not be administered if the client has an alteration in the renal function. If there is a complication with renal failure, then these medications should be discussed with the healthcare provider and may not be administered due to the risk of nephrotoxicity.

Prior to administering these medications, the nurse should assess the BUN and creatinine level. The creatinine level is a more accurate evaluation of the renal function than the BUN. The creatinine evaluates the end product of protein and muscle catabolism.

In addition to these drugs, radiology contrast media can also result in kidney tissue disease. This is not good for any client with renal disease or a geriatric client who already has an alteration in the glomerular filtration rate.

I CAN TESTING HINT: As individuals age, there is a decrease in the renal function resulting from a decrease in the number of nephrons that are functioning. The outcome is a decrease in the glomerular filtration rate. The geriatric client consequently may experience a decrease in the excretion of these drugs listed on the right page resulting in toxicity. If a geriatric client has an order for a potentially nephrotoxic drug, the priority of care is notify the healthcare provider to verify if the order is appropriate. For any client with a new order for these medications, it is important to review the BUN and serum creatinine to determine if it is safe to administer one of these drugs to the client. If these values are elevated, then the healthcare provider must be notified, since it would be unsafe to administer any of these drugs.

Normal value ranges:
Serum BUN: 10-20 mg/dL
Serum Creatinine: 0.6-1.2 mg/dL

DRUGS THAT CAN CAUSE NEPHROTOXICITY

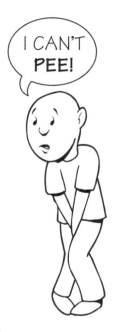

acetaminophen (high doses, acute)
acyclovir, parenteral (Zovirax)
aminoglycosides
amphotericin B, parenteral (Fungizone)
analgesic combinations containing acetaminophen, aspirin or other salicylates in high doses, chronically
ciprofloxacin
cisplatin (Platinol)
methotrexate (high doses)
nonsteroidal anti-inflammatory drugs (NSAIDs)
rifampin
sulfonamides
tetracyclines (exceptions are doxycycline and minocycline)
vancomycin, parenteral (Vancocin)

Diagnostics For The Renal System

Specific Gravity (sg) of Urine: shows concentrating/diluting ability of kidney. (e.g., reduced sg = excess fluid intake, diabetes mellitus or insipidus), (e.g., elevated sg = dehydration, sweating, SIADH). Range is 1.003-1.030 g/mL.

Renal Scan: Evaluates renal blood flow and function. ACE Inhibitors should not be administered 48 hours prior to procedure. Assess for hypotension; hydrate client well.

IVP: (*intravenous pyleogram*) of the kidney. *Refer to "Priority Plan Prior to a GRAM" for specifics; Cardiac Chapter.*

Renal arteriogram (angiogram): *Refer to "Priority Plan Prior to a GRAM" for specifics; Cardiac Chapter. Refer to "Priority Plan After a GRAM" for specifics; Cardiac Chapter.*

Radiography: X-ray of the kidneys, ureters, and bladder (KUB) to visualize these structures. Ask female client if she is pregnant. Remove clothes and jewelry over the area to have an x-ray. *Refer to "Priority Plan Prior to a GRAM" for specifics; Cardiac Chapter.*

Cystoscopy: Examines the bladder for abnormalities and/or occlusions of the ureter or urethra. Client is usually under mind anesthesia/consent needed. Assess for signs of bleeding and infection. After procedure, urine may be expected to be pink tinged and client presenting with urgency, burning, and frequency. Assess for infection for first 72 hours following procedure. (Refer to "Assessments After Any Test That Ends in SCOPY" for specifics; Respiratory Chapter.)

CT Scan: Provides cross-sectional images of the kidney to evaluate the kidney size and to evaluate for cysts, obstruction, or masses on the kidney. *Refer to radiography (KUB) above for plan.*

Excretory urography: Used to assess for obstruction, size of the kidney, and/or for a parenchymal mass. *Refer to KUB for plan.*

Ultrasound: Evaluates kidney size or for an obstruction in the lower area of the urinary tract. Risk is minimal to client.

Renal biopsy: Removal of a tissue sample for cytological exam. Nursing Care: "**BLEED**" will assist you. **B**leeding disorders or uncontrolled hypertension are always contraindications. **L**ook at coagulation values and hold antiplatelet and anticoagulants. **E**valuate for bleeding and maintain a pressure dressing over site. **E**ducate about positioning (on affected side for 30-60 min. after procedure and bed rest 24 hours. **D**etermine if there are any complications with bleeding, ↓ BP, and pain after procedure.

LABORATORY TEST	NORMAL VALUE RANGE	INDICATION
*Serum BUN	10-20 mg/dL	↑ in renal failure
Serum Creatinine	0.6-1.2 mg/dL	↑ in renal failure
**24-hr Urine Creatinine Clearance	80-140 mL/min	↓ in renal failure

*****BUN** may also be elevated if client is dehydrated or has an increase in protein intake.

******Urinary Creatinine Clearance:** Evaluate GFR; 24-hour-urine collection; start procedure with discarding the first voided specimen in the AM, and then begin timing the test; collect all of the urine for the next 24 hours and keep it cool or refrigerated.

DIAGNOSTICS FOR THE RENAL SYSTEM

"DIAGNOSTIC" exams can be hazardous to the health of our clients.

It is our mission to keep them safe!

The designated NCLEX® standards are outlined below to assist you in organizing the assessments, nursing interventions, and evaluation that must be incorporated into our critical thinking and clinical reasoning for clients experiencing a diagnostic procedure, treatment, or laboratory procedure.

D iagnostic test results—monitor; intervene for complications.

I njury and/or complications from procedure should be prevented.

A ssist with invasive procedures (e.g., thoracentesis, bronchoscopy).

G lucose monitoring, ECG, O_2 saturation, etc. may be performed.

N ote client's response to procedures and treatments.

O btain specimens other than blood (e.g., wound, stool, etc.).

S igns and symptoms of trends and/or changes-monitor, and intervene.

T each client and family about procedures and treatments.

I dentify vital signs and monitor for changes and intervene.

C omplications should be noted and followed immediately with an action.

This image is to remind you that "Sure Look" Holmes is looking into the hippo's mouth to assure he is safe! Just as "Sure Look" Holmes, the nurse is not responsible for ordering these tests, but to maintain client SAFETY prior to, during, and after these diagnostics have been completed.

©2014 I CAN Publishing®, Inc.

Lab Changes With Chronic Renal Failure

The kidneys regulate fluid, acid-base, and electrolyte balance, while also eliminating wastes from the body. The filtration occurs in the glomerulus via a semipermeable membrane. When the pressure gradients from the glomerular capillaries across the semipermeable membrane to the glomerulus are altered, changes in the GFR occur. GFR < 15 mL/min. indicate kidney failure. Refer to the trampoline on the right page. Notice, the majority of the semi-permeable membrane is colored in, indicating it is not working effectively. This will result in the lack of ability to regulate the acid-base and fluid and electrolyte balance.

As a result of changes in the semipermeable membrane, these values are jumping up which can lead to physiological complications from the changes in the acid-base balance and electrolyte imbalance The calcium and hemoglobin/hematocrit look as if they are falling off the trampoline. **Calcium** can get low. Hyperparathyroidism causes hypocalcemia and hyperphosphatemia resulting in demineralization of the bones (renal osteodystrophy). **Creatinine clearance** is decreased in renal disease. **Anemia** is a problem for clients in renal failure, since there is impairment in the erythropoietin. Erythropoietin may be administered to stimulate production of the red blood cells to minimize complications with anemia (↓ Hgb).

Phosphorous (Ph) Remember when phosphorus is elevated, the calcium level is low, which is seen in renal disease. This occurs from the hyperparathyroidism. Hyperphosphatemia results in demineralization of the bones (renal osteodystrophy). Aluminum hydroxide gel (Amphojel) is a phosphate binder used to increase the elimination of phosphate. Stool softener should be used due to undesirable effect of constipation.

Potassium (K^+) certainly is jumping up on this trampoline. Monitor EKG pattern for spiked T waves. Sodium polystyrene sulfonate (Kayexalate) or Sorbitol: an osmotic cathartic: may be given with exchange resins to induce diarrhea to excrete potassium ions. With severe hyperkalemia, IV hypertonic glucose and regular insulin may be administered to move potassium into the intracellular space.

Metabolic acidosis is seen in chronic renal disease; there is an accumulation of acid.

Magnesium (Mg): Avoid magnesium (antacids) due to risk of toxicity. Monitor dietary intake of magnesium.

Serum Creatinine & BUN are ↑. Serum creatinine level is the end product of protein and muscle catabolism. This is elevated in renal disease. BUN is also used to diagnose renal problems.

Serum Sodium (Na^+) must be decreased in diet or regulated based on levels.

LAB CHANGES WITH CHRONIC RENAL FAILURE

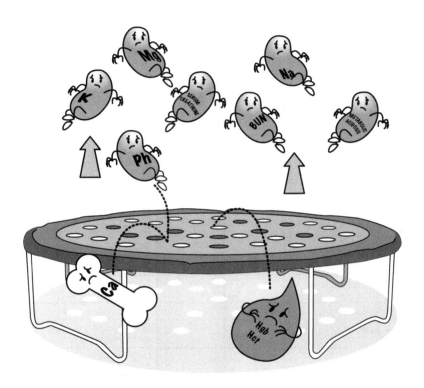

Chronic Kidney Disease (Chronic Renal Failure/CRF)

Chronic kidney disease is an irreversible reduction in the function of the renal system. The result is the kidneys are not able to maintain the body environment. Refer to the trampoline on the right page. *Notice the cement over the semipermeable membrane. There is no longer any ability to filter!* In the renal system, as well, the GFR decreases gradually as the nephrons become destroyed.

Multiple body systems are affected by chronic renal failure. *The EKG must be monitored due to changes in F&E; the edematous ankle is from fluid retention. The heart has failed (under trampoline) & pulmonary edema has become a problem. The sad brain may occur due to the altered mentation that may take place. The hand is scratching the arm due to pruritus, and the big toe has gout. The bone has broken due to hypocalcemia.* "**FAILURE**" will now also assist you in organizing these concepts.

Concepts	Increased	Decreased	Nursing Care
Fluid and Electrolytes			
Fluid overload	X		Weight, I&O, VS, etc.
Hyper/hyponatremia			(*Refer to p. 206-209*)
Hyperkalemia	X		Monitor dysrhythmias; (*Refer Hyperkalemia on pgs. 210-211*); No foods high in K+.
Metabolic Acidosis	X		Sodium Bicarb may be administered per order; Monitor dysrhythmias
Anemia (Erythropoietin)		X	Administer Erythropoietin (bleeding precautions)
(Leukocytosis)	X		Infection control precautions!
Immobility	X		ROM, Protective devices, stool softener, bran.
Integumentary	X		Decrease irritation from Pruritus; assess bruising
Lethargy/Depression	X		Emotional support
Ulcers (GI)	X		Assess for bleeding. Avoid magnesium-based antacids.
Respiratory System		X	Evaluate breath sounds, O_2 sat. (could progress to Pulmonary edema; T,C, DB
Review nutritional needs: Sodium, Potassium, Protein			Decrease in diet
Carbohydrates and Fats			Increase in diet for energy source
Total parenteral nutrition/ enteral nutrition			May be necessary to help heal
Endocrine System Calcium		X	Careful with bones!
Serum glucose / lipids	X		Monitor and plan care

CHRONIC KIDNEY DISEASE

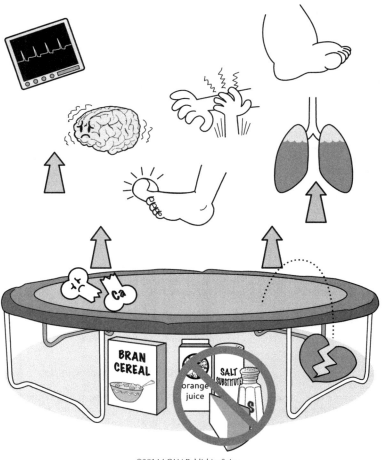

Dialysis

Di is heading into dialysis (shower) to get her toxins washed off. Water, by osmosis, moves toward the solution in which the ion concentration is the greatest. *The power of the water from the shower through the semipermeable membrane around the showerhead allows for Di to have her waste products washed off, so they can go down the drain.* Due to the size of the membrane (drain), it is too small for the blood cells and protein molecules to pass through, consequently they will not go down the drain. *Di sure looks better after her dialysis, although she is still lethargic and tired due to her lack of erythropoietin that develops new red blood cells. She will continue taking her iron and monitoring her activity level to conserve energy. She is on the scales to evaluate the change in fluid overload from prior to dialysis. Her nurse held her antihypertensive medications prior to the dialysis to prevent complications.*

Dialysis is a process to initiate the passage of particles (ions) from an area of increased concentration to an area of lower concentration across semipermeable membrane. In hemodialysis, the semipermeable membrane used has pores that are large enough for waste products and water to transport through. These pores are, however, too small for blood cells and protein molecules to pass through. In peritoneal dialysis, a similar process occurs; however, the intra-abdominal peritoneal membrane of the client is used, and due to the pore size protein is lost.

Note: In hemodialysis, the role of the nurse is to assess for patency and provide safe care to the access site (*i.e, external arteriovenous shunt, graft, etc.*). Remember, to evaluate patency, you feel (palpate) a thrill and/or hear (auscultate) a bruit. No BPs, blood samples, or IV fluids in the access site or the extremity with the vascular access site. Assess pulses distal to the access site.

Indications: Just remember, that if you were out in the woods and got any bug bites like mosquitos, etc., then you would want to get your skin washed off! Dialysis is actually washing off the blood cells. Indications for starting dialysis are outlined below!

- **B**   **BUN** > 120 mg/dL
- **U**   **Uncontrolled** hypertension, uremia, and metabolic acidosis
- **G**   **GFR** < 15 mL/min
- **S**   **Serum** potassium level > 6 mEq/L; serum (fluid) volume overload

Nursing care includes assessing baseline weight, vital signs, and electrolytes.

Since dialysis does not manufacture RBCs, the hemoglobin will not increase following procedure, where as, the electrolytes should improve from the procedure.

SIDE EFFECTS

Hypotension; postural hypotension
Muscle cramps
Bleeding form the access site; if bleeding from the site occurs, apply pressure, and notify the dialysis unit.

COMPLICATIONS

Disequilibrium Syndrome: Caused by too rapid a decrease of BUN and circulating fluid volume. It may result in cerebral edema and increased ICP, headache seizures; nausea, vomiting. Other problems may include blood loss, hypotension, sepsis, hepatitis B & C.

DIALYSIS

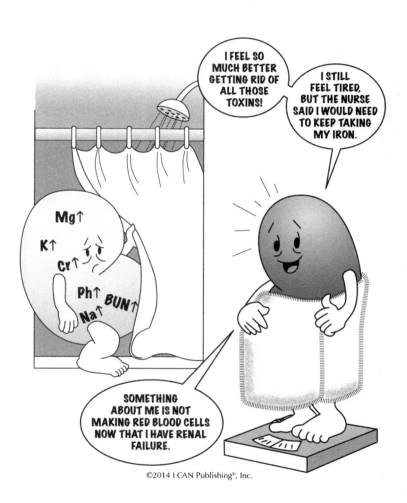

"Raise your words, not your voice. It is the rain that grows flowers, not thunder."

RUMI

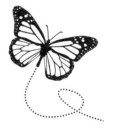

ENDOCRINE

Diagnostics For The Endocrine System

PITUITARY
Osmolality Urine: Normal range–250 to 900 mOsm/kg of water
Osmolality Serum: Normal range–285 to 295 mOsm/kg of water
These two tests evaluate ADH.

> **I CAN TESTING HINT:** Syndrome of Inappropriate Antidiuretic Hormone (SIADH)–Serum osmolality dilute and urine osmolality is high. Diabetes Insipidus: Serum osmolality high and urine osmolality is dilute.

THYROID
Thyroid-stimulating hormone (TSH): Normal range: 0.4–6.15 microunits/mL. This hormone stimulates the thyroid hormones release from the anterior pituitary gland. No special care is required.

> **I CAN TESTING HINT:** TSH may be ↑ in hypothyroidism; ↓ in primary hyperthyroidism.

Triiodothyronine (T_3): Normal range – 70 to 205 ng/dL
Thyroxine (T_4): Normal range – 4.0 to 12.0 mcg/dL
When the thyroid gland is stimulated by TSH, thyroid hormones will be released. When T_3 and T_4 are low, TSH increases secretion. T_3 and T_4 are evaluated to confirm abnormal TSH. No special care is required; random blood samples are required.

> **I CAN TESTING HINT:** T_3, T_4 ↓ in hypothyroidism; ↑ in hyperthyroidism

Radioactive iodine uptake (RAIU): Normal range < 35% of injected amount of radioactive iodine (^{123}I). This test measures the amount of ^{123}I that is absorbed by the thyroid gland. An absorption of > 35 % of ^{123}I indicates a complication with hyperthyroidism. This test is contraindicated if client is pregnant. Thyroid medication can interfere with test results. If client had another test that used an iodine-containing dye, then this test would be contraindicated.

PANCREAS
Fasting blood glucose (FBG) (*also referred to as Glucose fasting blood sugar (FBS and fasting plasma glucose (FPG)*): Normal range: 70-110 mg/dL; Levels > 126 mg/dL is diagnostic for diabetes mellitus. Teach client to be NPO 8 hours prior to exam. No antidiabetic agents prior to exam.
Oral glucose tolerance test: Normal range: 1 hour levels < 200 mg/dL; 2 hours levels < 140 mg/dL; Levels > 200 mg/dL = diabetes mellitus. At the start of the test a FBS is drawn. Client then drinks a specific amount of glucose. Serum glucose levels are then drawn every 30 min. (or designated intervals by HCP) for 2 hours. Monitor for hypoglycemia during procedure. Teach client to continue with balanced diet for 3 days prior to exam, and then remain NPO 10-12 hours prior to test.
Glycosylated hemoglobin (HbA1c): Normal range for a nondiabetic: 4%-6%; target goal < 7%. This is the best indicator for control of diabetes, since it measures glucose attached to hemoglobin.
Adrenal Cortex: Serum ACTH-A.M. values, 25-200 pg/mL; evening, 0-50 pg/mL. If suppression of the ACTH is normal, Cushing's Syndrome is ruled out.

DIAGNOSTICS FOR THE ENDOCRINE SYSTEM

"**DIAGNOSTIC**" exams can be hazardous to the health of our clients.

It is our mission to keep them safe!

The designated NCLEX® standards are outlined below to assist you in organizing the assessments, nursing interventions, and evaluation that must be incorporated into our critical thinking and clinical reasoning for clients experiencing a diagnostic procedure, treatment, or laboratory procedure.

D iagnostic test results—monitor; intervene for complications.

I njury and/or complications from procedure should be prevented.

A ssist with invasive procedures (e.g., thoracentesis, bronchoscopy).

G lucose monitoring, ECG, O_2 saturation, etc. may be performed.

N ote client's response to procedures and treatments.

O btain specimens other than blood (e.g., wound, stool, etc.).

S igns and symptoms of trends and/or changes-monitor, and intervene.

T each client and family about procedures and treatments.

I dentify vital signs and monitor for changes and intervene.

C omplications should be noted and followed immediately with an action.

This image is to remind you that "Sure Look" Holmes is looking into the hippo's mouth to assure he is safe! Just as "Sure Look" Holmes, the nurse is not responsible for ordering these tests, but to maintain client SAFETY prior to, during, and after these diagnostics have been completed.

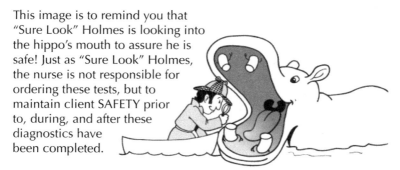

©2014 I CAN Publishing®, Inc.

SIADH

"Soggy Sid" has SIADH (syndrome of inappropriate antidiuretic hormone), a condition that continually releases the antidiuretic hormone (ADH). With increased ADH, the body retains water and gets so Soggy that water intoxication may occur.

Sid's cap is hiding his bandaged head from a head injury, which is a major risk factor for SIADH. Due to his cerebral edema, he is prone to seizures. Notice his limbs are small. There is no obvious edema, yet he has gained weight in his body. The intake and output record will document low urinary output because he's keeping it all on board. The urine specific gravity will be high. The serum sodium will be decreased (dilutional). Limit Soggy Sid's fluid intake. He may be given diuretics to assist with fluid excretion, especially if he has respiratory or cardiac problems. Keep Soggy Sid's bed flat or only slightly elevated. This position of his head will decrease the secretion of ADH. Keep the neuro checks going. Soggy Sid is in serious condition! Do you see a link here with the previous reviewed concept of "Hyponatremia" on page 216-217?

I CAN Testing HINT: Urine = **CONCENTRATED**
↑ Urine Sodium
↑ Urine Osmolality

Blood = **DILUTE**
↓ Serum Sodium
↓ Serum Osmolality

These labs would be just the opposite for "Diabetes Insipidus"! See how EASY this is!

SOGGY SID

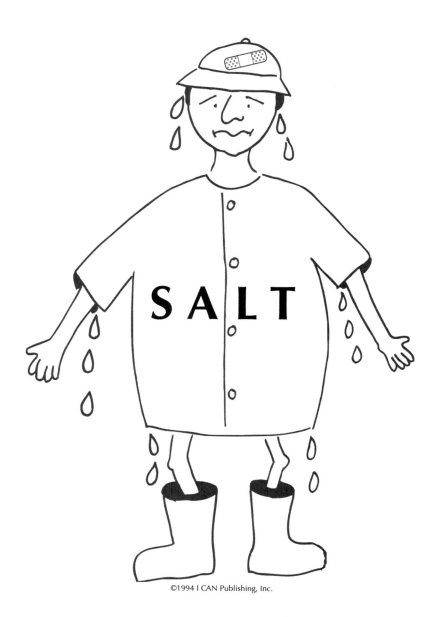

Diabetes Insipidus

Due to a lack of pitressin excretion from the Pituitary gland, our poor dried-up California prune is shriveled up because he urinates a lot (polyuria). This loss of body fluids will cause him to be very dehydrated and have a low specific gravity in his urine. To monitor Mr. Prune, the nurse will need to keep accurate daily weights and watch his vital signs.

Offer him plenty to drink and keep a watch on his specific gravity. He may require IV fluids for rehydration. This guy can get dehydrated in a hurry and must be watched closely. Do you see a link here with the previous reviewed concept of "Hypernatremia" on page 214-215?

S-I-A-D-H
(Syndrome of Inappropriate Antidiuretic Hormone)
Lyrics © (Sing to tune: BINGO)

Chorus
S-I-A-D-H,   S-I-A-D-H,   S-I-A-D-H,
This hormone stops the PeePee.

Verse 1
Brain tumors, trauma, and bad bugs
A complication might be—
S-I-A-D-H,   S-I-A-D-H,   S-I-A-D-H,
This hormone stops the PeePee.

Verse 2
Low output, sodium; gained weight
And high S. gravity (specific gravity)
S-I-A-D-H,   S-I-A-D-H,   S-I-A-D-H,
This hormone stops the PeePee.

Verse 3
But, Diabetes Insipidus
The opposite you'll see
Pee, Pee...Give IVs...
Pee Pee...Give IVs...
Pee, Pee...Give IVs...
Vas-o-pressin they need!

Verse 4
High output, sodium; pounds lost,
And low S. gravity (specific gravity)
Pee, Pee...Give IVs...
Pee Pee...Give IVs...
Pee, Pee...Give IVs...
Vas-o-pressin they need!

Used with permission: Created by Darlene A. Franklin, RN MSN

DIABETES INSIPIDUS

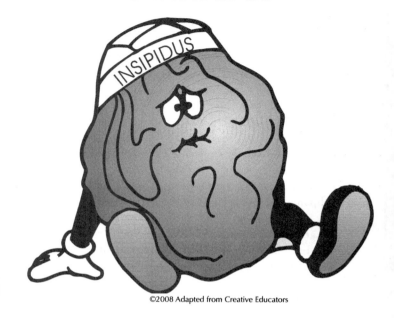

D

I + O, daily weight

L ow specific gravity

U rinates lots

T reat = pituitary hormone

r **E** hydrate

Hyperthyroidism

"**GO GETTER GERTRUDE**" will help you remember the major symptoms of hyperthyroidism. Her last name, of course, is Graves. Graves' disease is the result of hyperthyroidism. One look at this visually stunning creature, and you can see how thin she is and how her eyes "bug out" (exophthalmus). Everything is running except her menstrual periods. Her HEART is running fast (increased pulse), her BLOOD PRESSURE is running UP, and her basal metabolic rate (BMR) is running, therefore the metabolism of drugs will be faster. She can eat a whole chocolate cake without ever gaining an ounce. She is running so much that she is cleaning out closets that don't need cleaning at 3:00 in the morning. Notice she is wearing short sleeves and pants because it takes a lot of energy to run, and she is hot all the time. While planning her nursing care, lower the room temperature and get rid of all those excess blankets. A quiet room will be great! Well-balanced meals (high in calories and vitamins) are a must. Due to the eye changes, protect cornea from drying. "GO GETTER'S" diagnostic tests would reveal an increase in the following reports: T_3 and T_4, BMR and uptake of ^{123}I. Serum Thyroid Stimulating Hormone (TSH) will be decreased in hyperthyroidism. Normal: 0.4-4.2 mIU/L.

I CAN TESTING HINT:

TSH ↓, T_3, T_4 ↑ = Hyperthyroidism

TSH ↑, T_3, T_4 ↓ = Hypothyroidism

GO GETTER GERTRUDE

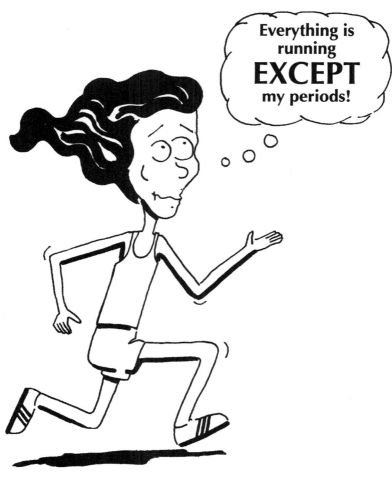

Thyroidectomy

The **BOW TIE** is around his neck because the hyperactive thyroid gland has been removed. Post-op can be a crucial period for these folks because they may **BLEED**. Often the blood collects behind the neck, being pulled by gravity if he is lying on his back. Place him in semi-Fowler's position to avoid tension on the suture line. Observe the **AIRWAY** due to potential swelling from being traumatized during surgery. Vocal chords may be swollen. Assess frequently for noisy breathing and increased restlessness. Evaluate **VOCAL** changes; increasing hoarseness may be indicative of laryngeal edema. If these people get into trouble they can lose their airway fast. It's advisable to have a **TRACHEOTOMY SET** available to open an emergency airway. The **INCISION** needs to be observed for swelling which can occlude the airway. Watch for normal wound healing. We don't want an infection. Evaluate calcium levels; parathyroids may have been damaged or accidentally removed. Since calcium potentiates the movement of electrolytes across the cell membrane and electrolyte balance is imperative for the heart cells to work, low levels could create an **EMERGENCY**. Have calcium gluconate available! Refer to "Hypocalcemia" on pages 224-225.

POST-OP THYROIDECTOMY

Bleeding
  Beware Thyroid Storm

Open airway

Whisper

Trache set

Incision

Emergency

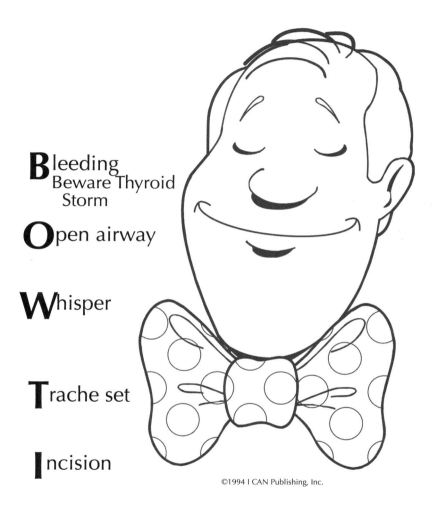

Hypothyroidism

This vision of loveliness is "**MORBID MATILDA**." Her last name, as you've probably guessed, is Myxedema (Hypothyroid). She has a slow deterioration of the thyroid function. It occurs mostly in older adults and five times more frequently in women than in men.

As you can see, Matilda has the family "bug-eyes" and she has no menstrual period like her sister Gertrude, but that's where the resemblance ends. (Refer to **Hyperthyroidism**.) Matilda is not thin. In fact, she can look at a piece of chocolate cake and gain weight. She had rather sleep at 3:00 in the morning than clean closets. She may also be sleeping at 3:00 in the afternoon because of her lack of energy. Her long pants and putting her hands in her pocket will keep her warm. Increasing the room temperature may be necessary.

Matilda will be placed on lifelong thyroid replacement, and will be on a low-calorie, low cholesterol diet to help with her weight loss. Morbid Matilda does not like these changes. She is definitely not a very happy camper!

MORBID MATILDA

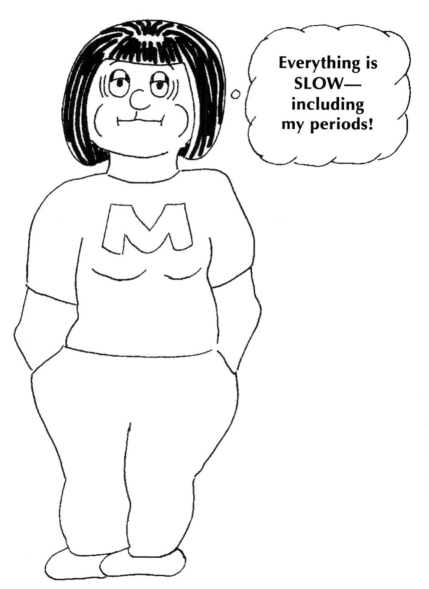

Diabetes Mellitus

"**FIDO**," the diabetic dog, is exhibiting all of the signs and symptoms of hyperglycemia. Sugar is floating around in his blood stream because there is no insulin to take the sugar into the cells.

Since the cells are starving for lack of sugar, Fido is dreaming of food. He has a huge appetite. His food bowl in front of him remains empty because he keeps trying to feed those starving cells (**POLYPHAGIA**). The high sugar content in his blood is pulling fluid from the cells which makes him very thirsty (**POLYDIPSIA**). Since his kidneys are compensating by dumping extra fluid and sugar out onto the street (**POLYURIA**), he has totally wet down the fire hydrant. Look at Fido's pants! They don't fit any more. The sugar and the fluid that he has taken in have not gone into his cells, since there is no insulin to assist in crossing over into the cell. As a result, poor Fido has **LOST WEIGHT**. What medication would you plan to have available? Insulin of course.

WHAT'S WRONG WITH FIDO?

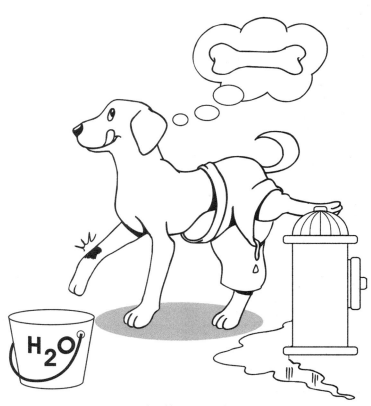

©1994 Adapted from Creative Educators

Insulin

Do you have difficulty remembering the onset, peak, and duration of the various types of insulin? Let us help simplify this for you, so it will be easy!! In your mind it will be helpful to categorize the rapid, short, intermediate, and long-acting insulin. The onset of the rapid-acting insulin (ultra-short acting) is < 15 minutes. The onset of the short acting (regular insulin) is 30–60 minutes. If you can recall this time frame being fast, then you will be able to remember the other insulins. For the intermediate insulin, multiply 60 x 2 and the onset is 60-120 minutes. For the long acting insulin, multiply 60 x 2 and 120 x 2 and the onset is 120-240 min.

As you can see on caps on the next page, the peak has a general progression. The rapid acting starts at 30-60 min. Regular starts with a peak of 3 hours. Take 3 + 1 = 4 and also multiply 3 x 4 = 12 to get a peak of 4-12 hours for the intermediate insulin. As you can see, the long acting insulin has NO peak.

The duration of the rapid-acting insulins (i.e., Lispro (Humalog), Aspart (Novolog), Glulisine (Apidra) are 4 hrs. The remainder of the times are in increments of 6. The regular insulin's duration is 6 hrs. Multiply that by 3 and the intermediate insulin is 18–24 hrs. The long acting insulin has the longest duration of 24 hrs. *Refer to* **"HYPOGLYCEMIA"** *for additional information regarding signs and symptoms of an insulin reaction on p. 256-257.*

Lantus and Levemir are long-acting insulins. They have an onset of 2-4 hrs. There is no peak and it has a duration of 24 hrs.

Remember–Regular insulin is the only insulin which may be given IV.

I CAN TESTING HINT: Peak Times on the caps of the *"Insulin Crew on the right page"* are the priority critical assessment, since this is one of the times when hypoglycemic reactions are likely to occur. The client will be **"TIRED"** if experiencing a reaction. *(Refer to p. 256-257)*

PEAK TIMES FOR INSULIN

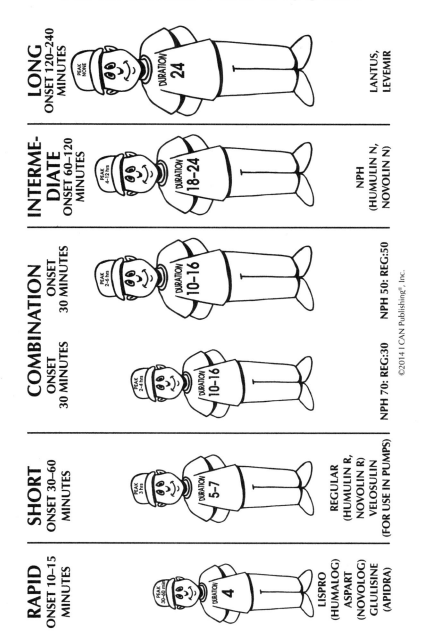

Hypoglycemia

People taking insulin may have hypoglycemic reactions. This is a fact. Some diabetics have them everyday; others rarely have this problem. Teach them the symptoms, so they recognize their situation. Some of the signs and symptoms to observe are they may get suddenly **TIRED** and run out of steam. **TACHYCARDIA** (rapid pulse) occurs as a warning. **TREMORS** or nervousness are other warning signs. They often become **IRRITABLE** and **RESTLESS**. They may mow anyone down in the coke line to get some food due to **EXCESSIVE HUNGER**. They know if they don't, they may be out! **DIAPHORESIS** is common, and is an excellent guideline for determining if the client is asleep versus having a hypoglycemic reaction. If the client is unconscious, administer glucagon IV. Encourage them to eat carbohydrates or drink milk if they are awake.

*If ever in doubt of a diagnosis of hypoglycemia versus hyperglycemia, give carbohydrates—severe hypoglycemia can result in permanent brain damage.

Remember this jingle to help recall the differences:

*COLD AND CLAMMY MEANS YOU NEED SOME CANDY
HOT AND DRY MEANS YOUR SUGAR IS HIGH.*

Jingle reprinted with permission, NEC, Dallas, Texas

SYMPTOMS OF HYPOGLYCEMIA

Tremors
Tachycardia

Irritability

Restless

Excessive hunger

Diaphoresis
Depression

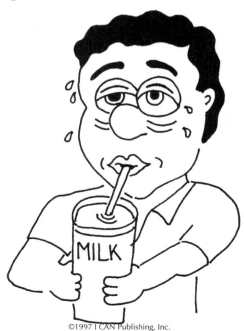

Cushing's Disease/Syndrome

One look at "**CUSHY CARL**" and you see his problem. He has an overproduction of hormones from the adrenal cortex. As you see, he's holding a "twinkie." These people may have a HIGH BLOOD SUGAR. The bag of chips he is holding indicates his INCREASE in SODIUM resulting in fluid retention. Increase in volume naturally will ELEVATE the BLOOD PRESSURE. Watch that POTASSIUM level, it will have a tendency to DECREASE and we certainly do not want his heart doing any strange dances (arrhythmias). Cushy's fat face also let's us know he's holding fluids. His "buffalo hump" probably scares him enough that his blood pressure goes up even higher. The sore on his leg won't heal because of his high blood sugar. (Would we want to protect him from INFECTION? You bet!)

Put 2 and 2 together. Would we want to give a diabetic steroids? Not if we can help it. Sometimes there are no options, so if this is the case, monitor the blood sugar. Now we know that cortisone (steroids) will increase the blood sugar even higher, increase edema, and increase the risk for infection. With all of this going on, Cushy will indeed need some assistance with his emotional state.

We know we would! What about you?

I CAN TESTING HINT: An easy way to remember the labs and organize the nursing care is to recall the saying, "**S**ome **P**eople **G**et **C**old"! Then take the first letter of this statement and convert to the following:

Some → Sodium ↑ *(Refer to p. 214 – 215 for hypernatremia.)*

People → Potassium ↓ *(Refer to p. 220-221 for hypokalemia.)*

Get → Glucose ↑ *(Refer to p. 252-253 for hyperglycemia.)*

Cold → Calcium ↓ *(Refer to p 224-225 for hypocalcemia.)*

There is a "**u**" in Cushing's to help remind you to start with the arrow in the **upward** direction and then each lab following will be in the opposite direction! The nursing care is reviewed with each of the designated concepts.

See how easy this is!! The great news is that there is a "**d**" in **Add**ison's and the arrow now will start down , so each of these labs are directly opposite for this disease. Yes, all you have to do is to understand this strategy and you will be able to answer many questions linked to these concepts!

Reference: *Pharmacology Made Insanely Easy*; Manning, Rayfield; p. 267; I CAN Publishing, Inc. ; © 2013.

CUSHY CARL

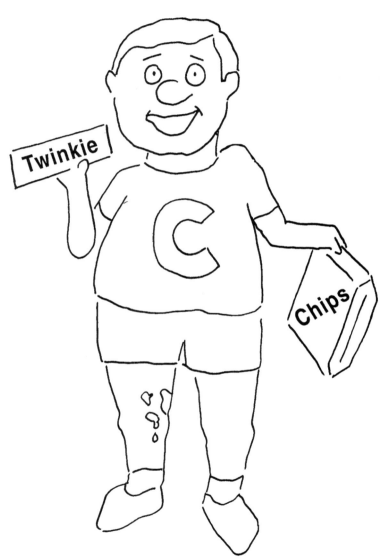

Addison's Disease

"**ANEMIC ADAM**," whose last name is Addison, is Cushy Carl's half brother. (*Refer to* **Cushing's Disease/Syndrome**.) The whole family thinks they have opposite characteristics. Adam has a disorder which is caused by a decrease in secretion of the adrenal cortex hormone.

Adam craves salt since he doesn't have enough. That is the reason he is out in the field at the salt lick. Hyponatremia has a tendency to cause low blood pressure. In addition, his potassium may be increased. He has hypoglycemia and complains of being tired and weak much of the time. This weakness is a cardinal complaint and usually is more severe in times of stress. Occasionally, Adam stays in bed. After his anorexia, nausea, vomiting and diarrhea, he is dehydrated and has a serious loss in weight. After all of this, who wouldn't be tired and weak? His skin has turned bronze, and it is not due to too much sun. This is caused by increased levels of melanocyte stimulating hormone (MSH). To prevent addisonian crisis, corticosteroids will have to be replaced.

ANEMIC ADAM

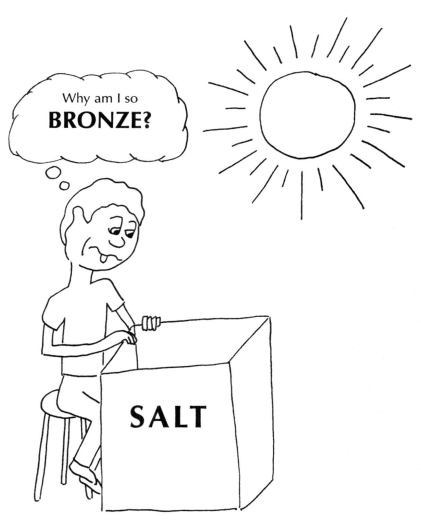

"Intuition literally means learning from within. Most of us were not taught how to use this sense, but all of us know well that "gut" feeling. Learn to trust your inner feeling and it will become stronger. Avoid going against your better judgment or getting talked into things that just don't feel right."

DOE ZANTAMATA

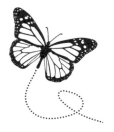

GASTROINTESTINAL SYSTEM

Diagnostics For The Gastrointestinal System

Upper Gastrointestinal Series, Barium Swallow: X-ray in which barium is used as a contrast material to diagnose complications of the stomach and esophagus. Nursing care will include: "**NPO**", Not performed on a client with acute abdomen until perforation ruled out. NPO for 8 hours prior to procedure. Push fluids after procedure to prevent constipation. May need a stool softener or laxative to promote excretion of barium. Oral intake of barium; client swallows barium to coat the GI tract. 72 hrs–norm. color.

Lower Gastrointestinal Series, Barium Enema: The use of barium as a contrast medium to x-ray the colon; barium is administered rectally. Nursing care similar to above. "**NPO**", NPO 8 hours prior to test; may have clear liquids eve before. Push fluids after procedure and administer a laxative to assist in expelling barium. Out with the stool in colon; administer enemas and laxatives eve prior to procedure. May feel cramping or defecation during procedure.

Endoscopy (Gastroscopy, Colonscopy, Sigmoidoscopy, Capsule Endoscopy, Esophagogastroduodenoscopy (EGD)): Endoscopy is used to visualize gastrointestinal tract (GI) using a fiber optic, flexible and lighted scope. A biopsy or clipping of a benign polyp may be performed. Upper GI: identifies tumors, ulcerations, inflamed areas, and esophageal varies treatment. Lower GI: identifies polyps, tumors, hemorrhoids; evaluation of diverticular disease or irritable bowel syndrome, etc. **Prior to procedure:** Upper GI-NPO; Lower GI-bowel prep, enemas, cathartics, clear liquid diet 24 hours prior to test; "**NSAIDs**": NSAIDs should be avoided, aspirin, iron supplements, etc. or any food such as gelatin with red coloring that may result in false positive results; Sedation (conscious) is used frequently for upper and lower GI studies or a colonscopy. Assess client's mouth for dentures and remove bridges if appropriate prior to upper GI studies; Insertion of the scope (prior to), a topical anesthesia will be used to anesthetize the throat; Decrease oral secretions by relaxing through a pre-op med for relaxation. Side-lying (left), knee-chest position (Lower GI) and explain need to take a deep breath during the insertion of the scope; client may feel urge to defecate as scope is inserted. **During procedure:** "**ABCDs**" Airway precautions during sedations; Bleeding (GI) and notify HCP; Consent verified prior to initiating procedure; Determine level of sedation; Safety- client identification, positioning. **After Procedure:** *Refer to "SCOPY"; Respiratory Chapter.*

Paracentesis: A catheter is inserted into the peritoneal cavity to determine causes for acute abdominal problems, assess for ascites, and/or to determine impact of abdominal trauma. During procedure, a NG tube may assist with maintaining gastric decompression. **Prior to procedure:** To prevent risk for bladder perforation, have client void. Assess coagulation labs if client has chronic liver problems. Position in semi-Fowler's; maintain sterile field for procedure. Do not drain more than 1 L if a client has ascites. **After procedure:** Monitor for complications including the "4 P's": Perforation of the bowel; Peritonitis; Pain referred to right shoulder from introduction of air into abdominal cavity; Pressure too low from too much fluid being removed. Exam should be contraindicated if pregnancy or possible bowel obstruction and coagulation problems.

Stool Examination: Evaluated for consistency, form, presence of blood, parasites, etc. Nursing Implications: "**STOOL**"–Stool in sterile container if evaluating for organisms; The stool must be fresh and warm for evaluating parasites or organisms. Occult blood is positive when paper turns blue; Over-the-counter drugs and general meds client is taking should be documented. No red meat, beets, etc. Look at size; specimen–should be approximately 30 mL.

DIAGNOSTICS FOR THE GASTROINTESTINAL SYSTEM

"DIAGNOSTIC" exams can be hazardous to the health of our clients.

It is our mission to keep them safe!

The designated NCLEX® standards are outlined below to assist you in organizing the assessments, nursing interventions, and evaluation that must be incorporated into our critical thinking and clinical reasoning for clients experiencing a diagnostic procedure, treatment, or laboratory procedure.

D iagnostic test results—monitor; intervene for complications.

I njury and/or complications from procedure should be prevented.

A ssist with invasive procedures (e.g., thoracentesis, bronchoscopy).

G lucose monitoring, ECG, O_2 saturation, etc. may be performed.

N ote client's response to procedures and treatments.

O btain specimens other than blood (e.g., wound, stool, etc.).

S igns and symptoms of trends and/or changes-monitor, and intervene.

T each client and family about procedures and treatments.

I dentify vital signs and monitor for changes and intervene.

C omplications should be noted and followed immediately with an action.

This image is to remind you that "Sure Look" Holmes is looking into the hippo's mouth to assure he is safe! Just as "Sure Look" Holmes, the nurse is not responsible for ordering these tests, but to maintain client SAFETY prior to, during, and after these diagnostics have been completed.

©2014 I CAN Publishing®, Inc.

Priority Plans For Infant With Severe Diarrhea

Diarrhea is the rapid movement of intestinal contents through the small bowel. Infants are susceptible to complications of dehydration and hypovolemia.

> Infants < 2 years of age have more than 50% extracellular fluid. This is 2–5 times greater than adults. SAFE care is all about PREVENTING alteration in fluid and electrolytes. *Refer to the image "CALLING THE SHOTS IN ACID VS. BASE," an easy strategy for an infant with diarrhea!*

Acute diarrhea is most often caused by an infection. Rotavirus is the most common pathogen in young infants and children hospitalized for treatment of diarrhea. Other precipitating factors may include: salmonella, clostridium difficile, malabsorption problems such as celiac disease and cystic fibrosis.

Weighing the infant daily will assist the nurse with identifying one early sign of dehydration. A weight loss of 3–5% will indicate mild dehydration, 5-10% will be moderate, and > 10% will be severe. Focus on preventing the progression of dehydration. Remember daily weight should be at the same time and same scales with no clothes.

Evaluate electrolytes (especially sodium and potassium), urine specific gravity. The infant can develop hypokalemia, hypernatremia, dehydration, hypovolemia, progressing to shock. A specific gravity of > 1.020 indicates mild dehydration. The key is for the nurse to monitor the trends with these values. Monitor for metabolic acidosis! *Remember, base (alkaline) comes out of bottom leading to metabolic acidosis.*

Intake and output; complete description of all vomitus and stools; inspect abdomen for distention; auscultate for bowel sounds; palpate for areas of tenderness all are included in the plan of care. Remember, 1 g diaper weight = 1 mL output. **Infection control** precautions: Standard and Contact Precautions (based on pathogen) are important to practice for prevention of infection transmission.

Give oral rehydrating solutions (ORS) as the first line of therapy; progress fluids and diet as tolerated; do not offer high-carbohydrate fluids (juices), carbonated fluids, broth, or sports drinks. If the infant is progressively getting more dehydrated, then IV fluids may be started.

Hydration status: Monitor for depressed fontanels if not closed, skin turgor, I&O, weight, etc. Keep the rectal area clean and use barrier creams to protect skin. **Health Promotion:** Hand hygiene is important to prevent the spread of the diarrhea. Teach parents and personnel the safe practice of personal protective equipment (PPE) based on the organism that is the cause of the diarrhea (Contact precautions for most infants with diarrhea). Demonstrate to the family how to properly dispose of the diapers and soiled linens close to the bedside. Instruct family how to keep clean and dirty areas in the room separate. Do not give antidiarrheal medications if causative agent is bacterial or parasitic. **The vital signs** should be monitored ongoing. RR and HR will continue to increase as dehydration worsens.

> **I CAN TESTING HINTS:**
> HR, RR, specific gravity, serum sodium, hematocrit values all ↑ with moderate dehydration.
> Weight, output, fontanels (sunken), capillary refill, serum potassium all ↓.
> Monitor the **TRENDS** with the VS, labs, & assessments for infants with diarrhea and intervene with the priority plan.

INFANT WITH SEVERE DIARRHEA

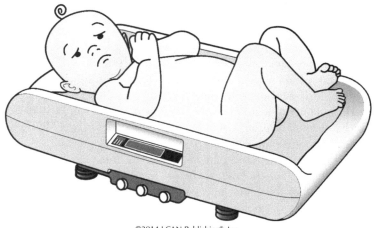

W eigh daily

E valuate electrolytes (especially calcium, sodium and potassium), urine specific gravity

I ntake and output; complete description of all vomitus and stools; inspect abdomen for distention; auscultate for bowel sounds; palpate for areas of tenderness

G ive oral rehydrating solutions

H ydration status—monitor (i.e., fontanels if not closed, skin turgor, etc.); hygiene (oral and rectal); Health Promotion

T he vital signs should be monitored ongoing

Peptic Ulcer Disease

Old "**PUD**" is a fine specimen of a man. He's standing there tapping his foot waiting impatiently on that bus, smoking his cigarette with a vengeance and checking to see if it's time for another NSAID (Nonsteroidal Anti-inflammatory drugs may cause GI bleeding). Just the kind of behavior that might precipitate peptic ulcer disease. When you think ulcers (except stress ulcers), think pain. Imagine a drop of hydrochloric acid on your open hand! First, the hand will hurt or burn, and once the acid has eaten the skin away, the hand will bleed. If the hand could be protected by a glove (food or drugs) the HCL might not eat through enough to bleed.

Drug timing is important in preventing this pain and bleeding. Generally, use anticholinergics before meals. (Refer to **Anticholinergics**.) Tagamet and zantac may be given with or after meals. Consider coating the stomach lining with the "white chalky stuff" such as maalox, titrilac, gelusil, or amphojel 1 hour after meals. Avoid giving within 1 to 2 hours of other medicines. Remind clients on sodium restriction to check the labels for sodium content. Amphojel, titralac, and digel have high sodium content. These clients will also need assistance in dietary modifications.

The Heliocobactor Pylori (Helicopter) organism is prevelent in PUD and can be treated with drugs.

ULCERS

Pain

Ulcers bleed

Drug timing

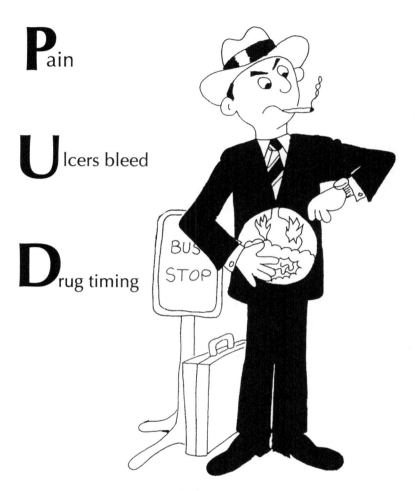

Gastric Reflux

As you can see, "**GERD**" is holding his stomach due to his problem with gastroesophageal reflux disease (GERD). He is also covering his mouth due to his discomfort with regurgitation of fluid and food particles. GERD is experiencing **REFLUX** of the stomach and duodenal contents into the esophagus leading to a spectrum of clinical manifestations predominated by inflammation of the esophagus.

REFLUX is most often related to inadequate relaxation of the lower esophageal sphincter (LES) that allows reflux of gastric acid and pepsin into the distal esophagus. Agents such as alcohol, benzodiazepines, calcium channel blockers, chocolate, peppermint, and narcotics cause LES relaxation.

REGURGITATION can be decreased by weight reduction if client is obese. The head of the bed may also be elevated. Alterations in the amount of **FOOD** eaten at one serving can also be effective in decreasing reflux. GERD should avoid large meals and sit upright 30–60 minutes after eating. GERD should **X** out carbonated beverages particularly 3 hours prior to going to bed. **ESOPHAGEAL SPASMS** may be relieved by avoiding agents that cause LES relaxation as indicated in the previous paragraph. As you can see, GERD's **LIFESTYLE** must be modified.

Remember GERD must manage this reflux, so he doesn't develop complications with nocturnal aspiration, recurrent pneumonia or bronchospasm, difficulty swallowing, or iron deficiency anemia.

REFLUX

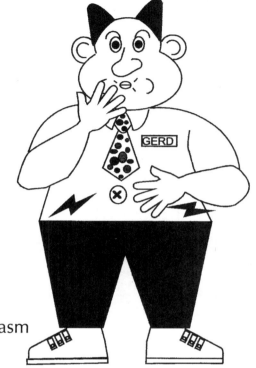

R egurgitation

E sophageal spasm

F ood—small meals

L ifestyle must be modified

U se of Prilosec, Prevacid, Nexium, Reglan, antacids, H_2 histamine antagonists

X out colas, milk to decrease acid production, peppermint

Anticholinergics

The major side effects of these medications are easily seen on the next page. Some examples of these medications include: Atropine, Methantheline (Banthine), Propantheline (Pro-Banthine), and Dicyclomine hydrochloride (Bentyl). Of course these drugs are given because of the desirable effects of decreasing salivation, lacrimation, urination, diarrhea, and GI motility. Blurred vision and dilated pupils are also side effects. It's when we get too much that we get in trouble. These medications are contraindicated in closed and open angle glaucoma, prostatic hypertrophy, and obstructive bowel disease.

Remember–Other current common medications often used for GI symptoms include: Rolaids, Tums, H_2 Antagonists, Proton pump inhibitors, and Helicobacter Pylori agents. Some of the agents are aluminum based and some magnesium based.

ANTICHOLINERGIC MEDICATIONS

Can't pee

Can't see

Can't spit

Can't sh*t

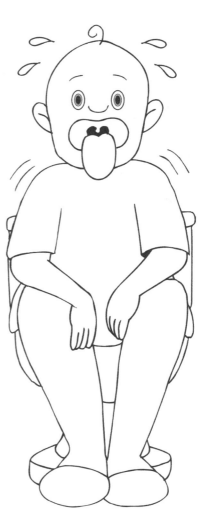

Antacids

Mag has had a history of an ulcer, but feels much better now since antacids coat her stomach lining. She, however, has developed another serious problem with DIARRHEA!!!! This is a major side effect of antacids containing magnesium such as Milk of Magnesia. The diarrhea must get under control or she will need to meet Alkali, a cousin, which will assist her in correcting the metabolic acidosis which may occur as a complication from the diarrhea. **Mag** should be monitored for dehydration, hypokalemia, and hyponatremia. If **Mag** were to remain on magnesium oxide for prolonged therapy, the magnesium level should be monitored periodically.

Al is also in the family and is taking an aluminum antacid such as amphogel for his ulcer symptoms. As you can see, **Al's** problem is constipation. He is so full of it that he can't get rid of it. CONSTIPATION is a major side effect of antacids containing aluminum.

Remember–Teach clients to take antacids one hour after meals and to refrain from taking other oral medications within 1-2 hours of any antacid.

AUNT ACID'S FAMILY

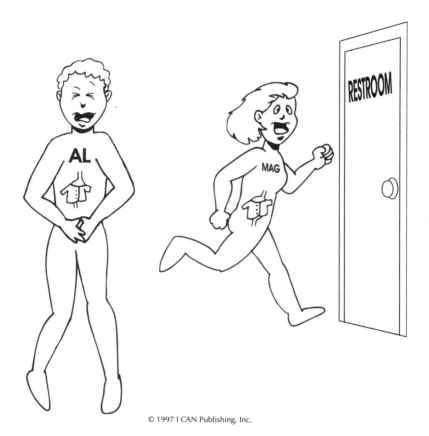

ALUMINUM   **MAG**NESIUM

Treatment of Ulcerative Colitis and Crohn's

Cathy Crampy has inflammatory bowel disease. She is bent over with the **CRAMPS** due to the inflammation. This is treated with steroids and a low fat and low fiber diet. Poor Cathy has her legs together to hold in that **DIARRHEA**. She is taking some antidiarrheal medications to decrease this problem.

Her **PAIN** is being relieved through her diet, **ANTICHOLINERGICS** and corticosteroids. Cathy may be NPO to decrease bowel activity; FLUIDS are introduced gradually. She will receive IV fluids and may even require hyperalimentation to restore the deficiencies.

Sulfasalazine (**AZULFIDINE**) is one of the **ANTIMICROBIALS** used to prevent exacerbations.

Her MEALS are modified to correct the deficiencies. She is on a high protein, high caloric and high vitamin diet. Cathy may live a very stressful life. She is always a day behind her deadlines.

COUNSELING will help her to identify how this life style can contribute to this condition. Emotional **SUPPORT** will assist Cathy Crampy in decreasing the stress in her life and help her to learn "To slow down and stop and smell the flowers in life."

CRAMPS

Control diarrhea
Control inflammation

Relieve pain
Restore fluid

Anticholinergics
Antimicrobials

Meals—correct nutritional deficiencies

Psychological counseling

Support emotionally/coping

© 1994 I CAN Publishing, Inc.

Colostomy

Clients with ulcerative colitis, Crohn's disease or other disease process in the lower gastrointestinal tract may require surgery that brings fecal elimination to an opening on the outside of the abdominal wall.

Connie Colostomy says that her colostomy is just like her **ANUS**.

A **ABLE** to regulate her stool through regular irrigations; therefore a colostomy bag is not required. Irrigations should be the same time frame daily.

N **NOT** watery. The stools are formed and do not leak on her clothes.

U **U** can do all you can do without the colostomy. Some foods will liquefy stools or cause noisy problems.

S **SWIMMING** is OK! Showers and tub baths are also acceptable.

This is probably NOT the case for Connie's friend ILLE who has an ileostomy.

Ille's stool is liquid. Bags are attached to the skin and skin breaks down easily. She must be taught about cleaning, removing the adhesive that holds the bag in place and cleanliness of the bag. She is usually not able to regulate the ileostomy because it is watery. She may lose fluids and electrolytes and need replacement. Some foods may also cause noisy (flatus) and "smelly" problems for Ille, which is embarrassing and hard to control.

Remember—Both Connie and Ille will have to live with these ostomies. The nurse's best approach is psychological support and education. They will need support through excellent therapeutic communication. The more they know about caring for themselves, the more "normal" they can be.

CONNIE COLOSTOMY

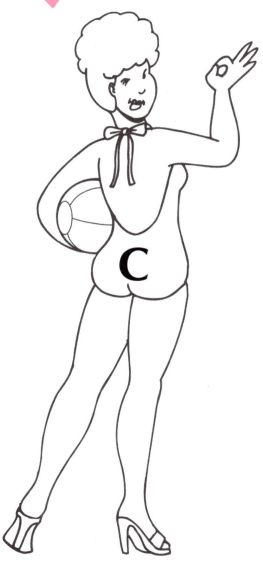
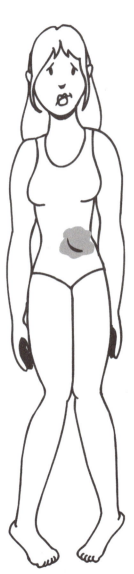

CONNIE COLOSTOMY **ILLE OSTOMY**

© 1997 I CAN Publishing, Inc.

Dumping Syndrome

This is a complication that can occur after gastric resection when stomach contents enter the intestine. The image that will pull this concept together for you is the DUMP TRUCK. Imagine that you are in a dump truck on the edge of a mountain. How would you feel? We know we would be nervous as kittens, sweaty and our heart would beat very rapidly. On a mountain edge, we are sure we would be dizzy and very weak. We may also have some abdominal cramping with some distention. These signs are, of course, because we are in the **HIGH** position. (Think of TOO MUCH, TOO SOON = TOO HIGH) Too much carbohydrate, salt, liquid, refined sugar, and in the high position on top of all of that is going to make us (excuse the expression) poop! The gastric contents high in carbohydrates rapidly enter the jejunum.

To remember how to prevent this from occurring, think of the dump truck in the **LOW** position. Think LOW. Teach clients to think small (LOW) meals. The carbohydrates, salt intake, and sugar need to be LOW (small amounts). No fluids with meals or for one hour following the meal. Lie client down for 20 to 30 minutes after meals to delay stomach emptying.

DUMPING SYNDROME

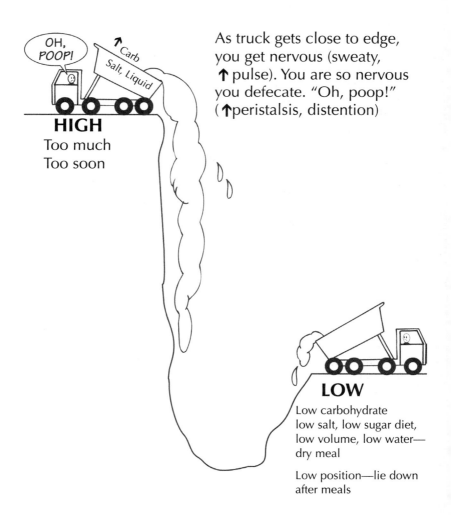

HIGH
Too much
Too soon

As truck gets close to edge, you get nervous (sweaty, ↑pulse). You are so nervous you defecate. "Oh, poop!" (↑peristalsis, distention)

LOW

Low carbohydrate low salt, low sugar diet, low volume, low water—dry meal

Low position—lie down after meals

© 1994 I CAN Publishing, Inc.

Tubes

First think about the concept of tubes in general. Remember, fluid or air can flow either way in the tube. Usually it is crucial for clients that the material in the tubes flows only the way that it is designed to flow. If it does not, then there can be disastrous results. This disaster most often takes the form of an INFECTION.

Look at a JP (Jackson Pratt) tube for example. This tube is a suction tube designed to suck out or pull off drainage from a specific area. It is imperative that the nurse know the reason for the tubes placement so that she can do some clinical reasoning. We want to be very careful that none of the drainage that it is coming out of the JP tube returns to the wound as this is likely to cause the clinical symptoms of infection in the client.

Let's just take a chest tube for example. The chest has a negative pressure (less than atmospheric). When a sharp knife or other trauma punctures the chest, air is sucked into the chest cavity and causes the lung tissue to collapse. The chest tube is placed into the cavity to renew the negative pressure, but unless the distal end of the tube is under water, the air can still go back into the chest allowing further lung collapse. If we know this, we will do all possible to see that the end of that chest tube stays under water and that we know what emergency measure to take if the water container gets broken.

Another example is the Foley catheter that indwells in the urinary bladder. The urine is "supposed to" flow into a collection bag that is below the level of the bladder. If for any reason that collection bag is moved higher than the level of the bladder, the old collected urine goes back into the bladder and causes an INFECTION.

Clients who are hospitalized and many at home have many tubes inserted into various orifices. It is our responsibility to know the placement and purpose so that we can reason how to care for them.

Remember **NAVEL** *can go into an endotracheal tube!*

Narcan
Atropine
Valium
Epinepherine
Lidocaine

TUBES

T rach (nasal, oral) medication

U rinary (foley, supra pubic) medication

B ronchial (chest) medication

E pigastric (nasogastric, JP, feeding, peg) medication

S urgical (drains, CSF drains)

Post-Operative GI Assessment

Back in the operating room as a client is being prepared for abdominal surgery, drapes are used over the body to help maintain sterility. Let's use the word **DRAPES** to look at the concept of postoperative GI assessment.

D **DRESSING**–Evaluate amount and characteristics of drainage.

R **RESPIRATORY SYSTEM**–Listen for those breath sounds! Get in some T, C & DB (turning, coughing and deep breathing) to prevent atelectasis.

A **ABDOMINAL ASSESSMENT**–Watch for abdominal distention. Normal bowel sounds should be heard every 5 to 20 seconds. The abdomen should remain soft. If it becomes hard, this may indicate bleeding, paralytic ileus, or peritonitis. If in doubt, measure abdominal girth.

AMBULATE–Will decrease blood clots caused by pooling of blood in extremities. Will decrease the development of a paralytic ileus.

P **PAIN MEDICINE**–Keep them comfortable. If they have a patient-controlled analgesia (PCA) pump in place, teach them how to use it.

PATENCY OF TUBES–This can be done through irrigations and monitoring the suction of drains and tubes.

E **ELIMINATION**–Keep an I & O record.

S **SPLINT**–Splint abdominal incision during T, C, and DB.

GI ASSESSMENT

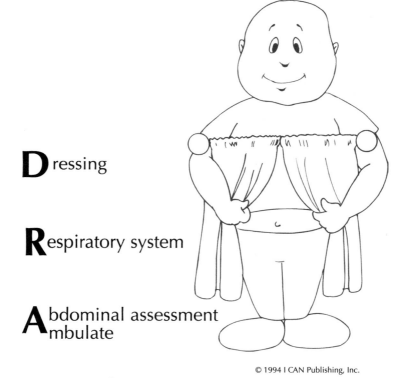

© 1994 I CAN Publishing, Inc.

Dressing

Respiratory system

Abdominal assessment
Ambulate

Pain medicine
Patency of the tubes

Elimination

Splint

Diverticular Disease

Diverticulitis is known as a diverticulum (a pouch-like herniation of superficial layers of the colon through weakened muscle of the bowel wall) that becomes inflamed. Multiple diverticula are referred to diverticulosis. Children who have a diverticular disease of the ileum are diagnosed with Meckel's diverticulum.

Risk factors for this disease include low-fiber in diet; high intake of processed foods, constipation, indigestible fibers (corn, seeds, etc.) may precipitate diverticulitis, but they do not contribute to the development of diverticula. Constipation and inactivity may also contribute to the development of diverticular disease.

Diverticular disease is typically asymptomatic. The degree of inflammation will result in various symptoms. Diverticulitis can result when undigested food and bacteria become trapped in the diverticula. The client will present with left lower quadrant pain. "**LEFT**" will assist you in organizing the clinical findings.

- L **Left** lower quadrant pain; may be accompanied by nausea and vomiting
- E **Evaluate** for abdominal distention; increased pain on palpation
- F **Fever**
- T **The** symptoms may progress to abscess, intestinal obstruction, and/or perforation

"**FIBER**" on the right page will assist you in remembering the priority care for these clients. Remember, if client has any **abdominal distress, all fiber should be avoided** until healed and the tenderness resolves.

- F **Fiber** in diet should be high. (*also known as high-residue*) Foods allowed on this diet include raw fruits and vegetables; whole grains that are high in residue and fiber. Any fibers that are indigestible should be restricted. These may include corn; seeds such as sesame and poppy; foods with small seeds (i.e., strawberries).
- I **Intake** of fat and red meat should be decreased. Restrict egg yolks, whole milk, fried foods, processed cheese, shrimp, avocados, butter.
- B **Bulk laxatives**, stool softeners may be used to prevent acute episodes of diverticulitis but NOT during an episode. Avoid enemas and harsh laxatives.
- E **Encourage** a high intake of fluids to prevent complications with an exacerbation.
- R **Remember** to increase physical activity, walking, exercise to manage uncomplicated diverticulum. With clients with severe diverticulitis, clients may need pain management with opioids; avoid morphine (decreases peristalsis). Bowel rest: NPO; may have an NG tube; hydration with IV fluids.

DIVERTICULAR DISEASE

F iber in diet high

I ntake of fat and red meat should be decreased

B ulk laxatives, stool softeners

E ncourage a high intake of fluids

R emember to increase physical activity, walking, exercise to manage uncomplicated diverticulum

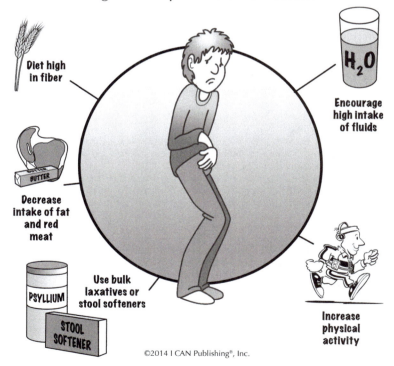

Diagnostics For The Hepatic And Biliary System

Serum Liver Enzymes: Elevated

Aspartate aminotransferase (AST): Normal range is 5-40 units/L; elevated in liver disease, acute hepatitis, pulmonary infarction, myocardial infarction.

Alanine aminotransferase (ALT): Normal range is 7-56 units/L; most definitive for liver tissue damage assessment.

Alkaline phosphatase (ALP): Normal range is 42-128 units/L; bone and liver are the primary sources for ALP. Liver or bone disease may be associated with extremely high levels, and must be correlated with specific clinical assessment findings.

Serum blood ammonia: Normal range is 15 to 110 mg/dL; If the ammonia is elevated, this indicates the liver is unable to convert ammonia to urea.

Bilirubin: Normal ranges are Direct-0.1–0.3 mg/dL; Indirect-0.1 to 1.0 mg/dL; Total-0.1 -1.0 mg/dL; the elevated bilirubin will occur as a result of an excessive destruction of the red blood cells or if there is an inability for the liver to excrete normal amount of bilirubin.

Albumin: Normal range is 3.5–5.0 g/dL; Liver impairment may affect the synthesis of protein and normal serum protein levels. Proteins are responsible for maintaining the colloid oncotic pressure in the serum.

Liver biopsy: Removal of a sample of tissue to determine the progression or extent of the liver disease by a needle aspiration. Nursing Care: "**BLEEDS**" will assist you in organizing the care for a client experiencing a liver biopsy.

- **B** Bleeding should be evaluated for after procedure. Immediately before biopsy, have client take a deep breath, exhale completely, and hold breath.
- **L** Look at coagulation results and have on chart before biopsy.
- **E** Educate client to be NPO for 6 hrs before biopsy. Educate to report excessive **bleeding**.
- **E** Educate client to lie on the affected surgical side for a period of time post-biopsy (approximately 2 hours or per protocol). Bed rest for 12-14 hrs postprocedure or per protocol.
- **D** Determine if there are any post-biopsy complications from bleeding such as HR ↑ or BP ↓. Assess for pneumothorax (*e.g., dyspnea, HR ↑, pleural pain, asymmetrical expansion of the chest wall, breath sounds ↓*). Assess for abdominal or referred shoulder pain; evaluate for bile peritonitis.
- **S** Signed informed consent from client prior to procedure.

> **I CAN TESTING HINT:** If you have any question about positioning the client after the liver biopsy, remember *"When you were younger, your mom would put a band aid on a cut or a sore to prevent bleeding"*. There you go, the same applies to this procedure! Position the client on the right side with a pillow under the coastal margin. This will facilitate compression of the liver.

Endoscopic retrograde cholangiopancreatograpy (ERCP): Uses a fiberoptic endoscope and fluoroscopy inserted orally to visualize any structure changes. **Prior to procedure:** Client will be NPO for 8 hours. Sedative will be given prior to and during procedure. *Refer to "Priority Care Prior to a* **GRAM***".* **After procedure:** Assess vital signs for infection or perforation. The most common complication is pancreatitis.

DIAGNOSTICS FOR THE HEPATIC AND BILIARY SYSTEM

"**DIAGNOSTIC**" exams can be hazardous to the health of our clients.

It is our mission to keep them safe!

The designated NCLEX® standards are outlined below to assist you in organizing the assessments, nursing interventions, and evaluation that must be incorporated into our critical thinking and clinical reasoning for clients experiencing a diagnostic procedure, treatment, or laboratory procedure.

D iagnostic test results—monitor; intervene for complications.

I njury and/or complications from procedure should be prevented.

A ssist with invasive procedures (e.g., thoracentesis, bronchoscopy).

G lucose monitoring, ECG, O_2 saturation, etc. may be performed.

N ote client's response to procedures and treatments.

O btain specimens other than blood (e.g., wound, stool, etc.).

S igns and symptoms of trends and/or changes-monitor, and intervene.

T each client and family about procedures and treatments.

I dentify vital signs and monitor for changes and intervene.

C omplications should be noted and followed immediately with an action.

This image is to remind you that "Sure Look" Holmes is looking into the hippo's mouth to assure he is safe! Just as "Sure Look" Holmes, the nurse is not responsible for ordering these tests, but to maintain client SAFETY prior to, during, and after these diagnostics have been completed.

Elevated Liver Enzymes

Remembering elevated liver enzymes is as easy as **ABC**. The next page will assist you with this. When the client has a history of alcoholism, the **ast** and **alt** will be elevated. If the client has a medical problem with biliary obstruction the alp will be elevated. Remember there is a **p** in **alp** and he is *"plugged up Paul."* In clients with a diagnosis of cirrhosis, the ast and alt will be elevated.

A note to remember: These liver enzymes are indicators of liver damage and are utilized as a system specific assessment.
 The AST/SGOT normal is 5-40u/L.
 The ALT/SGPT normal is 7-56u/L.

ELEVATED LIVER ENZYMES

Remember, elevated liver enzymes are as easy as **ABC**

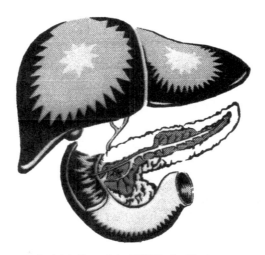

Reprinted with permission ©1994 Creative Educators

Alcoholism (ast, alt)

Biliary obstruction (al**p**) "plugged up Paul"

Cirrhosis (ast, alt)

Cirrhosis

Here is "Larry Leak Liver," who is no longer able to synthesize protein. This results in a decreased colloidal osmotic pressure. (COP holds fluid in the liver and blood vessels.) Since he no longer easily accepts blood from his unique dual blood supply, he also develops portal hypertension. This causes poor Larry to Leak fluid into the peritoneal cavity resulting in **ASCITES**. Too much swelling in the esophagus will cause Larry to get into **AIRWAY** trouble. To prevent complications from **SWELLING**, he may be started on diuretics along with potassium supplements. Salt-poor albumin will assist with hypoalbuminemia. An esophageal tamponade tube will provide compression of **BLEEDING** on esophageal **VARICES**. Prevent bleeding by soft, nonirritating foods. Let's not give him hot coffee to drink. **LABS** such as liver enzymes will be increased. Hypoalbuminemia, prolonged PT, and altered bilirubin metabolism will be seen in lab reports. Hepatic **ENCEPHALOPATHY** will result if Larry is unable to detoxify ammonia, the end product of protein metabolism. As waste products back up, Larry's **SKIN** will turn jaundiced. Decrease discomfort from pruritus. IS THERE HELP? Avoid cocktails (ETOH) and avoid over-the-counter drugs. Larry's liver is simply unable to detoxify them!

CIRRHOSIS

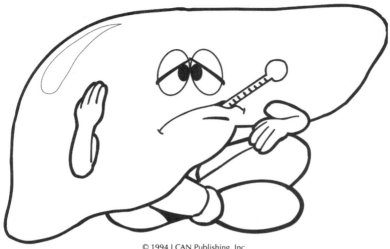

Airway—avoid ETOH and OTC drugs

Swelling

vari**C**es

Inspect lab work

To prevent bleeding

Encephalopathy

Skin

Tylenol (Acetaminophen) Overdose

A major undesirable effect of tylenol overdose is hepatic necrosis. It is like we have taken a hammer and beaten "the hell out of the liver." The dose of tylenol should not exceed 4g/day. Other side effects are negligible with recommended dosage. With acute poisoning, the following adverse effects may occur: **anorexia, nausea and vomiting, epigastric** or **abdominal pain, HEPATOTOXICITY, hypoglycemia**, and **hepatic coma**.

Tylenol (Acetaminophen) is a very useful drug for pain and fever. (Refer to Poison Control for more specific plans.)

Remember—Do not administer to clients with liver disease.

TYLENOL OVERDOSE

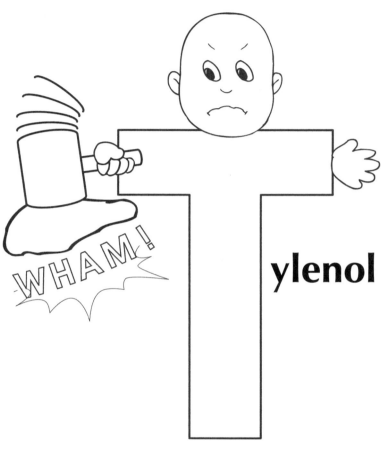

Pancreatitis

The Ace is the high card in a deck of playing cards. This will help you to remember that the "**ASES**" (enzymes of amylase and lipase) are elevated (HIGH) when pancreatitis is present.

- **P** **PAIN MANAGEMENT**–Nonnarcotic analgesics (aspirin, ibuprofen, acetaminophen) may be tried.

  PANCREATIC ENZYME replacement therapy may be indicated.

- **A** **ABDOMINAL PAIN**–Typically, acute pancreatitis produces constant epigastric, periumbilical, or left or right upper abdominal pain radiating to the back, often increased by food and decreased by upright posture. Abdominal tenderness, decreased bowel sounds, distention, and fever may be part of the assessment.

- **N** **NPO** initially–Nasogastric suction for exacerbations, Total Parental Nutrition (TPN) and fluid replacement as necessary. Initiate dietary and insulin therapy for diabetes mellitus secondary to pancreatic insufficiency.

- **C** **CALCIUM** may be low.

- **R** **RISK FACTORS**–Alcoholism, biliary tract disease, a penetrating duodenal ulcer and trauma are also associated with pancreatitis.

- **E** **EVALUATE** glucose, electrolytes, hematocrit, serum amylase and lipase, hypotension, and bowel function.

- **A** **ANALGESICS, ANTICHOLINERGICS, ANTACIDS**, *H2-receptor* **ANTAGONISTS, AND ANTIBIOTICS** are utilized.

- **S** **STIMULANTS** such as spices, alcohol, or coffee should be avoided.

PANCREATITIS

"ASES" HIGH

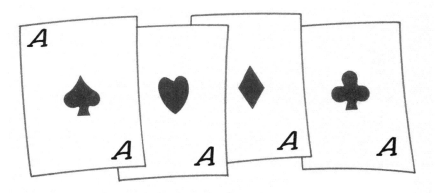

AMYLASE AND LIPASE ARE HIGH WHEN PANCREATITIS IS PRESENT

"Strength doesn't come from what you can do.
It comes from overcoming the things you once
thought you could not."

UNKNOWN

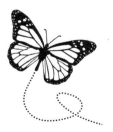

MUSCULOSKELETAL SYSTEM

Diagnostics For the Musculoskeletal System

Antibody Tests (Rheumatoid Factor): Used to determine presence auto-antibodies (rheumatoid factor). Clients with connective-tissue disease will present with Rheumatoid Factor. The higher the antibody titer, the greater degree of inflammation. **(Anti-CCP):** Measures antibodies to cyclic citrulline protein; early detection of RA.

Antinuclear Antibody (ANA): Evaluates the presence of antibodies that destroy the nucleus of body tissue cells (e.g., connective tissue diseases such as systemic lupus erythematosus).

Arthroscopy: The use of an arthroscope which is inserted into a joint for visualizing the structure. Procedure is performed in the OR with strict asepsis and with local or general anesthesia. Diagnoses knee abnormalities. ("SCOPY" earlier in the book does not apply here due to the location of the scope.) Revised for this procedure, "**SCOPE**": **S**epsis; assess/teach for signs of infection. **C**ompression bandage may be applied for 24 hours after procedure. **O**mit exercise for a few days following procedure–walking is permitted. **P**ost procedure–wound covered with sterile dressing. **E**ducate about vascular compromise, mobility restriction, and procedure for sterile dressing change.

Arthrocentesis: Samples of synovial fluid are obtained from an incision of a joint capsule. Local anesthesia is induced. Prior to aspiration of the fluid, aseptic preparation is completed. Synovial fluid is examined for infection and bleeding into the joint and to diagnose arthritis.

Myelogram: Dye is injected into the subarachnoid space and x-ray films of the spinal cord and vertebral column are obtained to evaluate for spinal lesions. *Refer to "Priority Care Prior to a **GRAM**" for specific; Cardiac Chapter*). Post procedure: HOB–30-50 degrees to decrease dispersion of the dye in the CSF and into brain. One difference for this "**GRAM**" is the need to evaluate for headache due to the irritation of the CNS.

Electromyelogram (EMG): This test evaluated the electric potential of the muscle with muscle contraction Electrical activity is performed after small needles are inserted into the muscle. The client needs to know that there is discomfort with the procedure. Client may need pain med due to the muscle stimulation. Assess and apply ice pack to needle sites to prevent and or relieve areas of hematomas.

X-ray: Non-invasive and most common diagnostic test. Used to: identify musculoskeletal problems; review the progress of condition or disease; or evaluate treatment effectiveness.

Computerized Axial Tomography (CAT) Scan: This scan will evaluate thin cross-sections of the brain to evaluate for tumors, edema, bleeding, etc. *Refer to "Priority Care Prior to a GRAM" for specific; Cardiac Chapter.* A few exceptions for this procedure include describing the CAT Scanner and removing all objects from client's hair. The client may only receive fluids four to six hours prior to this procedure.

DIAGNOSTICS FOR THE MUSCULOSKELETAL SYSTEM

"**DIAGNOSTIC**" exams can be hazardous to the health of our clients.

It is our mission to keep them safe!

The designated NCLEX® standards are outlined below to assist you in organizing the assessments, nursing interventions, and evaluation that must be incorporated into our critical thinking and clinical reasoning for clients experiencing a diagnostic procedure, treatment, or laboratory procedure.

D iagnostic test results—monitor; intervene for complications.

I njury and/or complications from procedure should be prevented.

A ssist with invasive procedures (e.g., thoracentesis, bronchoscopy).

G lucose monitoring, ECG, O_2 saturation, etc. may be performed.

N ote client's response to procedures and treatments.

O btain specimens other than blood (e.g., wound, stool, etc.).

S igns and symptoms of trends and/or changes-monitor, and intervene.

T each client and family about procedures and treatments.

I dentify vital signs and monitor for changes and intervene.

C omplications should be noted and followed immediately with an action.

This image is to remind you that "Sure Look" Holmes is looking into the hippo's mouth to assure he is safe! Just as "Sure Look" Holmes, the nurse is not responsible for ordering these tests, but to maintain client SAFETY prior to, during, and after these diagnostics have been completed.

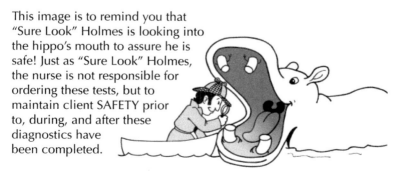

Osteoporosis

JOSEPHINE BONE-A-PART is working to prevent immobility in her "mature years." She is on a treadmill because weight-bearing exercise increases bone strength. She may also take Fosomax and calcium to decrease her risk of developing osteoporosis. ACTONEL is another prescription that may be used to prevent and treat osteoporosis in post-menopausal women. She knows that her drinking and smoking have got to stop if she doesn't want to be laid up with broken **BONES**.

- **B** **BONE** density studies are the noninvasive x-ray diagnostic tests that are commonly used. There is no prep, no pain and not much time involved in this x-ray. Just lie down and they'll shoot it.

- **O** **OUT** of calcium is an issue. Inadequate calcium intake early in life may have predisposed Josephine Bone-A-Part to the development of osteoporosis. Calcium supplemental therapy (about 1500mg per day) is usually recommended for post-menopausal women. Young women should be advised to have a daily dietary intake of at least 1000 to 1500 mg of calcium per day. Magnesium and Vitamin D may also need to be supplemented.

- **N** **NEED** Drugs **AFTER** osteoporosis has developed and to prevent further deterioration. The drugs on Josephine's table work in different ways. To decrease the GI side effects of most of these medications, drink with 8 ounces of water first thing in the morning. Stay sitting up and NPO for at least half an hour before eating or taking other drugs. Forteo, an expensive injectable drug, is currently used in the treatment of severe osteoporosis.

- **E** **ESTROGEN** given orally has demonstrated its ability to decrease the incidence of osteoporosis. In addition, estrogen improves the client's lipid profile (HDL cholesterol rises, LDL cholesterol falls) and overall cardiovascular risk declines. Weight bearing EXERCISE, such as walking, helps the BONES.
EDUCATION early in life will assist in preventing complications from osteoporosis.

- **S** **STRESS** fractures especially of the hip, waist or vertebra are common. Education and prevention of falls are important in minimizng fractures and maintaining independence for post- menopausal women.

Remember—Prevention is the BEST action!

JOSEPHINE BONE-A-PART

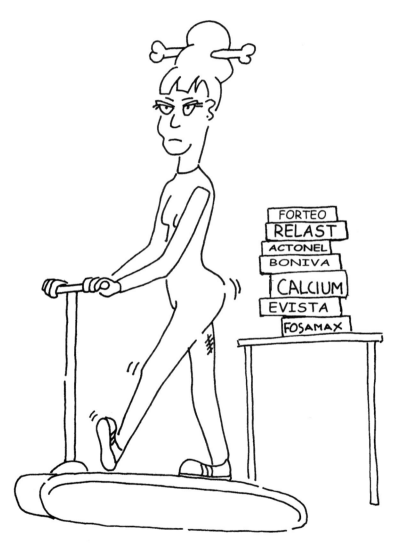

Arthritis

Arthur has osteoarthritis. He wakes up in the morning stiff and achy and finds it hard to reach his walking cane. His fingers are all swollen at the joints (Herberden's nodules) and other joints are affected. He may feel better after his shower as the hot water warms up those joints. Arthur has on his swim trunks because he is going to water therapy at the local spa. Water therapy is probably the best exercise, since it better protects his weight bearing joints. He will definitely need to rest after his swim.

Tylenol may be the medication of choice and Arthur will have to be reminded to keep his dosage at or below 4 gms/24 hours to prevent an overdose. (See **TYLENOL OVERDOSE**)

Remember—Arthur may not want to move because of his pain, but physical activity is imperative for him to retain his independence.

ARTHUR ITIS

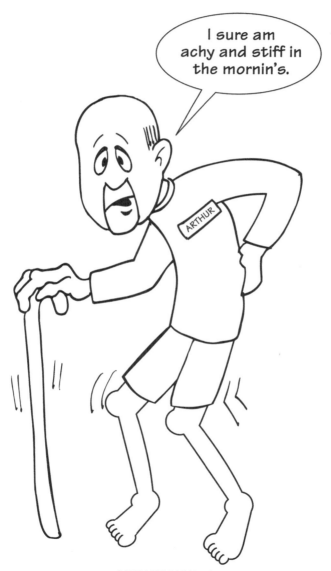

Nonsteroidal Anti-Inflammatory Drugs (NSAIDs)

NSAIDs are a group of medications that prevent prostaglandin synthesis. What does that mean? Prostaglandins contribute to the following: inflammation, body temperature, pain transmission, platelett aggregation, and other actions. These prostaglandins are not stored, but are released on demand.

What type of physical problems may benefit from NSAIDs? Fever and inflammation (ie. arthritis) can be reduced by these medications.

Are there any undesirable effects from NSAIDs? There are several undesirable effects that the nurse must assess and educate clients to report. These include GI upset or bleeding, **ototoxicity** (ringing in the ears), **hepatic necrosis**, or **nephritis**.

As a nurse, what should be included in the plan of care?

1. Administer medications with **food to decrease GI irritation**.

2. Teach clients about actions and side effects and report any dark, tarry stools, "coffee ground or bloody emesis", other **GI distress or ringing in the ears**.

3. Instruct client to inform healthcare providers about these medications prior to any dental or other type of surgery. NSAIDs should be discontinued approximately **5–7 days before the procedure** to prevent any complications with bleeding.

4. NSAIDs are not the drugs of choice if the client has any compromise in either the renal system or the liver.

5. Evaluate the effectiveness of the NSAIDs.

NSAIDS

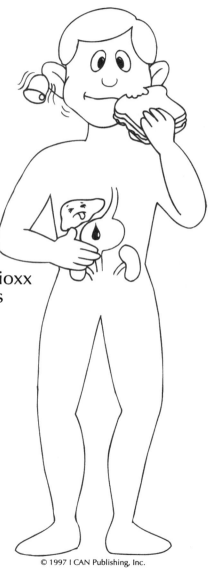

No alcohol

Side effects

Aspirin sensitivity—
do not give

Ibuprofen, Indocin, Vioxx
are a few examples

Do take with food

Stop 5–7 days
before surgery

Gout

Gout is generally presents rapidly with swelling and a painful joint. It is an arthritic condition that results from an alteration in the metabolism of uric acid (hyperuricemia). An end product of purine metabolism is uric acid. The diagnostic serum uric acid level would be greater than 6 mg/dL. Clients who are receiving chemotherapy may also develop hyperuricemia (secondary gout). Typically the uric acid crystals are in the large toe, but may also involve ankles and knees. During an acute attack, protect the affected joint by immobilizing the joint. Encourage gradual weight reduction. Instruct the client to avoid salicylates. Encourage **high fluid intake** (>3L / day) to increase excretion of uric acid and to prevent the development of uric acid stones.

The drug of choice to prevent GOUT decreases uric acid synthesis is allopurinol (Zyloprim). Uric acid is the end product of purine metabolism. Condition of hyperuricemia may also occur in individuals receiving chemotherapy (secondary gout). Medications for an acute attack may include colchicine, indomethacin (Indocin) or naproxen (Naprosyn).

Teach clients to avoid foods high in purines such as **organ meats**, shell fish, and preserved fish (anchovies, sardines) and avoid **alcohol**. We would like to see the urine output **increased** to 2 liters per day to help decrease the risk of stones.

Remember–Clients with renal insufficiency should receive a reduced dose of Allopurinol.

GOUT

Gulp 3 liters fluid per day

Organ meats or wines

Urine output increased to 2 liters per day

Teach

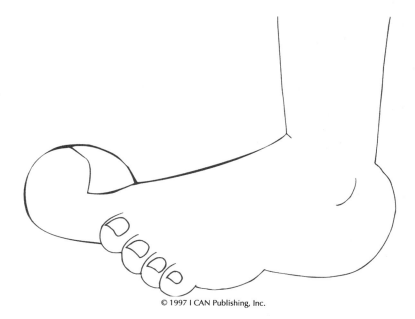

Care of Client in Traction

The purpose of traction is to immobilize fractures and maintain alignment until surgery or until injury is stable enough to allow for safe casting. Traction can also assist with preventing or decreasing muscle spasms. The two types of traction typically used are skin and skeletal. The skin traction works through a force of pull directly applied to the skin, thus working indirectly on the bone. The skeletal traction uses a metal pin or wire that is inserted in or through the bone. Another example of traction is a Halo. Priority nursing care includes assessing hardware for stability and signs of infection. It is important to cleanse around the pin sties using sterile technique. If there is an order, apply antibiotic ointment to the pin site, and continue to assess for signs of infection.

Let's now visit Ellie Elephant who is in skin traction on the right page, and review the priority nursing care.

Ellie Elephant gets in more trouble. She has fallen, **FRACTURED** her trunk, and is in traction. We will need a **FIRM MATTRESS**, and will probably need help putting her through **RANGE OF MOTION** exercises. Pay attention to those feet; we don't want a problem with **FOOT DROP**. Without good body **ALIGNMENT**, Ellie may get contractures and decubiti. **ALIGNMENT** will also help keep the traction pulling from both ends which is the reason for traction anyway. Let's get Ellie a **TRAPEZE (part of the equipment)**, so that she can help us turn her to keep the pneumonia away. Ellie needs to cough and deep breathe on regular intervals to prevent **RESPIRATORY COMPLICATIONS**.

If, like Ellie, the client is in skin traction, then skin integrity becomes an added concern. The skin requires ongoing assessment and preventive care to prevent any breakdown. One **COMPLICATION** of a fracture of long bones is a fat embolism. It can be transported to the lungs producing symptoms of acute **RESPIRATORY** distress. Now, what will we do about her **URINARY** retention? What about **CONSTIPATION** from immobility? Increase fluid intake will assist with both forms of alteration in elimination. In addition to the need for fluid increase, it will be important to add fiber to the diet to decrease risk of constipation. Ellie may need help with the bedpan. Be sure and **EVALUATE FOR CIRCULATORY IMPAIRMENTS**. The 5 P's will help. They are pain, pallor of skin, pulses (especially distal to the injury), paresthesia, and paralysis. Compartmental syndrome can be a major problem. **SKIN CARE** is important for all clients, but especially for the older adult. A diet high in protein will assist with both prevention of skin breakdown and healing. (*Assess renal function tests prior to starting a high protein diet.*) Maintain linens by keeping them dry and clean. Hygiene is very important for the prevention of skin breakdown. Remember, "*An ounce of prevention is worth a pound of cure.*"

While the nurse is responsible for the client in traction, a component of safe care is for the traction ropes and weight to hang freely from any obstructions. A client who has continuous traction should never have a traction weight removed or changed. There should never be anything, such as bed-rolls, pillows, or foot boards, between the client and counterweight. Traction applied in one direction requires counter-traction that is equal to be effective. The client's feet should not touch the end of the bed.

Safe nursing care is the hallmark to helping Ellie Elephant experience an Efficient recovery! *Good Luck! Elephants and people in traction can be a major challenge!*

CARE OF CLIENT IN TRACTION

Firm mattress
Foot drop

ROM—for unaffected extremities

Alignment

Complications

Trapeze

Urinary retention

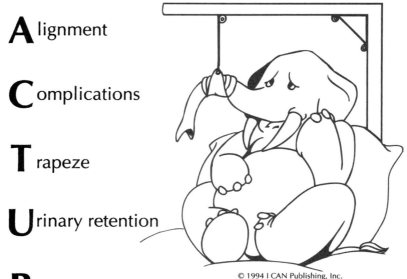

Respiratory complications

Evaluate circulatory impairments (5 P's)

Skin integrity

Adverse Effects of Immobility

It is **AWFUL** being immobilized! Have you ever tried it? The nursing goals are to prevent these potential complications from occurring.

A   **ATELECTASIS**–There may be a decrease in client's ability to cough and move those secretions which will result in a decreased oxygen exchange. Infections can lead to this complication.

Encourage turning, coughing and deep breathing. Putting the head of the bed up will help with breathing and coughing. Maintain adequate hydration.

W   **WASTING OF THE BONES**–Demineralization of bones leads to muscle weakness and atrophy. Range of motion exercises are mandatory. Maintain appropriate alignment while positioning.

F   **FUNCTION LOSS**–This can result from the above problem. Prevent by active contracting and relaxing large muscles.

U   **URINARY STASIS**–Increase those fluids and decrease the calcium intake. If possible, have client sit to void.

L   **LAST BUT NOT LEAST CONSTIPATION**–Encourage diet with adequate protein, bulk and liquids.

IMMOBILITY

Atelectasis

Wasting of bones

Functional loss of muscle

Urinary stasis

Last but not least, constipation

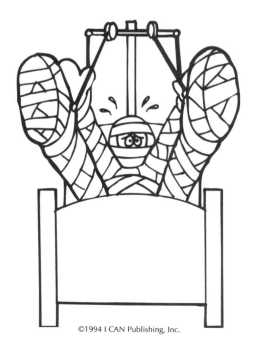

Crutch Walking

Measurement may be taken with client supine or standing

Evaluate in supine: measure the distance from the client's axilla to a point 6" lateral to the heel

Adjust hand bars so client's elbows are flexed approximately 30 degrees

Standing: evaluate distance from client's axilla to a point 4" to 6" to side and 4"-6" in front of the foot

U should be able to put 2 of your fingers between client's axilla and crutch bar

Remember, if client was measured while supine, assist to stand with crutches

Evaluate distance between client's axilla and arm

Four-Point Alternate Gait:

Partial weight on both feet

Arthritis or cerebral palsy are some examples of who would benefit from this gait

Real safe gait, in that there are 3 points of support on the floor at all times

The gait provides a normal walking pattern and makes some use of the muscles of the lower extremities

Three-Point Alternate Gait:

One foot should be able to bear total weight

Non-weight bearing for the affected foot or leg

Educate to move both crutches forward together with the affected leg while the weight is on the client's hands on the crutches. The unaffected leg is then advanced forward.

I CAN TESTING HINT: If you have a moment that you are unable to remember this information, notice the links to both walking with a cane and/or walker. Both of these assistive devices, in addition to the three-point alternate gait, moves the assistive devices first with the affected leg and then advances the unaffected leg.

CRUTCH WALKING

Four-Point Alternate Gait:

P artial weight on both feet

A rthritis or cerebral palsy are some examples of who would benefit from this gait

R eal safe gait, in that there are 3 points of support on the floor at all times

T he gait provides a normal walking pattern and makes some use of the muscles of the lower extremities

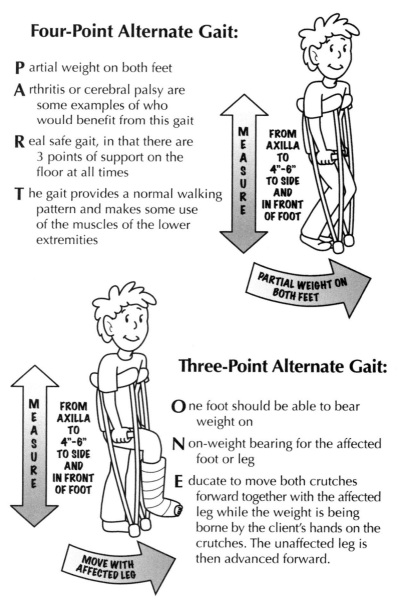

MEASURE FROM AXILLA TO 4"-6" TO SIDE AND IN FRONT OF FOOT

PARTIAL WEIGHT ON BOTH FEET

Three-Point Alternate Gait:

O ne foot should be able to bear weight on

N on-weight bearing for the affected foot or leg

E ducate to move both crutches forward together with the affected leg while the weight is being borne by the client's hands on the crutches. The unaffected leg is then advanced forward.

MEASURE FROM AXILLA TO 4"-6" TO SIDE AND IN FRONT OF FOOT

MOVE WITH AFFECTED LEG

Crutch Walking

Remembering how to instruct the client to use crutches while walking up and down the stairs is "INSANELY EASY". Just look at our friend, Charlie, with his crutches on the next page. He is putting his good leg up on the stair first "UP TO HEAVEN!" When he goes down, his bad leg will go first! Remember, "BAD GOES TO YOU KNOW WHERE."

CANE WALKING

These same principles work for the client walking with the cane. The difference is that the cane is used in the opposite hand of the affected limb.

Remember – Strong side leads!

CRUTCH WALKING

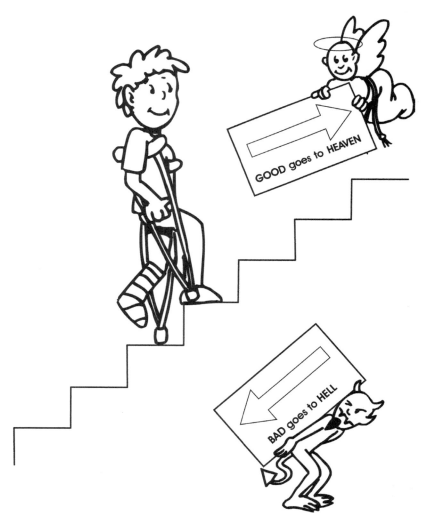

Cane Walking

The image is demonstrating an easy strategy for you to remember how to teach or evaluate walking with a cane. When measuring for the correct size of a cane, measure from the wrist to the floor. Notice the cane is positioned on the unaffected side and moved with the affected leg. Remember the saying, *"The goal is to go for the* **COAL**".

Cane is on the **O**pposite side of the affected leg and cane is advanced with the **A**ffected **L**eg!

This strategy will assist you in understanding safe practice when using a cane.

I CAN TESTING HINT: Recognize the need to teach your client about safe cane walking. This would be a great example of putting options in chronological order of how to use the cane properly.

CANE WALKING

C ane is used on the side opposite the affected leg.

A ffected leg and cane move together.

N ote that the cane should be advanced simultaneously with the opposite affected lower limb.

E valuate for correct size...measure from wrist to the floor.

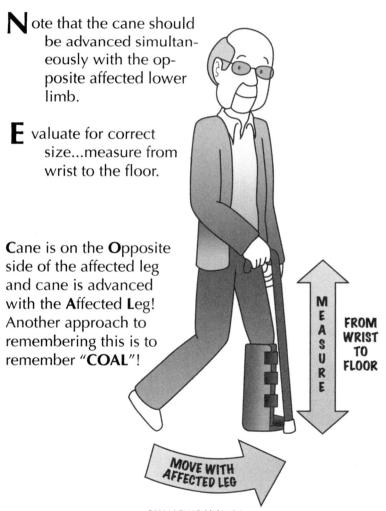

Cane is on the **O**pposite side of the affected leg and cane is advanced with the **A**ffected **L**eg! Another approach to remembering this is to remember "**COAL**"!

MEASURE FROM WRIST TO FLOOR

MOVE WITH AFFECTED LEG

©2014 I CAN Publishing®, Inc.

Walking With a Walker

The image is demonstrating an easy strategy for you to remember how to teach or evaluate walking with a walker. The principle that is consistent between the cane and walker is that both of these assistive devices are **advanced with the affected limb**.

Walker is advanced with the **affected lower limb** and cane is advanced with the affected leg!

Wear shoes when determining the correct size for the walker. Wrists of client are even with the hand grips on the walker when arms are dangling downward.

Advance the walker approximately 12 inches.

Lower limb that **is affected should be advanced with walker**.

Keep unaffected limb back, and then after affected limb has moved forward then move unaffected limb forward.

I CAN TESTING HINT: Remember, the walker is used to prevent clients from falling into the "**WALL**"! **W**alker advanced with **A**ffected **L**ower **L**imb!

WALKER

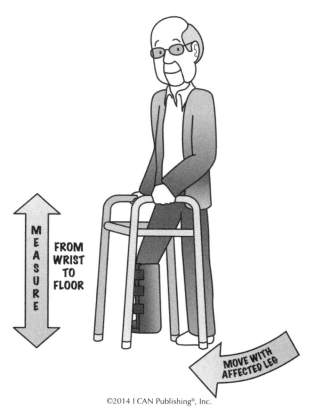

Wear shoes when determining the correct size for the walker. Wrists of client are even with the hand grips on the walker when arms are dangling downward.

A dvance the walker approximately 12 inches.

L ower limb that is affected should be advanced with walker.

K eep unaffected limb back; then after affected limb has moved forward, move unaffected limb forward.

"All that we are is the result of what we have thought. The mind is everything. What we think, we become."

BUDDHA

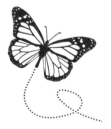

NEUROLOGICAL SYSTEM

Diagnostics For The Neurological System

Electroencephalography (EEG): A noninvasive procedure used to detect electrical activity of the brain. May also be used to detect metabolic disorders, sleep disorders, and encephalitis. Nursing care should include: "**HAIR**"

- **H** Hair should be washed prior to test. After test, wash electrode past out of hair.
- **A** Avoid caffeine, cola, tea, energy drink, other stimulants.
- **I** Identify from HCP if any meds should be held prior to procedure such as sedatives/tranquilizers.
- **R** Reinforce to client that there is no danger of electrical shock, and it is painless!

Computerized Axial Tomography (CAT) Scan: This scan will evaluate thin cross-sections of the brain to evaluate for tumors, hemorrhage, edema, etc. *Refer to "Priority Care Prior to a **GRAM**" for specifics; Cardiac Chapter.* A few exceptions for this procedure in contrast to the general care include describing the CAT Scanner. Four to six hours prior to this procedure the client may only receive fluids. Remove all objects from client's hair. Dye may be injected into the spinal cord for evaluation of intervertebral disks and the bone density.

Cerebral Angiogram: Injection of contrast material into the cerebral circulation. The flow throughout the cerebral circulation is followed by a series of x-ray films. *Refer to "Priority Care Prior to a **GRAM**" for specifics; Cardiac Chapte).*

Myelogram: *Refer to diagnostics in the Musculoskeletal System.*

Magnetic resonance Imaging (MRI): Records the signals from the cell nuclei in a manner that supports and provides information about soft tissue structures such as blood vessels and tumors.

- **M** Metal objects remove—hearing aids, buckles, jewelry.
- **E** Evaluate if client has a pacemaker—interferes with both the test and pacemaker! Not a candidate!
- **T** The insulin pumps or joint replacements on clients are not good candidates for MRI.
- **A** Avoid test if client is pregnant or obese.
- **L** Long magnetic tunnel for the procedure (assess for claustrophobia; may require sedative).

Lumbar Puncture: Spinal fluid is withdrawn and fluid pressure measured through a needle inserted into the lumbar area at the L4 –L5 level. If client has increased intracranial pressure (IICP), this is contraindicated. Nursing care is to assess for a spinal fluid "**LEAK**" following procedure.

- **L** Lateral recumbent with knees flexed is the appropriate position for exam.
- **E** Empty bladder prior to exam. Encourage high fluid intake following procedure.
- **A** Advise HCP if for a change in the client's neuro status before procedure. IICP-contraindicated.
- **K** Keep client flat at least 3 hours, and sometimes up to 12 hours, to ↓ occurrence of headache.
- **S** Spinal fluid leak from puncture site needs to be determined; if leakage occurs, a severe headache may occur.

Skull and Spine X-Ray Studies: Procedure done to detect fractures, calcifications, etc.

DIAGNOSTICS FOR THE NEUROLOGICAL SYSTEM

"DIAGNOSTIC" exams can be hazardous to the health of our clients.

It is our mission to keep them safe!

The designated NCLEX® standards are outlined below to assist you in organizing the assessments, nursing interventions, and evaluation that must be incorporated into our critical thinking and clinical reasoning for clients experiencing a diagnostic procedure, treatment, or laboratory procedure.

D iagnostic test results—monitor; intervene for complications.

I njury and/or complications from procedure should be prevented.

A ssist with invasive procedures (e.g., thoracentesis, bronchoscopy).

G lucose monitoring, ECG, O_2 saturation, etc. may be performed.

N ote client's response to procedures and treatments.

O btain specimens other than blood (e.g., wound, stool, etc.).

S igns and symptoms of trends and/or changes-monitor, and intervene.

T each client and family about procedures and treatments.

I dentify vital signs and monitor for changes and intervene.

C omplications should be noted and followed immediately with an action.

This image is to remind you that "Sure Look" Holmes is looking into the hippo's mouth to assure he is safe! Just as "Sure Look" Holmes, the nurse is not responsible for ordering these tests, but to maintain client SAFETY prior to, during, and after these diagnostics have been completed.

©2014 I CAN Publishing®, Inc.

Meningocele/Omphalocele

Both of these disorders have a sac on the outside of the body. The meningocele is a sac-like cyst of meninges filled with spinal fluid that protrudes through a defect in the bony part of the spine. A myelomeningocele is a sac-like cyst containing meninges, spinal fluid and a portion of the spinal cord with its nerves that protrudes through a defect in the vertebral column. The omphalocele is a protrusion of the intestines on the abdomen.

The nursing care is similar to a seal (**CELE**) in the water. We certainly do not want these sacs (**CELES**) to get too dry. Sterile, normal saline soaks may be used to prevent drying.

Correct positioning is also of paramount importance in preventing damage to the sac (**CELE**) as well as providing nursing care after surgery.

*BE KIND TO NATURE AND KEEP
THE SEALS IN THE WATER.*

MENINGOCELE/ OMPHALOCELE

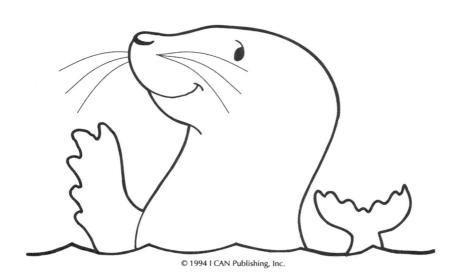

Hydrocephalus (PIES)

Hydrocephalus is caused by an imbalance in the production and absorption of cerebral spinal fluid (CSF) in the ventricles of the brain. This infant will present with an enlarged head. Visualize **PIES** as we refer to the assessments and plans for this condition.

- **P** **PROJECTILE VOMITING**–A symptom of increased intracranial pressure (IICP). Teach parents signs of IICP. Many of these infants are difficult to feed, so small feedings at frequent intervals are recommended.

- **I** **IRRITABILITY**–High pitched cry is characteristic of IICP with an infant. Evaluate the level of consciousness; it is frequently the initial symptom of IICP.

- **E** **ENLARGED HEAD AND FONTANEL**–Normally at birth, the occipital frontal circumference (OFC) is approximately 2–3 cm. larger than the chest circumference. A bulging fontanel is also a sign of IICP.

    EDUCATE family and refer to appropriate community agencies.

- **S** **SEPARATION OF SKULL**–As the CSF increases in the ventricles, there will be a separation of the cranial suture lines. They may have bulging "sunset eyes." If infant has a **SHUNT**, observe for infection and IICP.

HYDROCEPHALUS

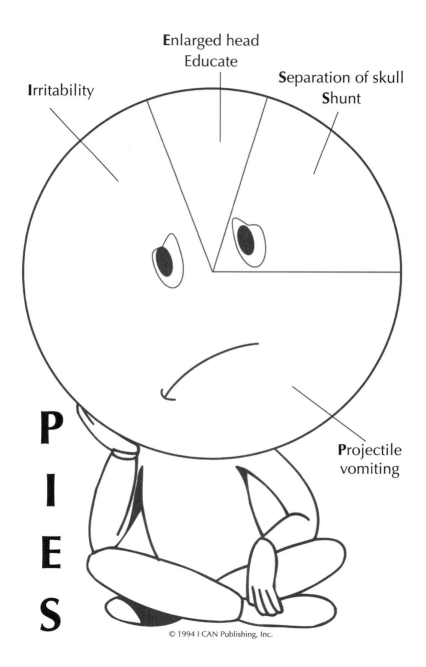

Glasgow Coma Scale

GLASGOW COMA SCALE is often found on both nursing exams and physician orders. In the past this scale has been hard to remember, but here's help. Notice that Glasgow is running (a motor runs, indicating **MOTOR** movements in the client). See Glasgow's **EYES** are open (the client can open eyes on command). The **VERBAL** indicator, like the newspaper comics, lets you know that Glasgow is talking (the client has clear verbal ability).

The score for this scale may range from 3–15. The less responsive, the lower the score; the more responsive, the higher the score.

This is a great scale to evaluate the client's level of consciousness! In summary, the Glasgow Coma Scale evaluates motor, eye opening, and verbal ability.

GLASGOW COMA SCALE

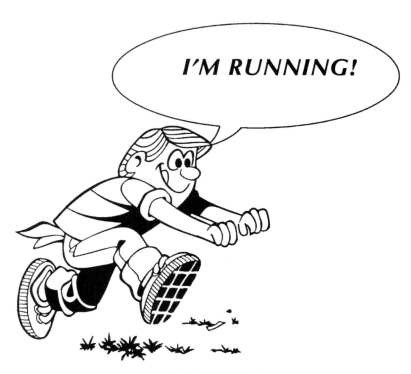

© 1994 I CAN Publishing, Inc.

1. MOTOR
2. VERBAL
3. EYES OPEN

Cranial Nerves (3, 4, 6, and 8)

This tool will help you to remember how some of the cranial nerves may be assessed.

3, 4, 6, makes my eyes do tricks!
Cranial nerves III, IV, and VI (oculomoter, trochlear, and abducens) assess extraocular movements.
Cranial nerve III is assessed by pupil constriction. Assess for pupils being equal and reactive to light.
Cranial nerve IV assesses eye movement.
Cranial nerve VI assesses lateral eye movement.

3, 4, 6, 8, how do we accommodate?
Cranial nerve VIII assesses hearing and balance. Check for hearing acuity.

3, 4, 6, 8

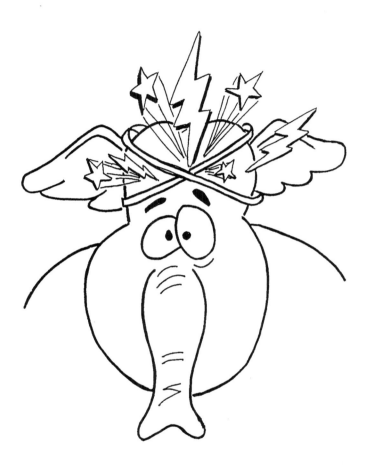

Cranial Nerves

Many students find it difficult to remember all 12 of the cranial nerves. This strategy has been developed to simplify the ability to easily remember all 12 of these nerves. Notice that on the next page we only have one nose (*olfactory*), which represents the 1st cranial nerve. God gave us 2 eyes to see with (*optic*), which is the 2nd cranial nerve. I always remember this cranial nerve by recalling "optic vision."

On the previous page, you may recall that cranial nerves 3, 4, 6 makes your eyes do tricks (*oculomotor, trochlear, and abducens*). The 5th cranial nerve is recalled by remembering 5 rhymes with tri (trigeminal).

The 7th cranial nerve (*facial*) can be remembered by visualizing placing the number 7 across your face with the top of the 7 going across your forehead and the bottom part going down over your face.

Think of the number 8 (acoustic) fitting nicely into your ear for remembering this nerve. Note that when you evaluate cranial nerves 9 and 10 this assessment is under your chin (*glossopharyngeal and vagus*). Notice these 2 nerves have a "**g**" in the spelling, and one of the assessments for these nerves is to check the **gag** reflex. As you progress to the 11th cranial nerve (*spinal accessory*), visualize a "1" on each shoulder that should remain in place as the client shrugs their shoulder. For the 12th cranial nerve (*hypoglossal*), visualize the client sticking their tongue out from side to side and saying "the end."

CRANIAL NERVES

1	2	3, 4, 6
God gave us one nose (olfactory)	God gave us 2 eyes to see with (optic)	Makes my eyes do tricks! (oculomotor, trochlear, abducens)
5	7	8
TRI Rhymes with Tri (for Trigeminal)	Can fit nicely across your face to help you remember the Facial Cranial nerves	Fits nicely into your ear to assist you to remember the acoustic
9, 10	11	12
Is under my chin. (glossopharyngeal, vagus)	Put a 1 on each shoulder and then shrug them, The 1's should not fall off (spinal accessory)	For tongue movement (hypoglossal)

©2008 I CAN Publishing, Inc.

Neurological Checks

There has been a lot of mystery around "neuro checks." The bottom line here is that the client remains alert and oriented, the pupils are equal and reactive to light, and all extremities can move on command. Of course, you want to compare with the last time the neuro checks were done. Were the pupils equal and reactive to light? Were all extremities moving spontaneously and to command? PERL MAE is just lying there in her oyster with one side waving her arm and leg while the other side is limp. Observe that one of her pupils is larger than the other.

These assessments are crucial for any neurological client. Observe the subtle differences! For example, is the client more difficult to arouse than earlier? Your response to this change in assessments can mean the difference between a successful or an unsuccessful recovery!

PERL MAE

Pupils **E**qual **R**eactive to **L**ight
Moving **A**ll **E**xtremities to command

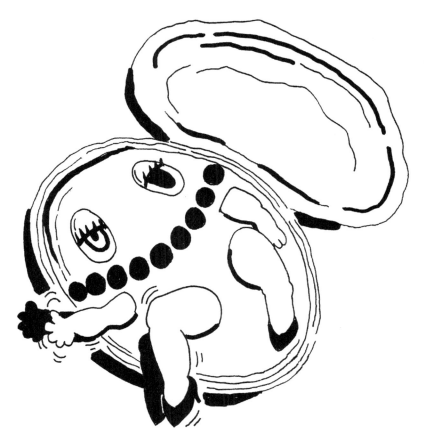

©1994 I CAN Publishing, Inc.

Vital Signs For Shock vs. IICP

Most of us have had the vital signs of shock drilled into our heads. We just have a hard time remembering how those vital signs change with increased intracranial pressure (IICP). Guess what? Vital signs in IICP change exactly opposite to changes in shock. All you have to remember are the vital sign changes in shock and you have the connection to recall the vital sign changes for IICP. Both shock and IICP have one commonality–both cause a loss of consciousness.

VITAL SIGNS FOR SHOCK VS. IICP

Shock	Vs.	IICP
↓	B/P	↑
↑	Pulse	↓
↑	Resp	↓
↓	Temp	↑
↓	Pulse Press	↑
↓	LOC	↓

©1994 I CAN Publishing, Inc.

Nursing Care For Increased Intracranial Pressure

Nursing care for the clients with increased intracranial pressure is focused on decreasing the pressure and assessing the level of consciousness. For this reason we use the image of **HEADS** as a memory tool.

- **H**   **HOB**–Maintain semi-Fowler's position to promote venous drainage and respiratory function. This would be contraindicated if the client had a spinal cord injury.

- **E**   **EVALUATE NEUROLOGICAL CHECKS**–The first sign of a change in the level of intracranial pressure is an alteration in the level of consciousness. Pupils also should react equally to light.

- **A**   **AIRWAY**–Evaluate current respiratory pattern. May require intubation and control on a volume ventilator.

- **D**   **DRAINAGE**–Drainage from the ears may be cerebral spinal fluid. A CSF leak would test positive for glucose. Apply a sterile dressing over ear and evaluate for signs of meningitis.

- **S**   **SAFETY**–Seizure precautions. No sedatives or narcotics. Restrict fluids. Control temperature, and avoid coughing.

NURSING CARE FOR INCREASED CRANIAL PRESSURE

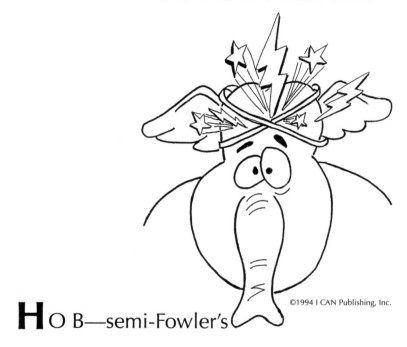

HOB—semi-Fowler's

Evaluate ICP

Airway—oxygen supplement

Drainage

Safety

Priority Clinical Assessment Findings For Meningitis

The child on the right page is experiencing complications from meningitis.

As you can see, the child is holding his painful "**NECK**" as he vomits. This abrupt vomiting is causing more pain to his neck from the inflammation of the meningeal tissue covering the brain and spinal cord. Pain in the **neck (nuchal rigidity)** is a classic symptom with clients who have meningitis. The **vital signs and neurological assessments** need to be done frequently based on hospital protocol. Keep in mind, the LOC is the earliest change that occurs with IICP, and the vital signs are one of the last changes. As the pressure increases the RR, HR may decrease in addition to deterioration in the Glasgow Coma Scale. **Intake and output** must be monitored ongoing. Cerebral edema may require limiting fluid intake. Due to the infection, the client will present with an **elevated fever**. The **heart rate (HR)** should be assessed for trends in changes that could indicate signs of shock or a complication with the ABCs (airway, breathing, circulation). (*Refer to Vital Signs for Shock vs. IICP.*) The heart rate goes up with oxygen and perfusion issues, but decreases with IICP. It is important to decrease the environmental stimuli due to the **headache and photophobia**. Monitor for any unusual **posturing**. Avoid abrupt manipulation of the child/adult(s) neck. **Chills** may be present due to the fever. Continue to assess the **cranial nerves and a change in the LOC**. The client may present with **Kernig's** sign that is resistance or pain at the knee and hamstring muscles when the client after thigh flexion attempts to extend the leg. Positive **Brudzinski's sign** occurs with neck flexion and the hips flex. This does not occur with the neonate, since they do not have a neck. The client should be monitored for purpura and petechiae. **Seizures** may occur, so assess and have appropriate equipment at the bedside to provide safe care.

"**OPISTHOTONIC**" will outline the assessment findings for the neonate and infant diagnosed with meningitis.

Neonate and Infant
- **O** Opisthotonos positioning: a dorsal arched position
- **P** Poor muscle tone and diminished movement
- **I** Irritability (change in sleep patterns)
- **S** Seizures; sucking poor–may refuse feeding
- **T** Temperature
- **H** Has apneic episodes
- **O** Observe a weak cry
- **T** The bulging fontanels
- **O** Observe vomiting
- **N** Note a change in sleep pattern with an increase in irritability
- **I** Increase in WBCs
- **C** Crying with position change

NECKS

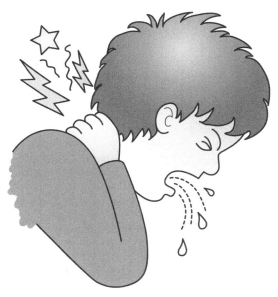

N uchal rigidity, Nausea and vomiting, Neuro checks and VS, I & O

E levated fever, HR, (signs of shock), airway, breathing, and circulation, Excruciating HA, eyes—photophobia, posturing

C hills, cranial nerves consciousness ↓

K ernig's/Brudzinski's sign positive

S eizures

Priority Nursing Interventions For Meningitis

Meningitis is an acute viral or bacterial infection that results in inflammation of the meningeal tissue. This infectious process increases permeability of protective membrane resulting in an elevated protein concentration in the CSF. Cerebral edema may occur as a result of the inflammatory process. Viral meningitis is more common than bacterial meningitis, but bacterial is more severe.

The assessment findings are outlined on the previous page. "**MENINGES**" will assist you in organizing the nursing care for these clients.

The diagnostics used for meningitis include a lumbar puncture, CT scan, and WBCs. If the client has ICP, then a CT scan may be done prior to the lumbar puncture. The WBCs will be elevated and the CSF and blood cultures will be evaluated for meningococcus bacteria.

Maintain client on bed rest with HOB ↑ 30 degrees. Avoid positioning or movement that contributes to the discomfort of the client. The client needs ongoing monitoring for signs and symptoms of complications such as increasing ICP and hearing and visual deficits. The client should have ongoing and frequent assessments of the *"NECK" (assessments on previous page for the child/adult) and "OPISTHOTONIC"(for the neonate and infant)*. Develop plans to prevent complications from immobility such as maintaining dry linens with no wrinkles. Monitor client's respiratory status and provide good respiratory hygiene.

Environmental stimuli should be adjusted to decrease the complication of a headache by dimming the lights and decreasing the noise in the room.

Nonopioid analgesics should be used for HA to avoid masking LOC.

Isolation precautions per protocol until antibiotics have been administered for 24 hours. Droplet precautions should be maintained until the organism has been identified. Preferably, the client should be in a private room. Implement fever reduction measures (cooling blanket if necessary). Intake and output should be monitored closely. Hydration should be maintained; however, cerebral edema may require limiting fluid intake.

Note: reporting meningococcal infections to public health department is a law.

Give antibiotics for bacterial meningitis. After the lumbar puncture has been completed, the CSF sample obtained, then the IV antibiotics should be started as prescribed. The IV infusion site should be assessed frequently for complications from the IV antibiotics. Assess for adverse effects from the medications.

Educate client, family and staff about infection control practice by adhering to droplet precautions, and standard precautions as nursing care requires.

Safety such as seizure precautions is important for these clients. Keep an airway, suction, oxygen, etc., at the bedside to support client if a seizure does occur.

MENINGES

M aintain bedrest with HOB ↑ 30 degrees; monitor "NECK" ongoing

E nvironmental stimuli ↓

N onopioid analgesics for HA to avoid masking LOC

I solation precautions per protocol until antibiotics have been administered for 24 hours. Implement fever reduction measures (cooling blanket if necessasry)

N ote: report meningococcal infections to public health department

G ive antibiotics for bacterial meningitis

E ducate client, family and staff about infection control practice, droplet precautions

S afety such as seizure precautions

Seizures

Caesar is experiencing an interruption of normal brain functioning by uncontrolled paroxysmal discharge of electrical stimuli from the neurons. **"CAESAR"** will outline the general nursing care for clients with seizures.

C COUNSELING is important for the family and the client to assist them in maintaining positive coping mechanisms.
CALM–After a seizure occurs, maintain a calm atmosphere and provide privacy.

A ANTICONVULSANTS–Phenobarbital (Sodium luminal), Primidone (Mysoline), Carbamazepine (Tegretol), or Phenytoin (Dilantin) are some examples of anticonvulsants.
APNEA and/or cyanosis must be monitored. Do not force anything into the client's mouth if the jaws are clenched shut. If the jaws are not clenched, place an airway in the client's mouth after the seizure. Artificial ventilation cannot be performed on a client during a tonic-clonic seizure.

E EVALUATE changes in the level of consciousness. After the seizure, evaluate client's orientation, activity, and any level of paralysis or muscle weakness.

S SAFETY–Protect the client from injuring himself by falling out of bed or striking himself on bedrails, etc. Loosen any constrictive clothing. Do not restrain client during seizure activity.

A AVOID ALCOHOL.
ACTIVITIES–Identify any activities that occurred immediately prior to the seizure. Describe any activity (movement) that occurred and body area affected.

R REDUCE STIMULI.
REMAIN with the client who is in seizure activity. Note the time the seizure began and how long it lasted.
REORIENT client after the seizure.

Remember–SAFETY is the biggest issue.

CAESAR (SEIZURES)

C
A
E
S
A
R

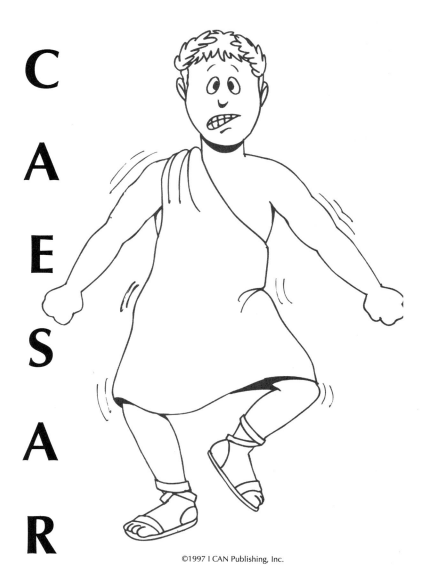

Dilantin (Dial at Ten)

Dilane has a seizure disorder and is taking the drug dilantin. She does not feel well and is calling the nurse at 10:00 A.M. Her therapeutic level for Dilantin should be 10-20 micrograms/mL. (EASY TO REMEMBER. THERE IS A TIN [TEN] IN DILANTIN.) Her adverse reactions from this medication include **gingival hyperplasia**, (see, she's showing you her big gums) **GI disturbances, hepatotoxicity**, (her liver is visible on her abdomen) **ataxia** (her legs are shaking), **hypocalcemia** and a decrease in the absorption of **vitamin D** (the milk on the table and the sunshine coming through the window will help this problem).

If Dilane's level becomes toxic, be sure and inform the healthcare provider. The medication will likely be decreased. If administered IV, then the only IV fluid that it should be mixed with is normal saline. During infusion, it is a good idea to always keep your eye on the cardiac monitor.

Remember—Teach good oral hygiene and nutrition.

DILANTIN (DIAL AT TEN)

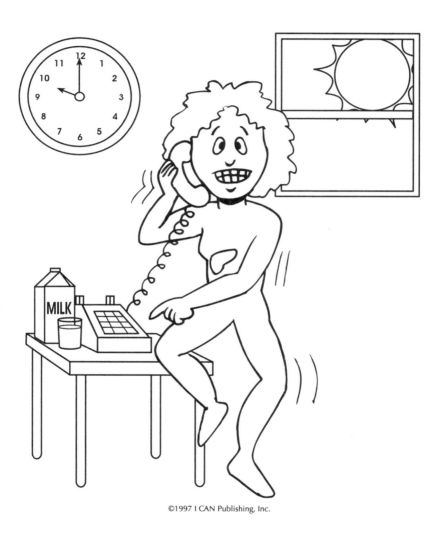

Parkinson's Disease

Meet "**PARK DARK**," our little old man with Parkinson's disease. This condition results from a depletion of, or an imbalance in dopamine and increased activity in acetylcholine.

Park's fingers want to "**PILL ROLL**" all the time. This tremor is rhythmic and rapid. Worse still, when he gets up out of the chair, his bottom is always trying to catch up with his head and never quite makes it, so he is often **ABOUT TO FALL**. **RIGIDITY** of the muscles results in jerky, uncoordinated "cogwheel" movements. Park is not always the fellow who wants to go to the restaurant for dinner because he "**KAN'T**" **SWALLOW WELL, DROOLS** his food and might get choked.

Park's last name is **Dark** because this is a dark, depressing disease, and he gets very sad about the whole thing. Medications used to enhance **DOPAMINE** secretion are levodopa (**L-DOPA**) and SINEMET. One of the latest drugs used for Parkinson's Disease is ropinirole (Requip), a non-ergot alkaloid dopamine agonist. **ARTANE** and cogentin are used to decrease effects of acetylcholine. Sometimes **COFFEE RESTRICTION** can reduce the pill rolling. Some **ANTIHISTAMINES** may be helpful to **KEEP MUSCLE TREMORS DOWN**.

"**PARK DARK**" bears watching. He unfortunately falls, spills hot food on himself and can get depressed to the point of harming himself. *He will need your support!*

PARK DARK

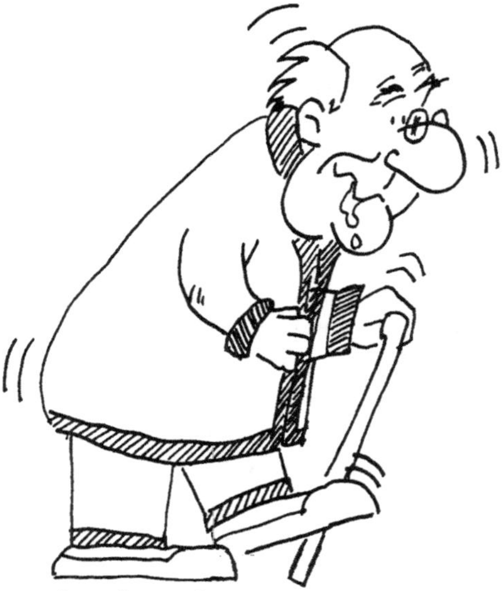

Pill rolling

About to fall

Rigidity

Kan't swallow/speak (drools)

Dopamine/L-Dopa/Sinemet

Artane—improves rigidity

Restrict coffee

Keep tremors down with antihistimine

Myasthenia Gravis

Why didn't somebody tell us that myasthenia gravis means grave muscle weakness? If they had, we would have asked ourselves where are the muscles? The heart is a muscle.

Muscles help move the chest for breathing and the legs for walking, to name just a few. If there is grave muscle weakness, we can see why **MYRA DYSTONIA** will get into deep trouble fast if she doesn't get her muscle strengthening medication (prostigmin or mestinon) on TIME! As you can see **MYRA DYSTONIA** has drooping eyelids and may even experience some difficulty moving her face. She will NOT have any sensory deficit, loss of reflexes, or muscle atrophy. This progressive weakness is caused from a failure in transmission of nerve impulses due to acetylcholine release. There are no cures at the present time. "**TIME**" is one of the most important factors.

- **T**   **TENSILON** is a drug with a short half life that will strengthen muscle weakness in Myra. This makes it a good drug for DIAGNOSIS and differentiating types of crisis (cholinergic crisis versus myasthenic crisis). It is not routinely given for treatment due to its short term effect.

- **I**   **INFECTION** and exercise make MYRA worse.

- **M**   **MUST** give medications on time. We sure don't want MYRA to go on that ventilator. We MUST avoid the use of sedatives and tranquilizers which cause respiratory depression. We MUST not give the client anything to eat or drink during a myasthenic crisis due to the risk of aspiration. After the crisis, remember to assess the ability to swallow and give a diet which is soft and easily swallowed.

- **E**   **EXACERBATIONS** and remission are part of this experience, but since the weakness is progressive it's likely to get worse with TIME.

MYRA DYSTONIA

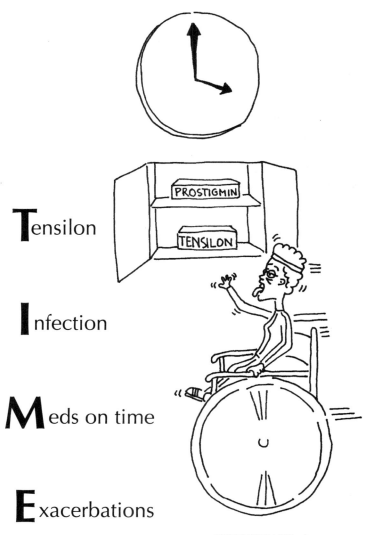

Tensilon

Infection

Meds on time

Exacerbations

Bell's Palsy

Ring the Bell for the Palsy that affects the seventh cranial nerve, resulting in muscle flaccidity on one side of the face. If the facial appearance is permanent, clients may need counseling assistance with maintaining a positive **IMAGE**. They may be ringing your call bell because of "pain" behind the ear, drooping of the mouth and an eyelid that won't close. **ANALGESICS** will be given to decrease the pain behind the ear. Ophthalmic ointment and eye patches may be needed at night to prevent drying of the cornea on the affected side. During the day, instilling **METHYLCELLULOSE** drops will help keep the eye moist (**GIVE EYE CARE**). Due to the discomfort, **EVALUATE** the client's **ABILITY TO EAT**.

Treatment may consist of corticosteroids and vasodilators. An inability to close the eyelid on the affected side, and a sagging mouth is scary; however, proper treatment and good nursing care will usually help clear up the problem with little residual.

BELL'S PALSY

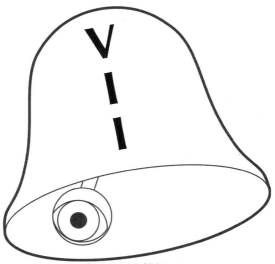

Image

Methylcellulose

Analgesics

Give eye care

Evaluate ability to eat

Trigeminal Neuralgia (Tic Douloureux)

This is a cranial nerve disorder affecting the sensory branches of the trigeminal nerve (cranial nerve V). Let us introduce you to Luke W. Arm. Luke says, "Hot food is painful!" He has a closed eye from frequent blinking and tearing. Facial twitching and grimacing are characteristic. The pain he experiences is usually brief and ends as abruptly as it begins. The word "**PAINE**" will help you remember the nursing care for Luke W. Arm.

The medical management of pain may be Dilantin or Tegretol, Dilantin, or Neurontin. The surgical intervention is a local nerve block or interruption of the nerve impulse transmission.

TRIGEMINAL NEURALGIA

Pain is excruciating

Avoid hot or cold

Increase protein and calories

Nerve, cranial V

Eye care

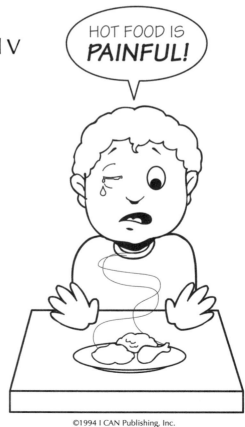

Botox

Botulinum is a dangerous organism that can give us food poisoning and can kill us. However, it has been found to be effective in the treatment of many medical disorders if given in very small doses.

The primary purpose of BOTOX is to relax muscles. This very positive action can work wonders in many areas. Because BOTOX allows muscles to relax usually within 3 days, it has become a very important product for cosmetic use in that frown lines and wrinkles disappear.

To be considered a safe practitioner of nursing, we must be aware of the dangers of administering the drug and of the side effects.

B **Botulinum** is a very poisonous substance and should be monitored carefully.

O **Occasional** headaches and nausea are side effects.

T **Target** muscles relax, deleting frown lines, wrinkles and some symptoms of dystonia.

O **Opening** of the eye may be affected and ptosis may occur.

X **X** out clients that already have muscle weakness (i.e., myasthenia gravis, cerebral palsy, etc.) as the Botox may affect or weaken non-targeted muscle groups.

Watch out for muscle weakness, especially that affects breathing and seeing! "The **Ox** Relaxing in the **Boat**" will help you remember that to promote client safety the nurse must monitor client for too much relaxation. If the client already has a medical condition that results in muscle weakness, then the medication should not be administered!

BOTOX

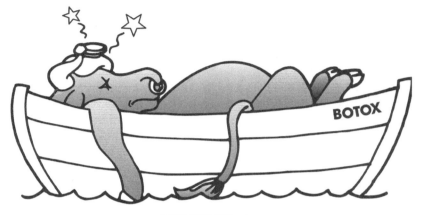

B otulinum

O ccasional headaches and nausea

T arget muscles relax

O pening of the eye may be affected

X out clients who have muscle weakness

Care of the Spinal Cord Client

"**PARALYZED POOCH**" has been out partying with the neighborhood dogs and has been in an automobile accident. He broke his neck and is unfortunately paralyzed from the neck down. The paramedic dog who came to the scene had to access his airway by a "jaw thrust" and log roll him to stabilize his neck. This will minimize further **CORD DAMAGE**. Assess Pooch's breath sounds for signs of hypoxia. Incentive spirometry and chest physiotherapy will assist in optimizing **RESPIRATORY FUNCTION**. Due to his loss of bladder function, **URINARY** retention is a problem. He will either have an indwelling catheter or require intermittent catheterization. Prevent urinary tract infections! Because Pooch is immobile watch for blood clots (**THROMBUS**). Compression stockings may help venous return. **CARDIOVASCULAR STABILITY** can be a problem due to SHOCK or autonomic dysreflexia. (*Refer to AUTONOMIC DYSREFLEXIA.*)

Pooch needs a **NEURO ASSESSMENT** for IICP (Refer to IICP visual). **FLUIDS AND ROUGHAGE** are necessary to keep bladder and bowels working. Calories and protein need to be increased. Watch for **SKIN BREAKDOWN**. An ounce of prevention is worth a pound of cure. Pooch is going to have a major life change. He will need **SUPPORT** in ventilating his feelings and establishing realistic short-term goals.

Remember, check for the tightness of those screws in the traction.

CARE OF SPINAL CORD CLIENT

Paralysis

Assess urinary/bowel

Respiratory depression/airway

Assess neuro/LOC

Log roll

Your circulation

Zap out thrombus

Encourage protein/fluid

Derma tone/dermatology

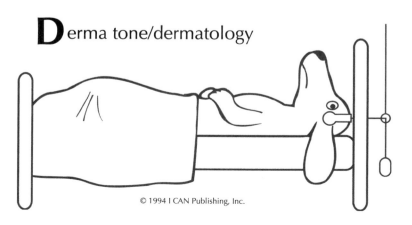

Anticoagulants

Coumadin, Heparin, and Lovenox are used to inhibit thrombus and clot formation. Clotting times will be prolonged which will assist in maintaining the flow or "stream of blood."

The key to successfully remembering the lab reports and antidotes for the appropriate anticoagulants are to think of (H) looking like 2 tt's in Heparin. The lab report necessary to evaluate while clients are on heparin is Ptt. The antidote also has 2 t's in it (protamine sulfate).

Coumadin's antidote is vitamin K. **C** and **K** sound alike which will help with association. The lab report which needs to be monitored is Pt.

Labs now report INR (international normalized ratio) values. The range for most clients on anticoagulants is 2–3. The exceptions are mechanical heart valves and recurrent thromboembolism clients who should be anticoagulated to an INR of 3–4.5.

ANTICOAGULANTS

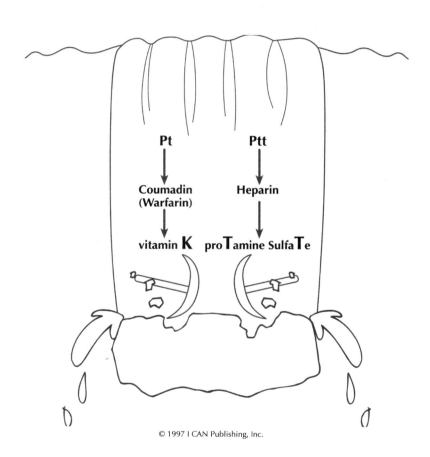

Autonomic Dysreflexia

This condition may occur in clients with a spinal cord injury at T_6 or higher. The stimuli below the level of injury triggers the sympathetic nervous system to dump catecholamines resulting in hypertension. Spinal injury blocks the normal transmission of sensory impulses. There is an exaggerated response to the sensory stimuli.

The most common causes are the 3 Fs: **FULL BLADDER, FECAL IMPACTION**, and a **FUNNY FEELING WITH THE SKIN**.

The assessments that occur as a result of these causes are: **FLUSHING** and **DIAPHORESIS, HEADACHE, HYPERTENSION,** and **BRADYCARDIA**. The priority treatment is to identify and REMOVE the CAUSE. Frequently the dysreflexia will subside. If possible, the head of the bed can be elevated. Watch the hypertension, so that it doesn't get out of hand.

These folks feel real badly and usually cannot tell you their problem. Once their bladder or bowel is emptied the sweating and bad feelings go away.

AUTONOMIC DYSREFLEXIA
(INJURIES AT T$_6$ OR HIGHER)

Causes
1. **F**ull bladder
2. **F**ecal impaction
3. **F**unny feeling with the skin

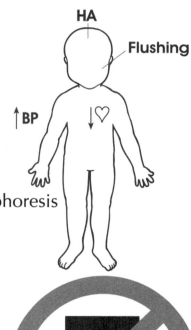

Assessments
1. Flushing & Diaphoresis
2. Headache
3. Hypertension
4. Bradycardia

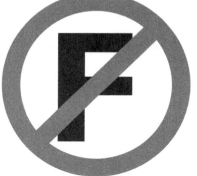

Stroke

When blood flow to the brain is interrupted, the assessment is an emergency. The American Heart Association utilizes the acronym "**FAST**" to help with the original assessment. If any of the assessments are deficient, the client must immediately reach medical help. Treatment that begins within 3 hours of the incident has the best chance for brain survival.

The treatment depends on the medical diagnosis of an ischemic incident or a brain bleed. If no hemorrhage is found, clot busting drugs such as tPA (tissue plasminogen activation) are usually administered. "**FAST**" becomes even more important when nurses realize the tPA is often ineffective if administered longer than 3 hours after the original incident.

Migraine headaches can mimic the symptoms of a stroke (CVA). Assessments are of paramount importance with these system specific assessments to prevent long range complications.

FAST

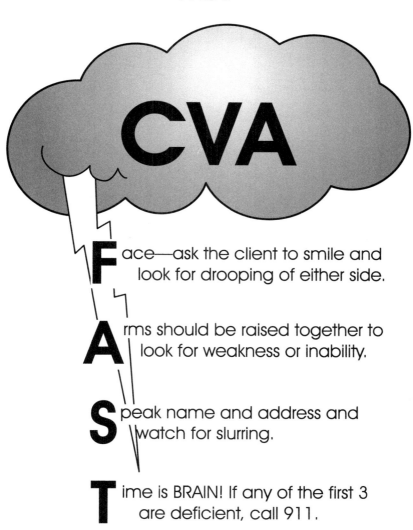

F ace—ask the client to smile and look for drooping of either side.

A rms should be raised together to look for weakness or inability.

S peak name and address and watch for slurring.

T ime is BRAIN! If any of the first 3 are deficient, call 911.

®2011 I CAN Publishing®, Inc.

*Remember, we only have 3 hours! Be **FAST** in assessments.*

"The pain you feel today is the strength you feel tomorrow. For every challenge encountered there is opportunity for growth."

UNKNOWN

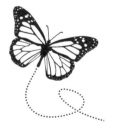

SENSORY PERCEPTION

Diagnostics For Ophthalmic and Hearing

Ophthalmic Diagnostics

Ophthalmoscopy: The examination in the back of the interior eyeball (fundus), including the optic disc, retina, macula, and blood vessels by using an ophthalmoscopy.

Visual Acuity Tests: These tests include the Rosenbaum and Snellen eye charts. The Snellen chart is placed 20 feet from the chart. The client is tested to determine what can be seen at a distance of 20 feet. A ratio between what client should see at 20 feet and what can actually be seen at 20 feet is the representation of the visual acuity. A ratio of 20/40 represents the client being able to see at 20 feet what should be seen at 40 feet.

Tonometry: Intraocular pressure (IOP) is measured by the tonometry. The normal IOP is 10 to 21 mm Hg; however, this is elevated in angle-closure glaucoma.

Hearing Diagnostics

Audiometry: Used to determine if hearing loss is conductive and/or sensorineural.

Rinne test: A tuning fork is held on the mastoid bone (bone conduction). After the client reports not being able to hear the sound, the vibrating tuning fork is then moved approximately 2 inches from the external ear (air conduction). The vibration will continue to be heard with normal hearing. This will be demonstrated with the client hearing the air conduction twice as long as the bone conduction (2:1 ratio). A conduction hearing loss would be suspected if the bone conduction was louder than the air conduction.

> **I CAN TESTING HINT:** Air > Bone = NORMAL; Bone > Air = Determines a conductive hearing loss. Just remember "**BAD**" hearing.

Weber test: A vibrating tuning fork is placed on top of the client's head or the middle of the forehead. Each ear should hear the sound equally well. If there is a conduction deafness, the sound will be heard better in the impaired ear. If the sound is heard only in the normal ear, then there is a sensorineural hearing loss.

Tympanogram: Used to measure the tympanic membrane's mobility and the structures of the middle ear relative to sound. Diseases of the middle ear can be diagnosed by this test.

Otoscopy: Used to examine the tympanic membrane and the external ear. The nurse needs to inform client that the auricles may need to be firmly pulled in order to visualize the tympanic membrane.

DIAGNOSTICS FOR OPHTHALMIC AND HEARING

"DIAGNOSTIC" exams can be hazardous to the health of our clients.

It is our mission to keep them safe!

The designated NCLEX® standards are outlined below to assist you in organizing the assessments, nursing interventions, and evaluation that must be incorporated into our critical thinking and clinical reasoning for clients experiencing a diagnostic procedure, treatment, or laboratory procedure.

D iagnostic test results—monitor; intervene for complications.

I njury and/or complications from procedure should be prevented.

A ssist with invasive procedures (e.g., thoracentesis, bronchoscopy).

G lucose monitoring, ECG, O_2 saturation, etc. may be performed.

N ote client's response to procedures and treatments.

O btain specimens other than blood (e.g., wound, stool, etc.).

S igns and symptoms of trends and/or changes-monitor, and intervene.

T each client and family about procedures and treatments.

I dentify vital signs and monitor for changes and intervene.

C omplications should be noted and followed immediately with an action.

This image is to remind you that "Sure Look" Holmes is looking into the hippo's mouth to assure he is safe! Just as "Sure Look" Holmes, the nurse is not responsible for ordering these tests, but to maintain client SAFETY prior to, during, and after these diagnostics have been completed.

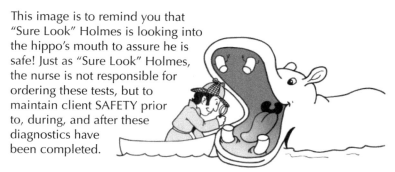

©2014 I CAN Publishing®, Inc.

Visual Changes

The images on the next page will help you recall the major eye disorders. **GLAUCOMA** is described by clients as seeing halos around lights. Tunnel vision is another common complaint resulting from an increase in intraocular pressure. Loss of vision can occur. Glaucoma is chronic and a major cause of blindness.

CATARACT is a complete or partial opacity of the lens. This disorder is described as a decrease in visual acuity. Imagine you had on your sunglasses, and we took a paint brush and painted white paint on the outside of your glasses. Could you see out? Of course not. Is it painful? No. That is similar to cataracts.

RETINAL DETACHMENT is described as a sensation of having a veil or curtain over the eye. This disorder is sudden in onset. Some clients may experience an area of blank vision. Retinal detachment occurs from a separation of the two layers of the retina. When separation occurs, vitreous humor seeps between the layers and detachment of the retina from the choroid occurs.

MACULAR DEGENERATION is described as a blind spot in the center of the field of vision. Peripheral vision is retained but client is unable to read, drive, etc. There is no cure at this time.

VISUAL CHANGES

Glaucoma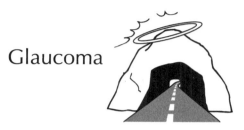

Halo tunnel

Cataracts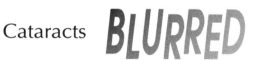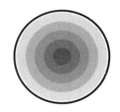

Blurred

Retinal detachment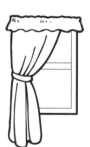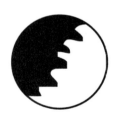

Curtain

Macular degeneration **BLACK SPOT**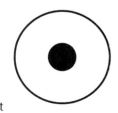

Black spot

©1994 I CAN Publishing, Inc.

Symptoms of Open Angle Glaucoma

The image on the next page shows a big cup (optic) in a tunnel (tunnel vision). The client with open angle glaucoma may occasionally see halos around lights. They experience a loss of peripheral vision, which creates this tunnel vision. The good news is that this is a painless condition. The bad news is that glaucoma is one of the leading causes of blindness. Although this condition is not an emergency, we want to help the clients prolong the effects of vision loss with medication. See the next page.

OPEN ANGLE GLAUCOMA

O ccasionally see halos around light

P eripheral vision (gradually lose)
ainless
rogressive vision loss

E arly stages asymptomatic
nlarged optic cup

N ot an emergency

Medications For Open Angle Glaucoma

Clients with glaucoma will experience an increase in intraocular pressure. They may feel as if there is a "**BAHM**" (a bomb going off in their eyes). Our bomb on the next page is pointed down because this is the direction that we want the intraocular pressure to go while our client is using these medications.

MEDICATIONS FOR OPEN ANGLE GLAUCOMA

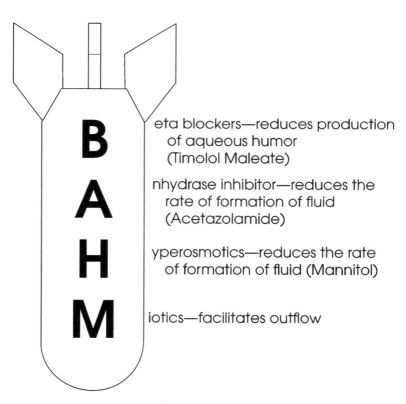

Beta blockers—reduces production of aqueous humor (Timolol Maleate)

Anhydrase inhibitor—reduces the rate of formation of fluid (Acetazolamide)

Hyperosmotics—reduces the rate of formation of fluid (Mannitol)

Miotics—facilitates outflow

©1997 I CAN Publishing, Inc.

Miotics

Miotics are given to people who have an elevated pressure in the eye due to glaucoma. The word miotics has a **C** in it for constrict. As a result of the constriction from these drugs, there is an increased flow of the aqueous humor. Interestingly enough, many of the miotic eye drops contain the word **CAR**. **CAR**pine, **CAR**bachol, and pilo**CAR**pine are all miotics.

Notice the tag on our friend's car. He *"KANT C"* well due to his tunnel vision. Clients with primary open-angle glaucoma experience a gradual loss of peripheral vision which is described as "tunnel vision."

Isn't that EASY?

CONSTRICT EYES: GLAUCOMA

MIOTICS
    O
    N O ATROPINE!!
    S
    T
    R
    I
    C
    T

GLAUCOMA

TUNNEL AHEAD

KANT C

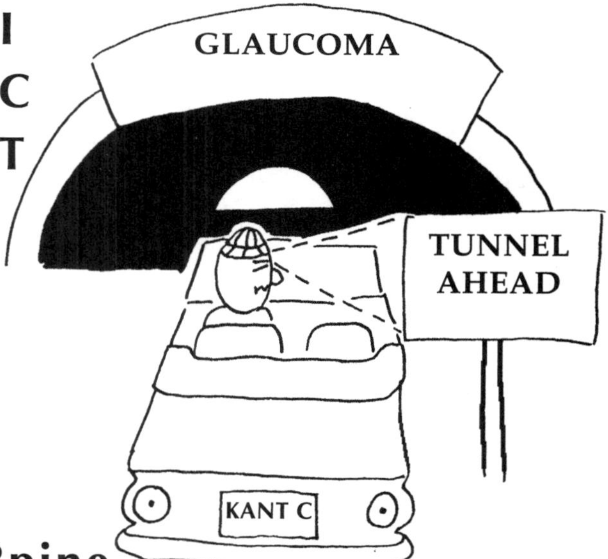

CARpine
CARbachol
pilo**CAR**

Ear Drops

Aren't these guys great! They epitomize Accelerated Learning.

The ear canal changes as we grow. To be sure that ear drops can get down into the ear, we need to remember how to hold the ear when we're putting in those drops. Notice the word *adult* has a **U** in it for **UP**. Hold the adult ear **UP** and back. Notice that the word *child* ends in a **D**. Hold the child's ear **DOWN** and back.

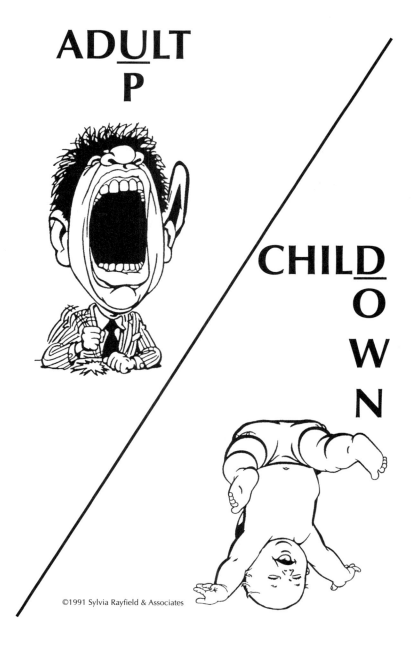

Priority Plan For Client With Hearing Impairment

H **Hearing aid**–Teach how to use and maintenance

E **Evaluate** how to remove ear wax if impacted cerumen is a problem; may need an ear irrigation

A **Assess** for dizziness, nausea, and vomiting if had a stapedectomy

R **Reassure** client during communication by standing in front of client at eye level to speak; speak slowly

I **Instruct** client not to wear hearing aid while bathing or swimming

N **No** hair spray, cosmetics, or oils around ear

G **Give** hearing aid a rest at night and turn it off and open the battery compartment to prevent battery drain

HEARING

H earing aid—Teach how to use and maintenance

E valuate how to remove ear wax if impacted cerumen is a problem; may need an ear irrigation

A ssess for dizziness, nausea, and vomiting if had a stapedectomy

R eassure client during communication by standing in front of client at eye level to speak; speak slowly

I nstruct client not to wear hearing aid while bathing or swimming

N o hair spray, cosmetics, or oils around ear

G ive hearing aid a rest at night and turn it off and open the battery compartment to prevent battery drain

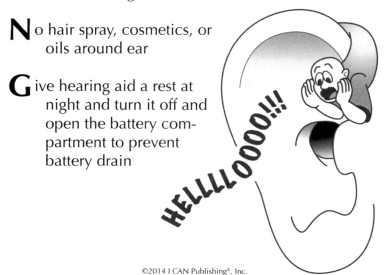

©2014 I CAN Publishing®, Inc.

"Keep your face always toward the sunshine and the shadows will fall behind you!"

WALT WHITMAN

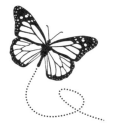

INTEGUMENTARY SYSTEM

Diagnostics For The Integumentary System

Culture and Sensitivity: A procedure to isolate a pathogen on culture media. Sensitivity indicates the response specific microorganisms from antimicrobial agents. If the organism is not killed by the medication, then it is resistant to the med. If it is killed by the med, then it is sensitive. A culture and sensitivity may be performed on a sample of drainage from a wound/lesion/pustule on the skin, sputum or urine specimen, and any other fluids from the body.

> **I CAN TESTING HINT:** Cultures should be done BEFORE starting antimicrobial therapy.

- **W** Wash hands prior to and after collecting specimen; encourage client to wash hands frequently.
- **A** A sufficient quantity of a specimen should be collected & placed in sterile container.
- **S** Standard precautions should be used when collecting specimen.
- **H** Have specimen labeled and delivered to lab promptly. Check protocol for delivery time. If report indicates client is not sensitive to prescribe antimicrobial agent, then notify HCP prior to administering additional doses.

Biopsy: Removal of a sample of tissue to determine diagnosis or malignancy by a needle aspiration. Biopsies can extract small amount of tissue not just from the skin, but from the liver, lung, renal, etc. These can be performed with local anesthesia or moderate sedation. These can also be done during scope procedures.

Nursing Care: "**BLEEDS**" will assist you.

- **B** Bleeding should be evaluated after procedure.
- **L** Look for bleeding; apply pressure and sterile dressing over site as appropriate.
- **E** Educate client to report excessive **bleeding and/or signs of infection**.
- **E** Educate client to check incision daily. Keep it clean, dry and intact.
- **D** Determine if there are any complications from bleeding such as HR ↑ or BP ↓.
- **S** Signed informed consent from client prior to procedure.

> **I CAN TESTING HINT:** Priority care prior following a biopsy is to immediately assess for signs of bleeding and continue ongoing assessment for signs of infection.

DIAGNOSTICS FOR THE INTEGUMENTARY SYSTEM

"DIAGNOSTIC" exams can be hazardous to the health of our clients.

It is our mission to keep them safe!

The designated NCLEX® standards are outlined below to assist you in organizing the assessments, nursing interventions, and evaluation that must be incorporated into our critical thinking and clinical reasoning for clients experiencing a diagnostic procedure, treatment, or laboratory procedure.

D iagnostic test results—monitor; intervene for complications.

I njury and/or complications from procedure should be prevented.

A ssist with invasive procedures (e.g., thoracentesis, bronchoscopy).

G lucose monitoring, ECG, O_2 saturation, etc. may be performed.

N ote client's response to procedures and treatments.

O btain specimens other than blood (e.g., wound, stool, etc.).

S igns and symptoms of trends and/or changes-monitor, and intervene.

T each client and family about procedures and treatments.

I dentify vital signs and monitor for changes and intervene.

C omplications should be noted and followed immediately with an action.

This image is to remind you that "Sure Look" Holmes is looking into the hippo's mouth to assure he is safe! Just as "Sure Look" Holmes, the nurse is not responsible for ordering these tests, but to maintain client SAFETY prior to, during, and after these diagnostics have been completed.

©2014 I CAN Publishing®, Inc.

Impetigo

Impetigo is a bacterial skin infection caused by invasion of the epidermis by pathogenic **Staphylococcus aureus** and/or group **A beta-hemolytic streptococci.**

The image of the honey bee on the right page will assist you in organizing the care for this infection and help you remember the assessment of **the pustule-like lesions with moist honey-colored crusts. These crusts are surrounded by redness.** The client will experience pruritus from the impetigo. This needs to be managed since the infection can spread to surrounding areas. This may appear anywhere on the body, but typically appears **on the face** and around the mouth.

The treatment may be topical. **Management** includes gently washing two to three times a day to remove the crusts. If only a few lesions are found, then mupirocin (Bactroban) antibiotic cream is the recommended treatment. If there are extensive lesions, a full course of systemic antibiotic therapy will be the treatment of choice. The full dose of antibiotics is important due to the risk in developing **glomerulonephritis.**

The Health Promotion Information information for a client with impetigo should begin with excellent **HAND WASHING! STANDARD/CONTACT PRECAUTIONS** will prevent transmission to other clients, the environment, and result in safe care! The client should be assured that the lesions heal without **scarring.**

IMPETIGO

H andwashing is a MUST!

O ral antibiotic therapy—treatment of course

N ot treated appropriately may lead to glomerulonephritis

E rosions—pustule-like lesions with moist honey-colored crusts surrounded by redness

Y es, these lesions may appear on body, but most commonly on face

B eta-hemolytic streptococci—cause; mupirocin (Bactroban) cream—if only a few lesions are found

E ducate family that lesions will not scar

E ncourage to take the full course of antibiotics

S taphylococcus aureus—cause

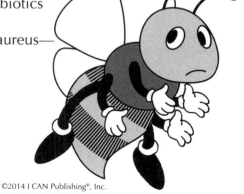

Parasitic Infestations: Pediculosis

There are several types of pediculosis.
Pediculosis humanus capitis: head lice.
Pediculosis humanus corporis: body lice.
Phthirus pubis: pubic lice or crabs.

The little "**LICE**" Man on the right page demonstrates the clinical manifestations for head lice. The **P's** below will assist you in organizing the key treatment plan for pediculosis.

Permethrin 1% liquid (Nix): With just one application this is effective against nits and lice. Instruct client to shampoo hair first, leave Nix on hair for 10 minutes, rinse off; may repeat in 7 days.

Pyrethrin compounds (e.g., Rid) for pubic and head lice.

Plan to treat all family members and close contacts and practice CONTACT PRECAUTIONS.

Plan to wash or dry-clean all bedding and clothing that may have lice or nits; vacuum or treat rugs/furniture

Plan to teach client and family the transmission of the head lice by sharing of personal items (e.g., caps, hats, etc.); advise not to share items.

Plastic bag should be used for nonwashable items and left for 14 days if item is unable to dry-clean or vacuum. Nits can hatch in 7 to 10 days when shed in the environment.

Place on and wear gloves when the nurse is examining scalp to prevent spread to others.

Place shampoo on hair and use a fine-tooth comb or tweezers to assist in removing the nits.

LICE

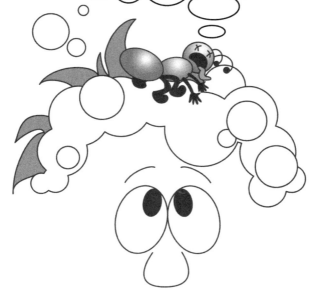

Priority Care For Decreasing Altered Skin Integrity

Nurses must not wait for a reddened area to occur prior to preventative measures are initiated. Prevention begins day 1 in preventing pressure ulcers. Clients high risk for developing complications with altered skin integrity may include clients who are immobile, inactive, experiencing shearing/friction; alteration and decrease in appropriate nutrition; have alteration in perception of pain; incontinence such as from urinary/fecal incontinence; and older adult clients who are experiencing loss of lean body mass, decreased elasticity of the skin, altered arterial or venous blood flow. One of the first interventions for these high risk clients would be to stimulate circulation and to prevent and relieve pressure to the skin by frequently altering the position. "**PRESSURE**" will review preventive care.

Position and turn every 1-2 hours.

Remember, one priority is that nutrition is important; increase carbohydrates, protein, vitamin C, and zinc; Intake - 2,000 to 3,000 mL/day. If serum albumin levels are < 3.5 mg/dL, this is a high risk for skin breakdown and may result in a decrease in healing and risk for infection. (Elderly: No lotions with perfume, No strong detergents. No skin products with alcohol.)

Eliminate pressure by special pressure relieving mattresses that provide for a continuous change in pressure across the mattress. **Silicone gel pads** placed under the buttocks of clients in wheelchairs; sheepskin pads can also protect skin. Maintain clean, dry skin and wrinkle free linens; sun protection factor (SPF) 15 or > when in sun can also be effective in preventing problems with altered skin integrity **Use** active and passive exercises to promote circulation.

Remositurize after bathing with lotion or protective moisturizer (NOT ELDERLY); remember to maintain head of the bed at or below 30° or at the lowest degree of elevation. Avoid wrinkles in sheets or clothing that my serve as a irritation to the skin. Rehydrate client.

Eliminate rubbing excessively and hot water with skin care. Use soft towel, especially following toileting to keep skin clean and dry. **Evaluate skin frequently**, especially over bony prominences. Two of the popular risk assessment instruments for evaluating pressure ulcers include the **Braden Scale** and the **P**ressure **U**lcer **S**cale for **H**ealing (**PUSH Tool**). *Refer to right page.* The Braden Scale scores six subscales: **sensory perception, moisture, activity-mobility, nutrition, friction, and shear**. The total range for this instrument is 6-23. A score of 19-23 indicates no risk. A score of 15-18 indicates client is at risk for skin breakdown. A score of 13-14 is moderate risk. A score of 10-12 indicates client is high risk for developing a pressure ulcer. This instrument is the most reliable and most used assessment scale for determining pressure ulcer risk. A score of 9 or below is very high risk.

The Pressure Ulcer Scale for Healing (**PUSH Tool**) was developed by the National Pressure Ulcer Advisory Panel (NPUAP) as a quick, reliable tool to monitor the pressure ulcer status over time. Ulcers are categorized according to **the wound size, exudates, and type of tissu**e. If the client gets a 0 on the monitor scoring the wound is healed. If the client gets a 17, the wound is not healed.

Great references are available at www.npuap.org.

PRESSURE ULCERS

Braden Scale
Sensory perception, moisture, activity-mobility, nutrition, friction, and shear

Pressure Ulcer Scale for Healing (PUSH Tool)
Ulcers are categorized according to size of the wound, exudate, and type of tissue

W ound
E xudate
T ype of tissue

Basal Cell Carcinoma

The basal cell carcinoma is **the most common type** of skin malignancy. The basal cell is rarely metastatic. The rate of recurrence is very high. Basal cell carcinoma is a cancer of the basal cell layer of the epidermis that can damage surrounding tissue and can advance to include underlying structures. However, because it can cause significant destruction and disfigurement by invading surrounding tissues, it is still considered malignant.

Statistically, in the United States approximately 3 out of 10 Caucasians may develop a basal-cell cancer within their lifetime. In 80 percent of all cases, basal-cell cancers are found on the face, head, and/or neck. It is typically found on the face between the hairline and the upper lip.

Clients present with a **pearly boarder** that is translucent. However, superficial basal-cell cancer can present as a red patch like eczema. Infiltrative or morpheaform basal-cell cancers can present as a skin thickening or scar tissue—making diagnosis difficult without using tactile sensation and a skin biopsy. This type of carcinoma is small, with a **waxy nodule with small**, superficial blood vessel surrounding it. This can progress to ulcer with bleeding and crusting. It is **irregular in shape**.

Just think of the formation of a bagel, and it will assist you in visualizing the appearance of the basal cell. Basal and bagel also sound alike. "**PIT**" summarizes the clinical presentation of this skin carcinoma.

PIT

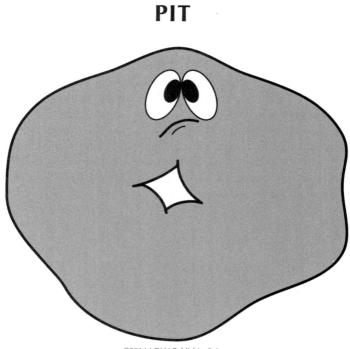

P early border that is translucent; appears as a small, waxy nodule

I rregular in shape

T he most common type of skin cancer; appears most on the face, usually between the hairline and upper lip

Malignant Melanoma

The malignant melanomas have the highest mortality rate of any form of skin cancer. This type of skin cancer is an aggressive, metastatic cancer that originates in the melanin-producing cells of the epidermis. These are caused by UV exposure without protection or overexposure to artificial light such as in tanning beds. The common sites for this neoplasm include back and legs in women; and trunk, head, and neck in men. These are frequently dark brown or black in color. They are characterized by a progressive or sudden change in the color, size, or shape of the mole. The right page outlines the A, B, C's for the malignant melanoma.

I CAN TESTING HINT: When studying for the NCLEX®, practice prioritizing which skin assessment would be most important to report or refer to the healthcare provider (HCP). Due to the high mortality rate, the melanoma is typically the option to select.

MALIGNANT MELANOMA

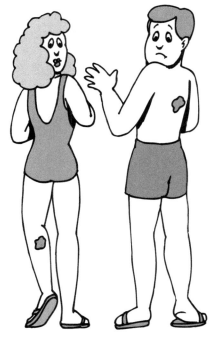

A symmetry

B order irregularity

C olor variegation

D iameter greater than 6 mm

E volving or changing in some way

Burns

Berny has been in a fire, and as you can see, he is wrapped up like a mummy. Berny "**BURNS**" will help us review burn care.

B   **BREATHING**–Keep airway open. Facial burns, singed nasal hair, hoarseness, sooty sputum, bloody sputum, and labored respirations indicate TROUBLE!

BODY IMAGE–Assist Berny in coping by encouraging expression of thoughts and feelings. This is tough and painful!

U   **URINE OUTPUT**–In older children and adults, urine output should be at least 30 to 45 mL per hour; in children weighing less than 66 lb., urine output should be 1 to 2 mL/kg/hr. Watch the K^+ to keep it between 3.5–5.0 mEq/L. Keep the CVP around 12 mm Hg. Urine output is the most sensitive indicator of fluid status.

ULCERS (Stress) – Administer intravenous H_2 blockes and/or proton pump inhibitors. Evaluate for complications from a bleeding ulcer due to the stress involved with the pain and altered image as a result of the burn.

R   **RULE OF NINE**– Used for adults to determine quick estimation of burn surface area. A more accurate determination uses charts that calculate the total body surface area burned and the depth of the burn based on age of the client.

p**ROTECTIVE ISOLATION**–Prevent client from getting infected. No flowers or plants with standing water should ever be in the room; eliminate fruits in the room. *Refer to "Infection Prevention: Positive Pressure" for more specifics on infection control.*

REPLACEMENT OF FLUIDS–Isotonic crystalloid solutions, such as 0.9% sodium chloride, or Lactated Ringer's solution are used during the first 24 hours. One-half of the fluid for the first 24 hours should be administered over the first 8-hour period, then the remainder is administered over the next 16 hours. First 24-hour calculation starts at the time of injury. Colloid solutions, such as albumin, or synthetic plasma expanders (Hespan) Plasma-Lyte, may be used after the first 24 hours of burn recovery. (Use large bore IV catheters if a large area of body is burned.) Fluid shift and edema occur within first 12 hours post burn and can continue 24 to 36 hours post burn. Mobilization of fluid and diuresis occur 48 to 72 hours post burn.

RELIEF OF PAIN–Analgesics are given intravenously; do not administer intramuscularly, subcutaneously, or orally since they will not be absorbed effectively.

N   **NUTRITION**–High protein and calories are components of the diet. (Determine by using daily caloric expenditure estimate.) Supplemental gastric tube feedings or hyperalimentation may be used in clients with large burned areas. Daily weights will assist in evaluating the nutritional needs.

S   **SIGNS OF SHOCK; SIGNS OF INFECTION**–Monitor alteration in sensorium (confusion), capillary refill time, HR, BP, CVP, renal function, spiking temperature WBCs.

REMEMBER THESE PEOPLE ARE AFRAID AND NEED SUPPORT!

BURNS

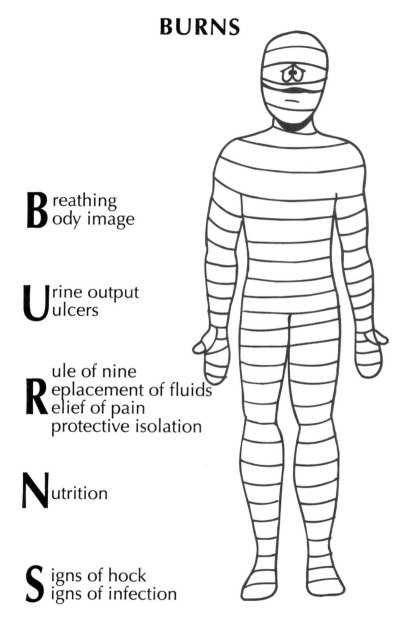

B reathing
  ody image

U rine output
  lcers

R ule of nine
  eplacement of fluids
  elief of pain
  protective isolation

N utrition

S igns of hock
  igns of infection

"The word 'encourage' simply means 'to urge forward.' Every one of us should have someone we believe in, someone we're urging forward, someone we're helping to achieve goals and dreams."

JOEL OLSTEEN

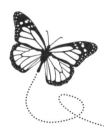

HEMATOLOGY

Diagnostics For Hematology

Bone Marrow Aspiration/Biopsy: A test used to diagnose the etiology of blood disorders or chromosomal abnormalities. Examples may include thrombocytopenia or anemia. Diseases such as some cancers or leukemia may be ruled out with this procedure. Nursing Care: "**BLEED**" will assist you. Typical site for bone marrow is the posterior iliac crest; alternative sites are sternum and anterior iliac crest. Biopsy site will be anesthetized with a local anesthesia, and client may also receive an analgesic or conscious sedation during pre-procedure care. Client may feel pressure while aspiration is being done. Look for bleeding, and as appropriate, apply pressure to the biopsy site to prevent bleeding. Apply a sterile dressing over site. Educate about being on bed rest for approximately 30 min. after the procedure. Educate client to avoid aspirin and any medication that affects clotting. Determine if there are any complications with bleeding and/or signs of an infection (e.g., temperature pain, swelling, WBC increase). Mild analgesics typically relieve the post-procedure discomfort.

Sickle cell test (SICKLEDEX): A test that is used for routine screening for sickle cell trait or the disorder. This test does not diagnose the difference between the trait and disorder. Up to 4 months following a transfusion of RBCs, a false-positive result can occur indicating client is positive for the trait.

Lab TEST	VALUE RANGE	INDICATION
RBC	Females: 4.2 to 5.4 million/uL Males: 4.7 to 6.1 million/uL	↓ may be anemia
WBC	5,000 to 10,000 /uL	↓ may be immunosuppression; ↑ may be infection
Platelets	150,000 to 400,000 mm^3	↓ may be a bone marrow depression, an autoimmune disease ↑ may be polycythemia or malignancy
Hgb	Females: 12 to 16 g/dL Males: 14 to 18 g/dL	↓ may be anemia
Hct	Females: 37-47% Males: 42-52%	↓ may be anemia (Note: Hgb x 3= Hct)
PT	11 to 12.5 seconds	↓ may be vitamin K excess; ↑ may be deficiency or clotting
aPTT	1.5 to 2 (desired range for anticoagulation)	Monitor if getting heparin; ↑ may indicate liver disease, disseminated intravascular coagulation (DIC), or hemophilia
INR	2 to 3 on warfarin (Coumadin)	Monitor if on warfarin

DIAGNOSTICS FOR HEMATOLOGY

"DIAGNOSTIC" exams can be hazardous to the health of our clients.

It is our mission to keep them safe!

The designated NCLEX® standards are outlined below to assist you in organizing the assessments, nursing interventions, and evaluation that must be incorporated into our critical thinking and clinical reasoning for clients experiencing a diagnostic procedure, treatment, or laboratory procedure.

D iagnostic test results—monitor; intervene for complications.

I njury and/or complications from procedure should be prevented.

A ssist with invasive procedures (e.g., thoracentesis, bronchoscopy).

G lucose monitoring, ECG, O_2 saturation, etc. may be performed.

N ote client's response to procedures and treatments.

O btain specimens other than blood (e.g., wound, stool, etc.).

S igns and symptoms of trends and/or changes-monitor, and intervene.

T each client and family about procedures and treatments.

I dentify vital signs and monitor for changes and intervene.

C omplications should be noted and followed immediately with an action.

This image is to remind you that "Sure Look" Holmes is looking into the hippo's mouth to assure he is safe! Just as "Sure Look" Holmes, the nurse is not responsible for ordering these tests, but to maintain client SAFETY prior to, during, and after these diagnostics have been completed.

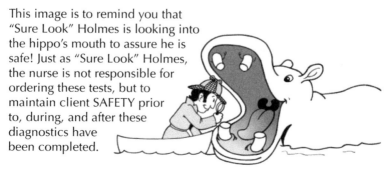

©2014 I CAN Publishing®, Inc.

Sickle Cell Anemia

Sickle cell anemia is characterized by the sickling effect of erythrocytes (red blood cells)–results in increased blood viscosity and increased red cell destruction. Increased viscosity eventually precipitates ischemia and tissue necrosis due to capillary stasis and thrombosis. The image for this condition is a rabbit on a bicycle (BiSICKLE). How do rabbits get around? Of course we know they "**HOP**"!

H HYDRATION–Viscosity may be decreased with adequate IV fluids. Monitor IV fluids and encourage fluid intake. Sluggish circulation may cause an electrolyte imbalance. Be aware of fluid and electrolyte imbalances caused by temperature elevations, vomiting and diarrhea, etc.

O OXYGEN–Administer oxygen. Adequate oxygen helps prevent sickling from occurring. Avoid fatigue, traveling to high altitude areas, aircraft travel or participating in a strenuous activity. Maintain rest if movement exacerbates pain. Promote respiratory health and tissue oxygenation. Avoid crowds and inhaling irritants. Routine exercise. Prevent infection; promote thorough hand washing.

P PAIN MEDICINE–Due to the client's extreme discomfort, analgesics will be given. Meperidine (Demerol) is not recommended; morphine, hydromorphone (Dilaudid), fentanyl (Sublimaze, Duragesic) may be used; patient-controlled (PCA) devices are frequently used to control pain.

PASSIVE RANGE OF MOTION–Passive range of motion may be beneficial. No active or passive range of motion if client is actively bleeding into joints.

S SUPPORT–Support the parents by encouraging genetic counseling. Child may be supported by providing normal developmental activities.

SICKLE CELL ANEMIA

H ydrate

O xygen

P ain medicine

S upport

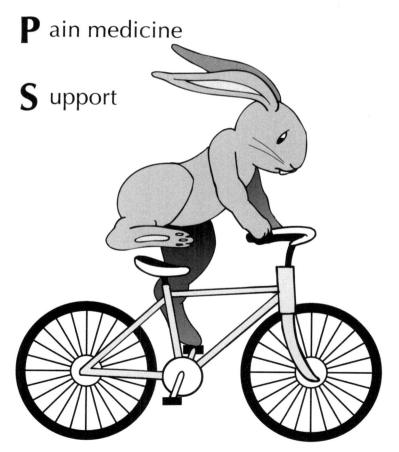

Polycythemia

Polycythemia Vera (Primary) is a blood disorder characterized by a proliferation of all red marrow cells. This disorder usually develops in middle ages. Several of the clinical manifestations and diagnostics are outlined below. To assist you in remembering this, just visualize "Mr. Ruddy" on the next page. His complexion looks as if someone had taken a red crayon and colored his face to give him a **ruddy complexion**. He may also present with an **enlarged liver**. Several diagnostics that are prevalent with polycythemia include: an **erythrocyte count that is elevated, excessive production of leukocytes and platelets**. Another clinical manifestation that may occur is a **decrease in the blood flow**. Treatment of care includes a phlebotomy and a **decrease in the iron intake**.

POLYCYTHEMIA

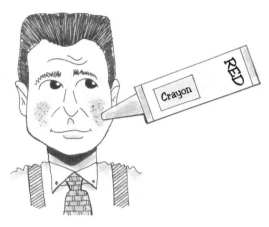

© 2004 I CAN Publishing, Inc.

Ruddy complexion

Erythrocytes increased
Excessive production of leukocytes and platelets
Enlarged liver

Decreased blood flow
Decreased iron intake

Priority Assessments For Leukemia

Leukemia is an uncontrolled proliferation of abnormal white blood cells. As a result of the infiltration of the leukemic cells into the body, eventually cellular destruction occurs. The strategy on the right page has been developed to assist you in remembering three primary consequences of leukemia that include infection from neutropenia, anemia from RBC destruction and bleeding (resulting in a decrease in the erythrocytes), and bleeding from decrease in the platelets (thrombocytopenia).

The image on the right page illustrates a lab tube with immature white blood cells. The way to remember the four main categories of clinical assessment findings is to visualize the "**NATS**" flying around you. *It is hard to get rid of these because they are so small and many. They are not mature and take extra energy to swat them away.* This strategy will assist you in organizing the clinical assessment findings within the structure of pathophysiology.

Let's begin with **neutropenia**. The definition of neutropenia is an abnormally small number of neutrophils. The mature leukocytes fight off infection, so consequently the outcome from neutropenia would be an increase in risk of infection. The assessment findings may be a sore throat, chills and fever, cough, anorexia, etc. Neutropenic precautions would be a priority nursing plan for this client. Never allow a child or adult with chickenpox to room with a child or adult who is immunosuppressed from leukemia or chemotherapy. Assess vital signs for a fever; administer medications as needed. Use acetaminophen rather than NSAIDs or aspirin. Do not administer Polio (IPV), varicella, measles-mumps-rubella, and influenza immunizations during immunosuppression.

Anemia may result from RBC destruction and bleeding causing the client to be lethargic and experiencing a feeling of being fatigue. These clinical findings would present as a result of a decrease in the hemoglobin. Remember RBCs transport oxygen, and with this reduction then the outcome would be a decrease in energy. The priority care would include rest and relaxation with organized nursing care to support the need for sleep.

Thrombocytopenia may result in bleeding tendencies due to the decrease in platelets. With this decrease, the client may present early on with petechiae, bruising easily, and/or epistaxis. Nursing care requires gentle handling with minimal needle sticks. Avoid strenuous activity when platelet counts are low and anemia are present.

Additional clinical **signs** the client could present with may include: swollen lymph nodes, loss of weight, CNS involvement, and/or splenomegaly/hepatomegaly. The CNS presentations may include a headache, confusion, or increased irritability. Nursing care for weight loss requires attention to nutrition that is appealing and will assist with healing. Encourage adequate protein and calorie intake, low-bacteria diet. Prior to chemotherapy, administer the prescribed antiemetic. Maintain adequate hydration to flush chemicals from the kidneys.

I CAN TESTING HINT: A key to successful testing is to understand the pathophysiology that occurs with the medical condition. This will assist you in organizing the clinical assessment findings, and will also be useful for prioritizing the nursing care.

PRIORITY ASSESSMENTS FOR LEUKEMIA

N eutropenia—Risk for an infection

A nemia—↓ hemoglobin

T hrombodytopenia—Bleeding

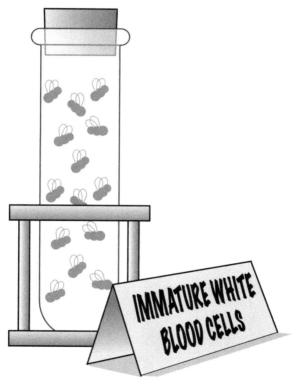

©2014 I CAN Publishing®, Inc.

Leukemia is numerous immature white blood cells like nats flying around you. Just remember they are so small it is hard to swat them away.

Multiple Myeloma

Meet "Mr. Bone" who will assist you in remembering the priority information for multiple myeloma. This disorder is a malignancy of the plasma cells, most common in men in their 60's. These malignant cells infiltrate into bones and soft tissues resulting in severe pain to the client.

Clients experience back and bone pain along with anemia and broken bones. Many clients will be on pain medication and comfort measures. Treatment consists of chemotherapy and palliative radiation therapy. Glucocorticosteroids are also included in the treatment plan. Clients need calcitonin to decrease hypercalcemia and reduce bone destruction.

To assist in maintaining physical equilibrium, clients must be encouraged to hydrate, ambulate, and medicate! Clients need to be evaluated for adequate hydration to prevent calcium from precipitating in the kidneys. Careful ambulation is helpful in decreasing hypercalcemia and improving pulmonary status.

Safety measures are necessary to prevent pathologic fractures!

MULTIPLE MYELOMA

Broken bones

On pain medication and chemotherapy

Need calcitonin

Evaluate blood and kidneys
(will show calcium loss)

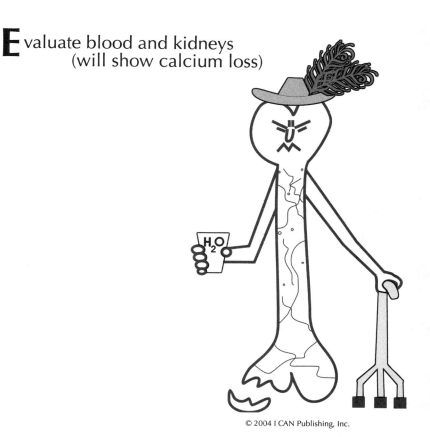

AMBULATE, MEDICATE, HYDRATE

"I always like to look on the optimistic side of life,
but I am realistic enough to know that
life is a complex matter."

WALT DISNEY

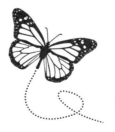

MEN & WOMEN'S CARE / CANCER

Benign Prostate Hypertrophy

The poor guy who has his "tubes" squeezed tightly due to an enlarged prostate gland will likely find himself going to surgery for a transurethral resection of the prostate (TURP). Prostatic tissue is removed through a resectoscope, so the urethra can once again pass urine easily.

When the guy comes back from surgery, he will likely have a triple lumen tube in his bladder to maintain continuous bladder irrigation (CBI) or Murphy drip. The **TUBE** will provide for **URINARY OUTPUT**, but it will contain bright **RED DRAINAGE**. If you see pieces of clots in the tube, it's time to increase the CBI to wash out the clots. Retained blood **CLOTS** may cause hemorrhage and we do not want that to happen! Unfortunately **CLOTS** may also cause bladder **SPASMS** that hurt. Belladonna and opium suppositories (B&O) are often ordered to help relieve the spasms. If the client complains of pain, evaluate the urinary drainage and make sure the catheter is patent.

Obstructions most commonly occur in the initial 24 hours due to clots in the bladder. Overdistention of the bladder can precipitate hemorrhage as well as bladder spasms.

TURPS

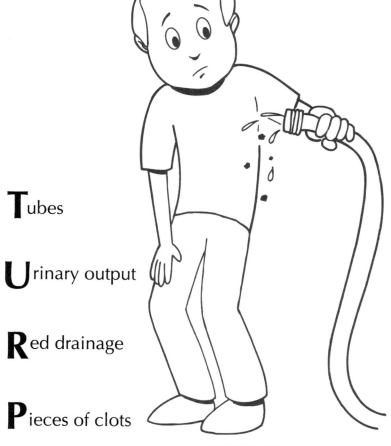

Tubes

Urinary output

Red drainage

Pieces of clots

Spasms

©1994 I CAN Publishing, Inc.

Care of Client After Mastectomy

Have you ever had a chicken without a breast? Well, this may be a first for you. Meet "Ester the breastless chicken." Ester had a mastectomy due to cancer. She has a family history with both her mother and sister having breast cancer. She refused to have the recommended annual mammogram after she turned 40.

After her mastectomy, no **BLOOD PRESSURES** or lab sticks were done on the affected side. She maintained the affected side in an **ELEVATED** position. Each joint was to be elevated and positioned higher than the more proximal joint to promote drainage. Ester met some wonderful women from **REACH FOR RECOVERY** who provided her with support. She was given pamphlets to read and phone numbers of some contact people who also had a mastectomy. After they left, she started her **EXTENSION** and **FLEXION** exercises. Squeezing a ball is a great exercise. **ABDUCTION** and **EXTERNAL** rotation should not be the initial exercises. Ester was taught how to do a SBE (self breast examination) once a month. The nurse recommended that she do it while she was taking her shower. The staff encouraged Ester to discuss her fears, concerns and anxieties in order **TO PROMOTE A POSITIVE SELF-IMAGE.**

CARE OF CLIENT AFTER MASTECTOMY

B P—not on affected side

R each for Recovery

E levate affected side
Extension and flexion exercises—initially (squeeze a ball)

A bduction and external rotation should not be initial exercise

S B E—once a month—about one week after period

T o promote a positive self-image

Safety With Radium Implants

"How do you feel today" is adopted from Sue Crow's book *Asepsis, The Right Touch*, an excellent down to earth book on infection control. Let's assume that the character in the bed has an internal radiation source (sealed source).

We want to plan our nursing care from afar! When you are in very close proximity to the client who has a radium implant, you get almost as much radiation as they do. Talk to them from as much DISTANCE as you can manage. Except when giving direct care, attempt to maintain distance of six feet from the source of radiation. Plan your care, so that you are in close proximity for the shortest period of TIME.

The client should be placed in a private room. Signs should be placed on the door warning of radiation source. SHIELD precautions are a must. Healthcare personnel should wear a dosimeter film badge that records the amount of radiation exposure. Visitors should be limited to 30-min. visits and maintain a distance of 6 ft. Pregnant individuals should not come in contact with client.

L Lead container should be kept in room if source can become dislodged.

E Educate client to remain in position to prevent dislodgement of radium implant; uterine implant–do not elevate head of bed past 20 degrees. Diet–low residue; urinary catheter; plan includes preventing complications from immobility.

A Ask client to notify nurse to assist with elimination.

D Distance of 6 feet from source of radiation.

Remember, these clients will get lonely because they are on bedrest and can't leave their room. *Be sure they can reach the telephone and the call light!*

RADIUM IMPLANTS

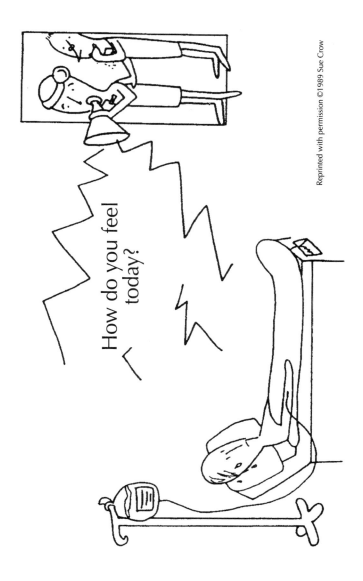

"Watch your manner of speech if you wish to develop a peaceful state of mind. Start each day by affirming peaceful, contented, and happy attitudes and your days will tend to be pleasant and successful."

NORMAN VINCENT PEALE

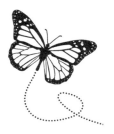

HEALTH PROMOTION

Levels of Prevention

Preventive healthcare is becoming more dynamic as people live longer! There is a focus on the enhancement and the promotion of health through daily exercising, dietary intake, stress reduction habits, etc. There are several levels of prevention that will assist with health maintenance recommendations. The focus is to educate the client actions for health maintenance and disease prevention such as providing information sessions, screening programs, and physical therapy.

The right page will assist you in associating which program is included in the three levels of prevention. Let's start with Primary prevention that incorporates programs to prevent disease. The "**P**" will assist you in remembering the plan is **prior to the onset of a disease**, and the plan typically includes **information** and/or **immunizations**. This is what we do daily in our life (at least we should!) such as *eat a healthy diet, follow a routine exercise program, maintain body weight, appropriate immunizations, etc.*

The second level of prevention includes early diagnosis and treatment. There is an "**S**" to remind you this includes screening and early detection of a disease such as having a routine pap smear. The goals for this level of prevention are to diagnose early and establish priorities for intervention. Some examples of this secondary level of prevention include: testicular self-examination, breast self-examination, glaucoma test, and/or colon-rectal cancer screening.

The third level of prevention has an "**R**" to assist you in remembering that there is a disease, and the goal is to **rehabilitate** the condition and/or **restore** to an optimum level of health. The key is the disease or condition has already occurred. Some examples of this level of prevention may include initiating physical therapy after a cerebrovascular accident or follow up with an ophthalmologist after the development of macular degeneration.

In summary, see how easy this is to remember! Primary has an "**I**" for immunization and a "**P**" for prior to onset, Secondary has a "**S**" for screening, and Tertiary has an "**R**" for Rehab!

LEVELS OF PREVENTION

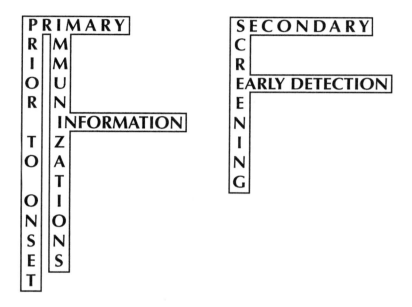

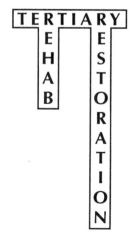

Client Education

Client education is vitally important for the client's safety, compliance with medications, reimbursement to hospitals, and the list is never-ending! The bottom line is that nurses need to effectively provide client education. Due to the importance of evaluating if the teaching has been successful, we have used the mnemonic "**TEACH BACK**" on the right page to help review a few principles for client teaching. "**RETURN**" in the box below will assist you with a few topics that should be consistently included in client education.

It is also very important for you to be able to apply the principles for education when you are answering questions about teaching. To simplify this, let's think of "**A PIE**" that is sweet and how much we enjoy the flavor after a nice meal. "**A PIE**" will assist you in recalling these principles and assist in making the teaching successful.

Assess–What does the client need to know and does the client perceive the need to learn the information? Are there any learning barriers? Assess the client's readiness to learn and understand their learning preferences and barriers to learning.

Planning–The nurse needs to develop objectives and a plan to teach the client this new information. This may include a demonstration, and then provide the client with the opportunity to return a demonstration. Other strategies may include a short video with hands on practice; written material for review; an interactive presentation including the new procedure or medication or any of the topics outlined on the right page.

Physical and Psychological Comfort–It is important for the nurse who is leading the teaching to always consider the physical comfort of the learner(s) (client). For example, if the teaching session takes place prior to lunch, and the client is hungry then minimal learning will take place. If there are distractions within the environment, then this will also affect the learning process. Many clients experience anxiety and fear when presented with new information. Always attempt to start the teaching session by identifying or assessing what the client knows about the topic. This will also decrease the anxiety prior to teaching.

Implementation–The information should be presented in a manner the client will understand. Provide opportunities for discussion, feedback; demonstrations, etc. The more active the learner (client) is the more they are likely to learn. Repetition is the mother of learning. Plan short sessions.

Evaluation–Return demonstrations are an excellent strategy for evaluating if a skill was accurately learned. A written quiz or verbal feedback are additional strategies that may be used for evaluation. It is not appropriate to simply document that teaching was completed. There MUST be evidence that client learned the information. Review "**TEACH BACK**" that will assist you in evaluating the outcomes from the teaching plan.

Topics for Client Education

- **R** Review medications (i.e., action, side effects, diet, etc.)
- **E** Equipment if being discharged with any (i.e., oxygen safety, glucometer, etc.)
- **T** The appropriate level of activity, procedures
- **U** Unexpected outcomes; undesirable effects, etc. that should be reported to HCP
- **R** Referrals; resources
- **N** Nutrition; needs any follow up

CLIENT EDUCATION

T The first step is to assess client's physiological needs are met; assess what client currently knows about condition.

E Evaluate evidence that learning took place (return demonstration); DOCUMENT.

A Assess literacy, learning levels, barriers to learning (language); readiness to learn, learning preferences.

C Clients want to apply learning immediately; choose vocabulary appropriate for client's understanding.

H Help older clients with sensory deficits (i.e., large-print books, etc.).

B Balance and empower client confidence to take charge of their health.

A Alleviate anxiety with practice and reinforcement; stimulate as many senses as possible. Use charts, equipment, etc. when appropriate.

C Communicate, communicate, communicate! Remember to include family!

K Keep teaching simple and short! Do NOT overwhelm client!

Growth and Development Throughout the Life Span

From infancy to elderly there are major issues regarding health promotion that the nurse needs to review with the clients. The word "**SPINE**" will help you remember these issues.

- **S** **STRESS MANAGEMENT** concerns clients throughout their lives. Children need to achieve various developmental milestones, which may be stressful during the growing process. As individuals age they must develop skill in adapting and coping to facilitate their stress management.
  SAFETY is an important part of clients' promotion of health. Safety includes anything from the toddler staying away from balloons to the elderly client watching for falls and drug/drug interactions.

- **P** **PHYSICAL ACTIVITY** for the child to develop, activity to increase cardiovascular health and decrease osteoporosis are vitally important in health promotion.

- **I** **INTERPERSONAL RELATIONSHIPS** are important to nurture. They prolong life and increase happiness. As the child grows into school age, their peers become increasingly more important in their life. During the working adult life, intimacy is an important developmental task.

- **N** **NUTRITION** is of paramount importance throughout the lifespan to promote health and prevent disease. It is important that the adult takes in an average of 3 servings of milk, meat, vegetables, and fruits and 6 servings of bread or rice a day.

- **E** **ENVIRONMENTAL SAFETY** is an important issue. We want to teach the importance of avoiding abuse, violence, poisoning, smoke inhalation, chemical spills and other noxious elements that put our life at risk.

GROWTH AND DEVELOPMENT THROUGHOUT THE LIFE SPAN

S tress
S afety

P hysical

I nterpersonal

N utrition

E nvironmental

©1997 I CAN Publishing, Inc.

Obesity

Obesity is an imbalance between the caloric intake and the energy expenditure resulting in an abnormal increase in fat cells. CDC has published that 66% of people in the United States over age 20 are obese. "**OBESE**" will assist in summarizing key facts.

- **O** **Obesity** is an imbalance between caloric intake and energy expenditure
- **B** **BMI**: 25 to 29.9 kg/m² is considered overweight
- **E** **Elevated** risk for cardiovascular, respiratory, musculoskeletal problems, & diabetes
- **S** **Sedentary** lifestyle
- **E** **Environment** is conducive to excessive caloric intake

> Risk Factors: ("**SIT**" *too long with minimal exercise*!)
> - **S** **Sedentary** lifestyle
> - **I** **Intake** of food exceeds energy expenditure
> - **T** **The** risks involved include: cardiovascular, respiratory, musculoskeletal, and diabetes.

The lady on the right, "DI," has been successful with her weight-loss program as you can see from the size of her pants. She did take Vitamins D, E, & K in addition to Beta Carotene daily while on orlistat (Xenical). "**SMALL**" will assist you in recalling these medication facts. Note, medications are NOT the priority with this condition; the priority is to change one's lifestyle and habits!

ORLISTAT (XENICAL) (also known as **tetrahydrolipstatin**) is a drug designed to treat obesity. Its primary function is preventing the absorption of fats from the human diet by acting as a lipase inhibitor, thereby reducing caloric intake. It is intended for use in conjunction with a HCP-supervised reduced-calorie diets.

The client should be advised to take this medication as directed by the HCP, by mouth with liquid sometime during each meal that contains fat or within 1 hour after the meal, usually 3 times daily. If client misses a meal or the meal contains no fat, skip that dose of the medication. To decrease the chance of unpleasant side effects, it is very important that no more than 30% of the calories in the diet come from fat. The daily intake of fat, protein, and carbohydrates should be evenly spread over 3 main meals.

Do not increase a dose or use this drug more often or for longer than prescribed. Since this drug can interfere with the absorption of certain vitamins (fat-soluble vitamins including A, D, E, K), a daily multivitamin supplement containing these nutrients is recommended. Take the multivitamin at least 2 hours before or 2 hours after taking orlistat (such as at bedtime).

If client is taking cyclosporine, take it at least 3 hours before or after orlistat to make sure the full dose of cyclosporine is absorbed into the bloodstream. If client is taking levothyroxine, take it at least 4 hours before or after orlistat.

The client should see some weight loss within 2 weeks after starting orlistat. Review importance of informing HCP if condition does not improve or gets worse. The key to a successful weight loss program is to BEGIN with a change in the lifestyle and habits in "**LIFE**".

> - **L** **Lifestyle** changes are the priority! Medications are NOT the priority, but safe medication administration is important for the client if this is the plan they pursue.
> - **I** **Increase** in exercise.
> - **F** **Food** selections (balanced diet consumed; www.mypyramid.gov).
> - **E** **Eliminates** risk factors with weight reduction.
> - **S** **Surgery** is an option: Bariatric surgery.

OBESITY

S upplement with multivitamin containing vitamins D, E, K, and beta-carotene should be taken daily

M anage by instructing client to take with meals as prescribed. If meals have no fat, can skip dose

A ction: Decreases the absorption of dietary fat by reversibly inhibiting enzymes (lipases)

L ook for undesirable effects initially such as flatus with discharge, fecal urgency, fecal incontinence

L oss of weight is the outcome when combined with a calorie reduction diet

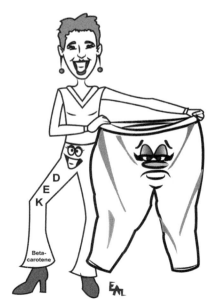

Infancy

Check out these kids and they will help you remember milestones for these ages. Developmental task is **TRUST** versus **MISTRUST** (Erikson).

0-3 months–Recliner is in the **RECLINING** position. His head lags. At two months lifts head and chest off bed. Totally dependent. Provide toys which are soft, cuddly and colorful.

3-6 months–**SITTER**–Starts rolling over. Six months of age can SIT for short periods of time leaning forward on hands. *This age is known as the High Roller.* They can turn quickly with their heads way up off the surface. Birth weight may double at 6 months.

6-9 months–**BOUNCER OR CRAWLER**–Can pull self to a sitting position. They start bouncing so much that they bounce out and start crawling by 8–9 months. Everything goes in the mouth. Safety precautions!

9-12 months–**CRUISER OR WALKER**–Walks with help. This age loves to cruise around furniture. The birth weight may triple and length doubled (12 months). Shows stranger anxiety; clings to mother. Continues in solitary play and can entertain self for short periods of time.

INFANCY

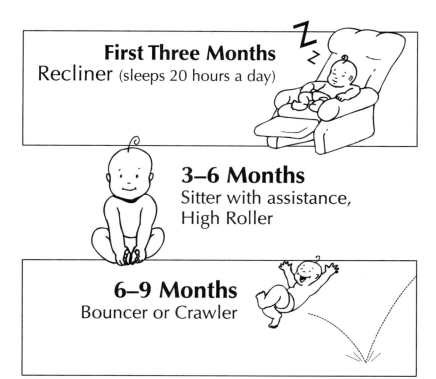

First Three Months
Recliner (sleeps 20 hours a day)

3–6 Months
Sitter with assistance, High Roller

6–9 Months
Bouncer or Crawler

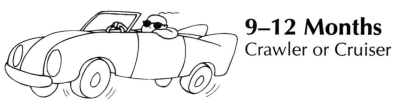

9–12 Months
Crawler or Cruiser

©1994 I CAN Publishing, Inc.

Toddler (1 to 3 years)

These children are "Into everything," have temper tantrums, and are called the "Terrible Two's." The typical words used with the toddler are "NO NO." Let's think of the opposite and consider that the nurse should "**PRAISE**" positive behavior. Refer to image for this explanation.

Notice in the image the child has a **PUSH-PULL** toy which is a favorite. Anything that will make them mobile so they can be **AUTONOMOUS**. These children like playing side by side (**PARALLEL PLAY**), but forget sharing!

The **R** is for the eyes because at bed time if certain **RITUALS AND ROUTINES** are not continued they will not close their eyes and go to sleep. Moral of that story is consistency! **REGRESSION** may occur during hospitalization. **PRAISE** appropriate behavior and ignore the rest. (*Easier said than done!*)

The **A** is for the body because toddlers are into **AUTONOMY**. They like to help dress and undress self. **ACCIDENTS** are a leading cause of death. They may have bruises on extremities from climbing and **EXPLORING** (**E** for feet). Keep poisons out of reach.

The **I** is for the arms, so they can be comforted by their parents. Allow parents to stay with child to decrease those **S**'s (tears) from **SEPARATION ANXIETY**.

ELIMINATION (toilet training) is one of the major milestones for the toddler.

PRAISE

P ush-pull toys
P arallel play

R ituals & routines
R egression

A utonomy versus shame & doubt
A ccidents

I nvolve parents

S eparation anxiety

E limination
E xplore

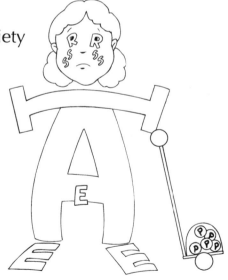

©1994 I CAN Publishing, Inc.

Poison Control

Tommy Toxin has crawled into trouble and ingested some substance that is toxic to his body. Mom and Dad must have the poison control number available! The **national number** that will route them to the local poison control center is **800.222.1222**. If mom is in California and is visiting in Georgia using her cell phone, she will be connected to the California center. If, however, she uses a local phone and calls this national number from Georgia, she will be connected to the center in Georgia.

For current practice, remember that the nurse's responsibility is to promote poison control or if poisoning does occur to prevent complications from occurring! Our initial focus for Tommy would be ABCs (airway, breathing, and circulation). "**POISON**" will assist you with Tommy's plan of care.

- **P** **PROMOTE STABILITY**–Assess the condition and provide airway support, obtain IV site if necessary.

- **O** **OFF/OUT**–Shower or wash **OFF** substance if it is radioactive. Remove clothing that has been contaminated, take them **OFF**! If Tommy has pills in his mouth, take them **OUT**! Eye may need to be flushed **OUT**. Antidotes may be necessary for heroin or drug overdose. Ingested substances may be taken **OUT** of the body by emesis, lavage, absorbents (activated charcoal), or cathartics. Inducing emesis by the use of syrup of ipecac is no longer routinely recommended for emergency or home treatment.

- **I** **IDENTIFY** the toxic agent. Do an accurate history and identify any available poison.

- **S** **SUPPORT** the client both physically and psychologically. Parents may feel guilty in regards to their parenting role. SUPPORT is imperative!

- **O** **ONGOING** safety education regarding poison control!

- **N** **NOTIFY** the poison control center, emergency facility, or provider of care for immediate care and consultation regarding treatment.

Remember the best solution to poisons is to keep them under lock and key.

TOMMY TOXIN

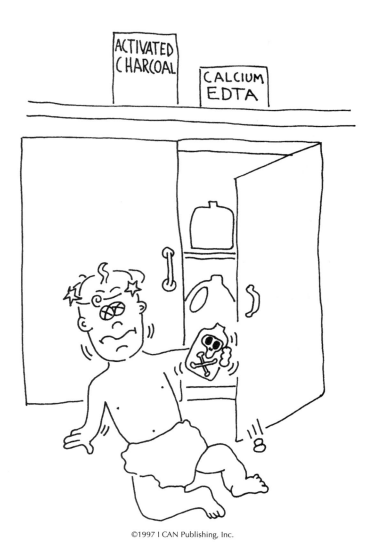

Preschool (4 to 5 Years)

Preschoolers have imaginations that don't stop. The word that is characteristic of this stage is "Why?" They ask questions frequently. "Why is the sky blue?" "Why do dogs have tails?" Due to their active imagination, we have selected the word **MAGIC** to describe this stage of development.

- **M** **MUTILATION**–They may fear mutilation. A typical statement is, "Cover my boo boo; don't let my blood run out!" Any invasive procedure is seen as mutilation (i.e., shot, I.V., enema, rectal temp., etc.).
- **A** **ASSOCIATIVE PLAY**–They progress from parallel play to more cooperative play. An active imagination is great while pretending they are the nurse, doctor, teacher, etc.

    ABANDONMENT–Children are afraid of being left.
- **G** **GUILT**–The feeling is that if I think something bad, the thought can cause a bad event to occur. This may cause guilt for the child.
- **I** **INITIATIVE** *versus* **GUILT**–Child is very creative and may have an imaginary companion. Imaginative toys and devices are favorites.
- **C** **CURIOUS**–Curious about factual information regarding the environment. They always ask, "Why?"

MAGIC

Mutilation

A ssociative play
bandonment

G uilt

I nitiative
maginary playmate
magination

C urious

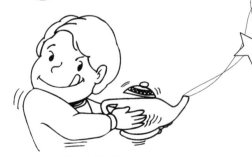

©1994 I CAN Publishing, Inc.

School Age (6 to 12 Years)

Can you see a big dimple in the chin of this child? When you look back over your school age photo albums, what do you often see in those pictures? Many of us see those crazy little **DIMPLES**!

This will help you to associate with this group.

- **D** **DEATH**–The bogeyman will jump out from under the bed to get them. Be honest about funerals and burials. Encourage ventilation of thoughts and feelings.
- **I** **INDUSTRY** versus **INFERIORITY**–"Chum" period. May enjoy collecting coins, cards, etc. May enjoy sports.

    IMMUNIZATIONS should be complete before entering school.
- **M** **MODESTY**–More concerned with modesty and privacy. Pull those curtains and close those doors.
- **P** **PEERS**–The younger children play mostly with their own sex. Older child is beginning to mix with the opposite sex and learn to use the computer early. They are skilled at texting.
- **L** **LOSS OF CONTROL**–Hospitalization is seen as a loss of control. Allow and encourage decision making.
- **E** **EXPLAIN PROCEDURES**–Use terms they can understand.

DIMPLE

Death

Industry versus Inferiority
  mmunizations

Modesty

Peers

Loss of control

Explanation of procedures

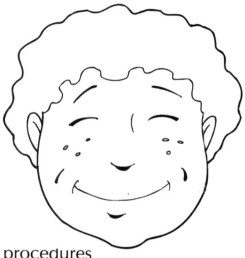

©1994 I CAN Publishing, Inc.

Adolescent (13 to 18 Years)

Adolescents are usually seen in groups or at least in **PAIRS**. Let's think about **PAIRS** while we review some milestones for the adolescent.

P **PEER** group is very important and connections are made through every social network and cell phone available. FACEBOOK and other networks allow this group to text, multitask, and collaborate in groups. Remember, carefully assess the diagnosis. Individualize the plan if client is on bed rest or in isolation.

A **ALTERED IMAGE**–They don't want to be seen as being different. Peer pressure may create problems with pregnancy, sexually transmitted diseases (STD's), substance abuse, and motor vehicle accidents. Piercings and tattoos are "IN," leaving infection as a possibility. Health Promotion programs should be developed to make adolescents aware of STD's, contraception, and the effect of drugs and alcohol on the body.

I **IDENTITY**–Adolescents may be struggling for a sense of identity. They are making important choices regarding college or career.

R **ROLE DIFFUSION**–Who are they and what are their goals? Educate families and schools regarding these struggles.

S **SEPARATION FROM PEERS**–Peer interaction may be encouraged during their hospitalization.

PAIRS

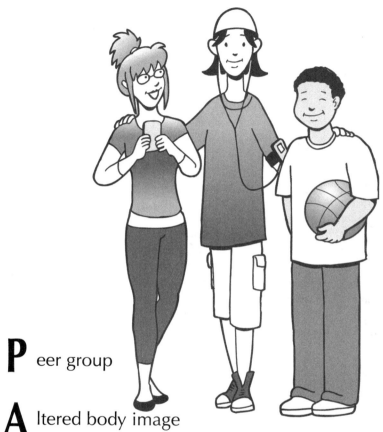

P eer group

A ltered body image

I dentity—Image

R ole diffusion

S eparation from peers

©2010 I CAN Publishing, Inc.

Young Adulthood (19 to 40 Years)

This developmental period includes adults from 19-40 years of age. **"INTIMACY"** has been developed as your strategy for organizing the major tasks for this age group based on Erikson's stage, *"Intimacy versus isolation"*. Typically during this period, **mates are selected** and intimate bonds are established. If there was inadequate resolution of the identify crisis during adolescence; however, there may be disturbances in the sex role identity.

As the career or vocation is established, **work takes on a new meaning**, and is important due to the connection with ego identity. Many young adults continue with **additional education tracts. The self-centered tendencies** that occurred in the previous developmental periods become less prominent. The young adult's sense of identity and self are based on appraisal by others. Young adults become more **independent from parents** and begin entering into adult relationships with them. They become more involved in the community working with the social network of peers, and **assume more civic responsibility**.

Health promotion and maintenance that are important for this period include **stress-related illnesses**; alcohol, and drug abuse. Pregnancy is, of course, another issue that would be important to include in the health promotion and maintenance plans of care. At this age, the young adult is fully physically mature and has full mental capacity.

INTIMACY

I ntimacy versus isolation

N ote: work is important due to connecting with ego identity

T he self-centered tendencies become less prominent

I ndependence from parents; Involvement with social network from community

M ates are selected and intimate bonds are established

A ssumes civic responsibility; Appraisals by others affect sense of identity and self

C areer or vocation is established; Conditions common—stress-related illnesses & substance abuse

Y oung adults continue educational tracts

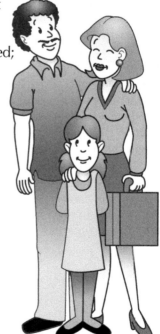

©2014 I CAN Publishing®, Inc.

Middle Adulthood (40 to 60 years)

This developmental period includes adults from 40-60 years of age. "**SANDWICH**" has been developed as your strategy for organizing the major tasks for this age group. Erikson's **developmental task is "Generativity versus Stagnation"**. This mnemonic and image were selected since middle adulthood is focused on assisting children to responsible adulthood while at the same time there is a role reversal with aging parents. This puts the middle adult exactly in the middle just like the meat is in a "**SANDWICH**". In addition to the **responsibility to both assisting children into adulthood** and experiencing a role reversal with **aging parents**, another major task during this period is reassessment of life goals.

Cognitive skills peak and creativity are at the maximum. While this is the stage where adults are at the **peak of vocational responsibilities, leisure time does begin to take on a new concern. Spouses and close friends** are the major companions in social activities. Many adults during this stage **conduct a vocational self-analysis**. During this period, retirement may occur. Community involvement increases due to the changes in the roles during this developmental period. The role of grand parenting may also be defined during this developmental period.

Health promotion and maintenance that are important for this period include menopause in addition to chronic health problems such as cancer and diabetes, etc. Many physiological changes **occur with organs. Special screening is important** (i.e., colon, breast, BP, mammograms, etc.) during this period. Regular physical exercise, regular dental visits, and immunizations as indicated should be included in the health promotion plan. A healthy life style including good nutrition, exercise, stress reduction, decrease in alcohol intake, and no tobacco should be encouraged.

SANDWICH

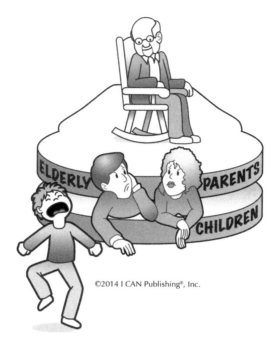

S pecial screening important (i.e., colon, breast, etc.)

A ffirms quality of relationships or lack of

N ote that this stage is at peak of vocational responsibilities

D evelopmental stage is Generativity versus Stagnation

W atch for many organ system changes

I nteractions (social) are rich due to life experiences

C onduct vocational self analysis

H obbies and leisure activities become more important; has responsibility of children and older parents

Older Adulthood (60 to 85 Years)

This developmental period includes adults from 60-85 years of age. "**ACCEPT**" has been developed as your strategy for organizing the major tasks for this age group based on Erikson's stage, "*Ego integrity versus despair*". Typically, if an older adult views life as worthwhile, then there will be a more positive response to aging, and will "**ACCEPT**" **the physical changes** that occur during this period.

Much of **the past time is spent on reminiscing over life** while **conducting a life review**! The favorable outcome with this process is wisdom that leads to an active concern, yet a feeling of being detached with life while in the face of death. Many older adults have lost a spouse, child, or family member. Death is realistic; however, older adults typically have a philosophic concept of death. This assists the older client with the **preparation for death**.

During this developmental period, the older adult accepts the many physical changes that occur such as alterations in all major body systems. Health promotion and maintenance that are important for this period include safety concerns such as the risk of falls due to alteration in the sensory input, polypharmacy, alterations in cognitive abilities, the use of canes, walkers, etc.

Family members and older adults need to be informed that acute **confusion may be indicative of medication reaction, infection, or fluid and electrolyte imbalance.** Older adults do not present the same as the younger adult. For example, since there is an altered pain perception, they may not experience dysuria if there is a urinary tract infection or discomfort if they have pneumonia. The first symptom may be acute confusion in contrast to fever or pain that would be the first symptom for the younger client.

The ultimate goal for this developmental period is to direct health promotion activities at supporting chronic conditions, promoting health, and promoting independence in activities of daily living and instrumental activities of daily living. This will assist the older client to "**ACCEPT**" the final changes that occur in life.

ACCEPT

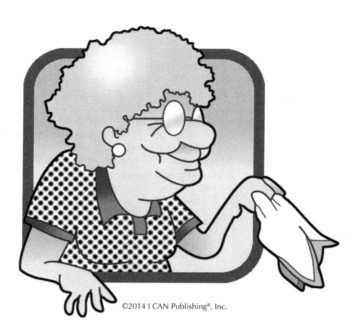

A ccepts physical changes

C onducts a life review

C onfusion that is acute may be indicative of medication reaction, infection, fluid and electrolyte imbalance

E go integrity versus despair

P reparation for death

T he past time is spent on reminiscing over life

Geriatrics (85 Years and Over)

This developmental period includes adults from 85 years of age and over. "**GERIATRIC**" has been developed as your strategy for organizing the major concepts that need priority attention during this age group.

One of the first concepts being a major concern for the adult who is over 85 years of age is the risk for **anxiety**. Many of these individuals are all alone. One ninety-five-year-old client I worked with said, *"Honestly, all of my friends have died and are in heaven. I have lived so long that I am afraid they must think I didn't get in!"* She had such a fun sense of humor. If we take time with our older clients, there is a lot to learn from them. Unfortunately, another challenge that can be a concern for this age is **abuse**. Elder abuse is very unfortunate, but it does occur. As a nurse practitioner, I can still remember elderly clients who had not been bathed for days brought in to the emergency room by their family members. In fact, they had not even had a warm meal for the same period of time. Their adult children who lived in the same neighborhood would not take them to their Dr's appointments consistently. This is abuse!! *What kind of message are we teaching our children, when we do not have time for our elders?*

A major risk for this developmental period is **falls**. This is such an important concept that we have a tool in this book dedicated to "FALL RISK."

Interdisciplinary collaboration is an important component of care for this developmental period. Many of these clients may be alone or going home after experiencing a life changing illness such as a cerebral vascular accident. The client may need assistance with dietary needs; occupational therapy to assist with independence; and/or physical therapy to assist with maintaining optimal level of activity, etc.

Assess skin integrity; plan to prevent skin breakdown. The difference in the skin assessment for the older adult is the skin is dry and flaking, and can develop excoriation from scratching. There may be a decrease in wound healing due to the alteration in the protein intake. There may also be evidence of bruising. Do not wait for the reddened area to occur prior to preventive measures being initiated. Risk factors include prolonged pressure caused by immobility, malnutrition, hypoproteinemia, vitamin deficiency, infection, excessive skin moisture, and/or equipment such as traction devices, restraints, etc. Due to the importance of this concept, we have included a strategy to assist you in, *"Priority Care for Decreasing Altered Skin Integrity."*

The nurse should **teach family and client** (e.g., care, activities, restrictions, medications, etc.) SAFE care is always the priority for these clients.

The nurse should be competent with **providing report (SBAR)**; reporting unsafe care; making referrals both while the client is in the hospital as well as during the discharge and at home. Refer to Management section to review *"Providing and Receiving Report," "Reporting Unsafe Care,"* and *"Making Referrals."*

The review for the impact **of infection, fluid and electrolyte imbalance and acute confusion for the geriatric client** will be reviewed on the page regarding the, **Priority Nursing Care for Geriatrics "FAN CAPES."**

GERIATRIC

G erontology organized around the framework of "FANCAPES"

E valuate for abuse/anxiety

R isk for falls

I nterdisciplinary collaboration

A ssess skin integrity, plan to prevent skin breakdown

T each family and client (care, activities, restrictions, medications, etc.)

R eport (SBAR); Unsafe care, referrals, discharge, etc.

I mpact of infection, fluid and electrolyte imbalance, etc.

C onfusion (Acute) - present

©2014 I CAN Publishing®, Inc.

Priority Nursing Care For Geriatrics

Adequate **fluid** intake can be difficult for the elderly, especially if they have dementia, are depressed, or physically unable to maintain good fluid intake. One of the aging changes is the perception of thirst declines. Many times the elderly will decrease their fluid intake to manage their urinary frequency. The elderly client should take in a minimal of 1500 mL of fluids daily unless there is a contraindication from a disease.

The adequacy of **aeration** should be assessed in the elderly client by reviewing the health history, vital signs, looking at the tissues and noting signs and symptoms such as dyspnea, tachypnea, etc. To ensure adequate ventilation, the nurse must help make respiratory exercises a daily routine and link them to other routines. Respiratory infections must be prevented by encouraging client to take the influenza and pneumonia vaccines; and avoiding exposure to individuals with respiratory infections. The elderly should be taught to report changes in the characteristics of the sputum. Yoga can also optimize the pulmonary and circulatory systems.

Nutrition is an important part of the care for the elderly client. The nurse should encourage a diet low in fat and high in fiber, iron, vitamin C, and thiamine with adequate sources of calcium. If bed rest is prescribed, it is imperative to increase fluids to as high as 3 or 4 L/day to prevent renal calculi, unless client has a condition such as congestive heart failure that would contraindicate this increase in fluids. Due to the alteration in taste and decrease in the digestive function, these may alter nutrition for the elderly client. The logical sequence of eating food is biting, chewing, and swallowing. New denture wearers should be encouraged to change the order to drink liquid first, then chew soft foods, and then bite into regular foods. Due to stress incontinence and nocturia, clients may restrict fluids intentionally. Constipation can be a chronic problem due to ↓ in peristalsis. The ↑ intake of fluids and ↑ fiber diet will assist with this discomfort. Poor nutrition may be as a result of depression and loneliness.

The ability to **communicate** is an essential ingredient for social interaction. Due to the intrinsic and extrinsic factors, older adults may experience obstacles in their interaction. Hearing and visual impairment may both have an impact on interaction. Nurses need to educate people not to shout, since it raises the frequency of the voice. Presbycusis and/or impacted cerumen can cause speech to be inaudible. Nurses need to develop supportive plans to facilitate communication. **Cognitive** function is highly individualized based on the health status of the client, experiences, and personal resources. Refer to *"Differences between Delirium/Dementia"* in the Psychosocial chapter.

Activities/abilities should be encouraged. Support in keeping the elder client's pain under control include guided imagery, warm soaks, yoga, and/or massage. If these do not work, begin with the weakest analgesic and gradually increase as necessary. **Polypharmacy** can be a major issue, so it is very important to review all meds and evaluate for interactions.

Due to alteration in **elimination** (renal function), potassium and protein intake should be evaluated and monitored. Caution should also be used with NSAIDS, aminoglycosides, etc. Metformin (Glucophage) may result in lactic acidosis for these clients.

Skin care will be addressed on several separate pages in the book. Nurses can demonstrate a caring attitude and attention to spiritual needs by asking the client about their desires such as arranging for a visit from the clergy, providing a Bible or rosary, offering to pray, etc. Nurses need to be aware that older clients can be easily awakened by noise and lighting associated with staff activities during the night. Regular exercise, exposure to sunlight during the day, and noncaffeinated herbal teas at bedtime are other measures to help elders fall **asleep**.

FAN CAPES

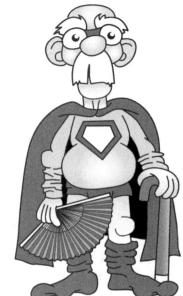

F luid

A eration

N utrition

C ommunication/Cognition

A ctivity/Abilities

P ain/Polypharmacy

E limination

S kin/Spirituality/Social support/Sleep

©2014 I CAN Publishing®, Inc.

Immunizations

Those immunizations! "Nurses think they are hot shots giving us babies those shots! Let me see if there is a way that I can delay getting these immunizations!"

I   **IMMUNIZATION STATUS** (what has been given before)

M   **MMR** made with eggs–do not give with allergy to eggs or neomycin

M   **MUST** be without fever

U   **UPDATE** with new vaccines available

N   **NEVER** give in gluteals (thighs and deltoids)

I   **IMMUNE SUPPRESSION** disqualifies attenuated live vaccine, MMR, varicella, and tuberculosis

Z   **"ZEIZURE"** disorders must be controlled before administration

E   **EVALUATE** sites for local reaction

D   **DOCUMENT**–site, lot number, parental consent, and RN signature

If child is diagnosed with leukemia, HIV infection, or is receiving a high dose of steroids, wait 3 months after therapy has stopped. Measles vaccine is recommended for asymptomatic HIV-infected children.

IMMUNIZED

I mmunization status

M MR made from eggs

M ust be without fever

U pdate with new vaccines available

N ever give in gluteals

I mmune suppression disqualifies

Z eizure disorders must be controlled

E valuate sites

D ocument

©1994 I CAN Publishing, Inc.

Diagnostics For The Maternity Client

Ultrasonography: The test is a noninvasive procedure that uses high-frequency pulse sound waves. These are transmitted via a transducer that is directly applied to the abdomen of the maternity client. This can also be done transvaginally. This is performed to assist in determining placental location for amniocentesis or placenta previa; gestational age; determine multiple gestations; evaluate fetal growth; or evaluate the volume of the amniotic fluid. There is no specific time for this procedure to be performed during pregnancy. The client needs to have a full bladder unless the procedure is being done to locate the placenta prior to an amniocentesis. The preferred position for the procedure is the supine position; the test takes approximately 20 to 30 minutes. A full bladder is not required for the transvaginal test. The client will be in the lithotomy position for this procedure.

Amniocentesis: An invasive procedure to obtain amniotic fluid. The indications for this diagnostic procedure are to evaluate for a chromosomal abnormality (i.e., neural tube defects such as spina bifida, etc). The procedure may be performed between 14 to 16 weeks. If the procedure is performed in the last trimester, it is to determine the lecithin/sphingomyelin (L/S) ratio (components of a protein that comprises surfactant). The ratio should be 2:1 or greater indicating sufficient surfactant. This typically would occur at approximately 35 weeks' gestation. Prior to the needle entry into the client's abdomen, the placenta is located by using an ultrasound; the needle site will be anesthetized, and amniotic fluid will be aspirated and sent to lab for testing. Complications are rare (less than 1%); however, they are possible. These would include discomfort at the needle site. Although a hematoma on the abdominal wall or risk for a miscarriage is very rare, the nurse should assess for these. If the mother is Rh-negative, Rhogam is administered after the procedure to minimize the risk of hemolysis of fetal blood cells. The fetal heart rate must be carefully assessed prior to and following the amniocentesis.

Nonstress test (NST) is done to observe the response of fetal heart rate to the stress of activity. Client may be in a semi-Fowler's position; the external monitor is applied to evaluate fetal activity; mother activates the "mark button" on the electronic fetal monitor when fetal movement is felt. If there is no fetal movement, the abdomen may be gently rubbed or palpated to stimulate movement; or the client may be asked to eat a light meal since blood glucose increases fetal activity. Any deceleration during the procedure must be reported to the physician.

> **I CAN TESTING HINT:** A NONREACTIVE NONSTRESS test is NOT good! A REACTIVE test is REAL good!

Contraction Stress Test (CST): This procedure is performed to assess the FHR response to the oxytocin-induced uterine contractions. Be on the outlook for late decelerations during this test. This test is all about evaluating potential hypoxia to the fetus. If the reading shows late decelerations (POSITIVE TEST) with at least two of the three contractions, this may indicate the possibility of insufficient placental respiratory reserve, indicating fetal hypoxia! The breast self-stimulation contraction stress test may be done instead of administering the oxytocin. This will produce endogenous oxytocin as a result of the stimulation of the breasts or nipples.

> **I CAN TESTING HINT:** A CST that is positive and the NST is nonreactive are most likely indicating fetal hypoxia! The desired outcomes for these tests would be a NEGATIVE CST with a NST that is REACTIVE!

DIAGNOSTICS FOR THE MATERNITY CLIENT

"DIAGNOSTIC" exams can be hazardous to the health of our clients.

It is our mission to keep them safe!

The designated NCLEX® standards are outlined below to assist you in organizing the assessments, nursing interventions, and evaluation that must be incorporated into our critical thinking and clinical reasoning for clients experiencing a diagnostic procedure, treatment, or laboratory procedure.

D iagnostic test results—monitor; intervene for complications.

I njury and/or complications from procedure should be prevented.

A ssist with invasive procedures (e.g., thoracentesis, bronchoscopy).

G lucose monitoring, ECG, O_2 saturation, etc. may be performed.

N ote client's response to procedures and treatments.

O btain specimens other than blood (e.g., wound, stool, etc.).

S igns and symptoms of trends and/or changes-monitor, and intervene.

T each client and family about procedures and treatments.

I dentify vital signs and monitor for changes and intervene.

C omplications should be noted and followed immediately with an action.

This image is to remind you that "Sure Look" Holmes is looking into the hippo's mouth to assure he is safe! Just as "Sure Look" Holmes, the nurse is not responsible for ordering these tests, but to maintain client SAFETY prior to, during, and after these diagnostics have been completed.

©2014 I CAN Publishing®, Inc.

Normal Discomforts During Pregnancy

- **B** **B**ackaches–Advise the client to maintain correct posture and wear shoes with low-heal. Teach client to do pelvic tilt exercises.
  Breast tenderness–Advise client to wear a well-supportive bra. Discuss the need to avoid using soap on the nipple and areola area.
- **A** **A**norexia, nausea & vomiting may occur in the first trimester. This morning sickness can be supported by frequent small meals. Recommend client to eat crackers in between meals with no fluid. The client should also take vitamin B_6 supplement. Assess weight, UO, and signs of hyperemesis. Teach to notify HCP if unable to eat/drink for > 24 hours, urine becomes dark and decreases, and/or heart rate pounds, or client experiences vertigo.
- **C** **C**onstipation may be relieved by increasing fluid intake of 6-8 glasses/day, and eating foods high in roughage including fruits. Review the importance of exercising daily and may use prescribed stool softeners.
- **K** (**C**)ontractions–Braxton Hicks indicate false labor. They may become uncomfortable, especially at night. The discomfort is typically located in the abdomen. True labor is where the contractions occur at regular intervals and increase with walking. This pain is in the back and radiates around to the abdomen.
- **A** **A**nemia (*pseudoanemia*) may occur due to the increase in blood volume during pregnancy. There is an increase in the blood volume starting in the first trimester and peaking in the middle of the third trimester at about 40% to 50% above pre-pregnant levels. This extra volume serves as a reserve for the loss of blood during labor. The stimulation of the bone marrow leads to a 20% to 30% increase in the total red blood cell volume. As a result of the plasma volume increase being more than the red blood cells, this may result in hemodilution, typically referred to as physiologic anemia of pregnancy (*pseudoanemia*). A multi-vitamin with iron is included in the plan of care for this change during pregnancy. The client is also advised to eat foods high in iron. Review with the client the importance of taking frequent rest periods during the day to support the feeling of fatigue.
- **C** **C**ramping in legs is a common discomfort during pregnancy. Recommended plans for the discomfort include: dorsiflex foot; stretch affected muscle and hold until cramping subsides; discuss applying warm packs; maintain appropriate calcium intake.
- **H** **H**eartburn is a discomfort that can be relieved by avoiding fried and fatty foods. Discuss the importance of eating small meals; maintaining appropriate posture by sitting and standing upright. The pregnant client has urinary frequency. Recommend that client voids frequently; decrease fluid prior to going to bed; avoid caffeinated or carbonated beverages. The client could use a perineal pad for leakage. Teach client Kegel exercises. Assess for UTI. Review the importance of voiding frequently and the need not to decrease fluids throughout the day. Discuss the importance of notifying HCP if client develops dysuria, foul-smelling or cloudy urine, and/or flank pain.
- **E** **E**dema in lower extremities is a frequent discomfort. (Cardiovascular; varicose veins): Avoid prolonged sitting or standing; apply support stockings before getting up. When sitting, elevate feet.
- **S** **S**hortness of breath (SOB) in last trimester may be relieved by correct posture; encourage periods throughout the day to rest. Position while resting in semi-Fowler's. Rise slowly from a supine position to minimize supine hypotension.

BACKACHES

B ackaches, breast tenderness

A norexia, nausea & vomiting in first trimester

C onstipation

K (C)ontractions (Braxton Hicks)

A nemia (Hemodilutional)

C ramping in legs

H eartburn, has urinary frequency, may experience hemorrhoids

E dema in lower extremities; epistaxis

S hortness of breath (SOB) in last trimester; supine hypotension

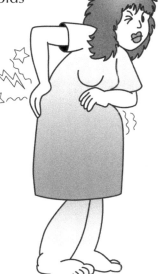

Danger Signs in Pregnancy

Visualize in your mind (or on next page) a pregnant woman who is experiencing some complications in her pregnancy. Her car will not start, so she calls a cab to take her to the hospital. The word "**CABS**" will help you remember these complications.

C **CHILLS AND FEVER**–Indicative of an infection, and is never normal during pregnancy.

CEREBRAL DISTURBANCES–Headaches during pregnancy can indicate severe preeclampsia.

A **ABDOMINAL PAIN**–Abdominal pain (epigastric area) may be due to edema of the liver capsule and may indicate a convulsion is impending. A rigid, board-like abdomen during the last trimester usually indicates abruptio placenta.

B **BLURRED VISION**–Visual disturbances may indicate hypertension elevated.

BLOOD PRESSURE ELEVATION is a complication with severe preeclampsia.

BLEEDING–Early bleeding could indicate a miscarriage, abortion, ectopic pregnancy or hydatiform mole. Bleeding in the last trimester may be indicative of placenta previa or abruptio placenta.

S **SWELLING**–Edema especially in the periorbital and digital areas is indicative of mild preeclampsia. Watch for **SUDDEN ESCAPE OF FLUID** (rupture of membranes)!

CABS

C hills and fever
cerebral disturbances

A bdominal pain

B lurred vision
blood pressure
bleeding

S welling
sudden escape of fluid

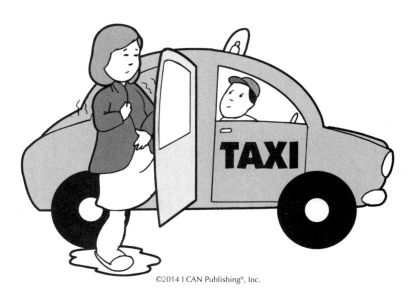

Pregnancy-Induced Hypertension

This condition is specifically associated with pregnancy, preeclampsia and eclampsia. When you think about the priority nursing care with this disorder, think about **PEACE**. It is of paramount importance to provide a peaceful environment to prevent seizure activity.

P **PROMOTE BEDREST, QUIET ENVIRONMENT**–These are crucial. In severe preeclampsia, absolute bedrest and sedatives (Valium) are important.

E **ENSURE HIGH PROTEIN INTAKE**–Due to proteinuria, protein intake should be increased in the diet. Sodium intake should remain normal. Avoid diuretics.

A **ANTIHYPERTENSIVE DRUG**–(Aldomet) methyldopa widely considered first line in pregnancy may be used to decrease the blood pressure. It's safe since it doesn't cross the placental membrane. Check maternal BP, pulse and FHR.

C **CONVULSION**–Prevent or control seizures. Administer IV Magnesium Sulfate. Have the antidote, calcium gluconate at the bedside for emergencies. Decrease the environmental stimuli.

E **EVALUATE PHYSICAL PARAMETER**–Evaluate for complications of magnesium sulfate toxicity.

PEACE

P romote bedrest, quiet environment

E nsure high protein intake (1g/kg/day)

A ntihpertensive drug: (Aldomet) methyldopa, widely considered first line in pregnancy

C onvulsions (Magnesium Sulfate)

E valuate physical parameters
    1. Blood pressure
    2. Urine output
    3. Respirations
    4. Patella reflex

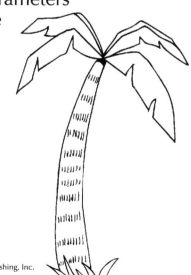

Magnesium Sulfate Toxicity

Magnesium Sulfate is the drug given to women to prevent seizures with the complication of pregnancy-induced hypertension (PIH). This medicine is a central nervous system depressant. The antidote is calcium gluconate. How can you remember the signs of too much of this medicine? Just remember that before a client has a seizure they may let out a loud **BURP**! (Do they do this in reality? Not usually; it is only a memory technique.)

Let me introduce you to Bonnie Burp. She has the following problems:

- **B** BLOOD PRESSURE DECREASED
- **U** URINE OUTPUT DECREASED
- **R** RESPIRATIONS DECREASED
- **P** PATELLA REFLEX ABSENT

Bonnie is predisposed to these side effects because magnesium sulfate is a central nervous system depressant. It acts by blocking the neuromuscular transmission.

Warning: Magnesium Sulfate cannot be used with some anesthetics as it paralyzes the client without sedation. In this situation, we must keep the client sedated.

MAGNESIUM SULFATE TOXICITY

B lood pressure decreased

U rine output decreased

R espirations < 12

P atella reflex absent

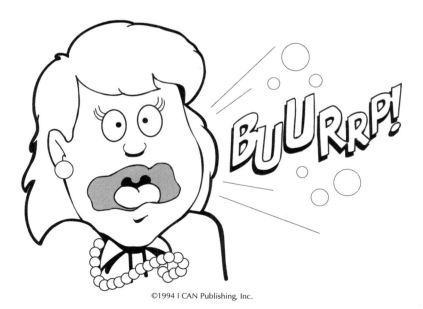

Gestational Diabetes

Gestational diabetes is classified as Type 3. The onset of this occurs during pregnancy and returns to normal glucose tolerance after delivery. The symptoms present as any client with diabetes where there is a significant increase in the 3 Ps: **polyphagia, polydipsia, and polyuria**. During the first trimester, hypoglycemia may actually occur; there is a decrease in the need for insulin during this trimester. Once the placenta is fully developed with active hormones that can make cells insulin resistant, then the client may **experience hyperglycemia in the second and third trimesters. Oral hypoglycemic agents are NOT used** to control diabetes in the pregnant client who had pregestational diabetes.

Antepartum period for GDM mother has a focus on monitoring **fetal and maternal well-being**. Home blood glucose monitoring; Diet: well balanced and no skipping of meals or snacks; exercise as prescribed.

Intrapartum period for GDM: As long as there is evidence of adequate placental function and the infant's response to stress is appropriate, the pregnancy will be **progress to term with an expected vaginal delivery**. During this period, the mother may need rapid acting insulin IV. Fetal monitoring will occur during labor.

In the postpartum period, metabolic and endocrine changes will occur rapidly after delivery. During this time, the insulin requirements for the mother will significantly decrease and will continue to fluctuate over the next few weeks. GDM mother's **glucose returns to normal after delivery**.

- **F** **Fetal** and maternal well being—monitor ongoing.
- **E** **Expect** insulin requirements to increase during 2nd and 3rd trimester.
- **T** **The** medication of choice is insulin. There is limited use of glyburide (DiaBeta) at this time.
- **A** **Anticipate** a vaginal delivery as long as there is adequate placental profusion.
- **L** **Look** for hypoglycemia during postpartum; insulin requirements will decrease.

FETAL

F etal and maternal well being—monitor ongoing

E xpect insulin requirements to increase during 2nd and 3rd trimester

T he medication of choice is insulin. There is limited use of glyburide (DiaBeta) at this time.

A nticipate a vaginal delivery

L ook for hypoglycemia during postpartum; insulin requirements will decrease

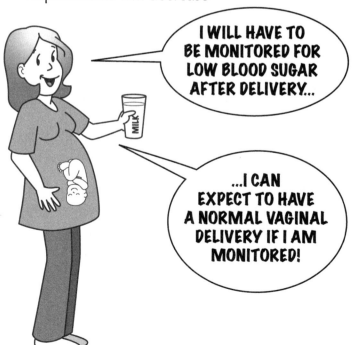

Decelerations

"**VEAL CHOP**" has been around for many years. It is a simple method to assist you in remembering which pathophysiology is occurring with each deceleration. Notice that the decelerations are outlined on the left spelling "**VEAL**" chop and the pathophysiology is on the right spelling veal "**CHOP**".

Each deceleration is outlined with the specific physiological changes that occur with the rhythm strips. The term and definition will be briefly reviewed below. The next few pages will provide you with another visual strategy to assist in reviewing each deceleration, the physiological implications to the fetus, and the priority nursing care.

V **Variable decelerations** indicate a complication with umbilical **cord compression**. The abrupt decrease of the fetal heart rate (FHR) is below baseline for greater than or equal to 15 seconds and less than 2 minutes.

E **Early decelerations** indicate a complication with **head compression**. This gradual decrease of the FHR will return to baseline associated with contractions. Onset, maximal fall, and recovery correlate with onset, peak, and end of contraction.

A **Acceleration** may occur during fetal movement and typically indicates fetal well-being and great **oxygenation**. The abrupt increase in FHR above the baseline rate of 15 beats/min or greater may last for 15 seconds or more.

L **Late decelerations** typically indicate **placenta/uterus insufficiency**. There is a gradual decrease (onset to lowest point {nadir} greater than or equal to 30 seconds) of FHR below the baseline. Typically, the onset, nadir, and recovery of the deceleration occur after the onset, peak, and recovery of the contractions.

Author of this powerful strategy is unknown.

VEAL CHOP

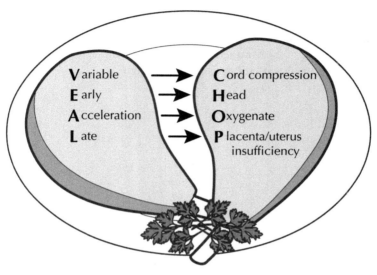

Fetal Heart Decelerations: Early Detections

What is happening? As you can see on the next page, there is pressure on the head of the fetus. The difference in this **EARLY DECELERATION** in contrast to a **LATE DECELERATION** is that the onset, fall and recovery of the heart rate coincide with the onset, peak and end of the contraction. This does not indicate a problem and usually occurs during the active phase of labor.

EARLY DECELERATIONS: HEAD COMPRESSION

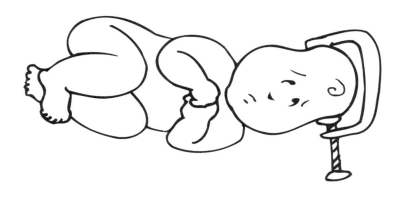

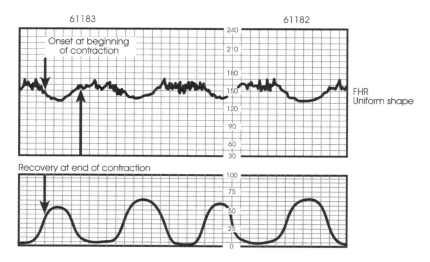

©2008 I CAN Publishing, Inc.

Fetal Heart Decelerations: Variable Decelerations

VARIABLE DECELERATIONS are usually shaped like a V or a squared U. These may occur any time during the contraction cycle or may be nonrepetitive. The pathophysiology is cord compression. The nursing care is to change the position of the mother. If it lasts more than one minute, attempt upward displacement of presenting part. Mother may be placed in the knee-chest position or Trendelenburg position. This pattern may indicate a prolapsed cord. If this is the case, prepare for immediate delivery. To assist with fetal oxygenation, the nurse may give the mother oxygen.

VARIABLE DECELERATIONS: CORD COMPRESSION

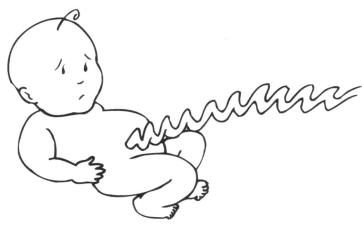

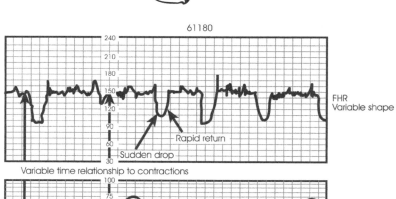

FHR
Variable shape

Rapid return
Sudden drop
Variable time relationship to contractions

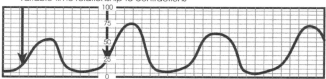

©2008 I CAN Publishing, Inc.

Fetal Heart Decelerations: Late Decelerations

LATE DECELERATIONS look similar to early decelerations but are offset to the right. They begin at about the peak of the contraction, and the nadir occurs well after the peak of the contraction. The cause of these is uteroplacental insufficiency. The focus will be on the nursing care on the pages following the rhythm strip.

LATE DECELERATIONS: UTEROPLACENTAL INSUFFICIENCY

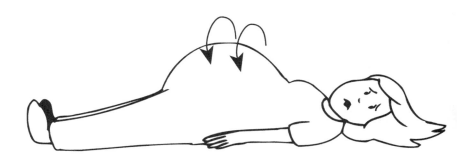

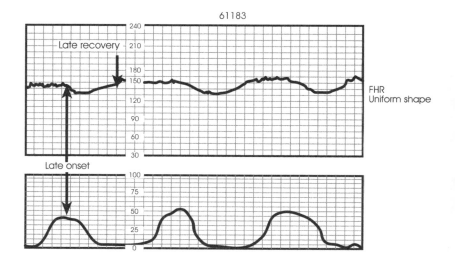

©2008 I CAN Publishing, Inc.

Late Decelerations

The Fire Department has come to the rescue of **FETAL DISTRESS**, and is planning to put out the problem. First, however, they must **UNCOIL** the fire hose. What does a late deceleration look like and what does it mean? It is a uniform shaped dip. The onset coincides with the peak of the contraction with the recovery occurring at the end or after the end of the contraction. It indicates uteroplacental insufficiency. If the fire department does not do something soon, the fetus is going to get into severe distress.

C **CHANGE POSITION**–Place mother in the left lateral position. For supine hypotension, change the maternal position.

O **OXYGEN**–Administer oxygen to mother to correct the uteroplacental insufficiency. If **OXYTOCIN** is infusing, stop the infusion. This may be causing uterine hyperactivity resulting in uteroplacental insufficiency.

I **IV FLUIDS**–Epidurals may cause dilation. Increasing hydration with IV fluids will increase the maternal blood pressure and the uteroplacental circulation.

L **LOWER THE HEAD OF THE BED** and elevate the feet to increase perfusion to the uterus.

LATE DECELERATIONS

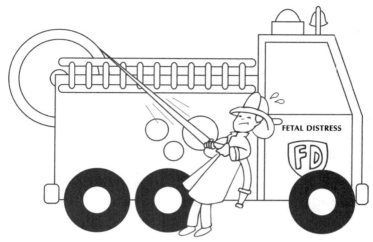

Reprinted with permission ©1994 Martha Eakes

U

N

C hange position (left side)

O xygen
xytocin—off

I V fluids

L ower head

Pitocin

"**Pitty Pitocin**," this pregnant woman, is slow to begin active labor, so the Doc decides to induce by using **PITOCIN**. Watch for those major side effects!

Visualize Pitty sitting in a row boat looking into a **PIT** watching the "TETANIC" sink into the "ocean" (**OCIN**). Complications of this drug are **TETANIC CONTRACTIONS**. Pitocin of course is a stimulant; so as Pitty watches the ship sink, her blood **PRESSURE** elevates! Just as a sinking ship takes in all that salty WATER, poor Pitty is left holding the excess fluid in her body (observe **INTAKE** and **OUTPUT**). She gets so nervous with all this happening that she goes into **CARDIAC ARRHYTHMIAS** causing Pitty's baby **OXYGEN** hunger and **FETAL HEART IRREGULARITIES**. This is so upsetting to Pitty that she gets **NAUSEATED** and **VOMITS** all over the row boat.

STOP THAT PITOCIN DRIP!!!!

SIDE EFFECTS OF OXYTOCIN (PITOCIN)

Pressure is elevated

Intake and output

Tetanic contractions

Oxygen decrease in fetus

Cardiac arrhythmia

Irregularity in fetal heart rate

Nausea and vomiting

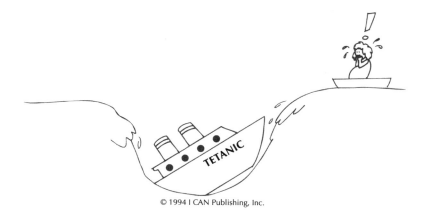

Regional Anesthesia

Regional anesthesia is used to anesthetize one **REGION** of the body; the client may remain awake and alert throughout the procedure. The image used will assist in recalling nursing care for the different **REGIONS** of the body.

- **R RESPIRATORY PARALYSIS**–Have ventilatory support equipment available. Avoid the extreme Trendelenburg position before level of anesthesia is set.

- **E ELIMINATION**–Evaluate the bladder for distention. When the epidural is done on a pregnant woman, labor may be delayed due to bladder distention.

- **G GASTROINTESTINAL**–Check when client last ate. Position to prevent aspiration. Antiemetics need to be available along with suction equipment.

- **I INFORM OF PROCEDURE**–Does the client understand the procedure? Check for drug allergies, make sure legal permit is signed and have client empty bladder.

- **O OBSERVE FOR HYPOTENSION**–Report B/P less than 100 systolic, or any significant decrease. Change client's position, administer oxygen and increase IV rate if client is not prone to CHF.

- **N NO TRAUMA TO EXTREMITIES**–Support extremities during movement. Remove legs from stirrups together.

ANESTHESIA

R espiratory paralysis

E limination

G I

I nform of procedure

O bserve for hypotension

N o trauma to the extremities

Inform of procedure

Respiratory paralysis

Observe for hypotension

G I

Elimination

No trauma to the extremities

©1994 I CAN Publishing, Inc.

Postpartum Assessment

If a parent's newborn is a daughter, the parent must "**BUBBLE**" the newborn during and after feedings. This will assist you with reviewing the postpartum assessment.

- **B BREAST**–Assess for and prevent mastitis. Teach how to cleanse breasts and nipples. Support with breast feeding.

  BLOOD PRODUCT, Rhogam, should be administered at 28 weeks, and within 72 hours after delivery.

- **U UTERUS**–Fundus should be firm and in the midline. Immediately after delivery, the top of the fundus is several finger breadths above the umbilicus. The fundus then descends into the pelvis approximately one finger breadth per day. Massage the fundus if it is boggy.

- **B BLADDER**–Observe for bladder distention; it may displace the uterus. Diuresis occurs during the first two postpartal days. Evaluate for UTI.

- **B BOWEL**–Stool softeners or laxatives may be necessary. By second or third day post delivery, normal bowel movements should occur.

- **L LOCHIA**–Should not have foul odor. Rubra (dark red first 3 days), serosa (pinkish, serosanguinous 3-10 days) and alba (creamy or yellowish after 10th day and may last a week or two).

- **E EPISIOTOMY**–Observe for infection and healing.

  EMOTIONAL–Support is a must!

POSTPARTUM ASSESSMENT

B reast
B lood product

U terus

B ladder

B owel

L ochia

E pisiotomy
E motional

Reprinted with permission ©1994 Martha Eakes

Neonate Assessments: "The 4 Hs"

The respiratory and circulatory systems for a neonate must rapidly adjust from being dependent to independent. The establishment of respiratory function with the cutting of the umbilical cord is the MOST critical extra-uterine adjustment as air inflates the lungs with the first breath.

With these extrauterine adjustments, the newborn must be assessed for signs and symptoms of complications, "**The 4 Hs**". The first "**H**" is "**HYPOXIA**", respiratory complications.

In order to assist the newborn with airway patency and oxygenation, the neonate may be positioned with the head slightly lower than chest. A bulb syringe may be used to suction the nostrils and oropharynx if needed.

Abnormal sounds–Expiratory grunting Respiratory distress (Hypoxia)– "**GRUNTS**": **G**runting, **R**etracting and **R**estless, **U**ninterested in feeding, **N**asal flaring, **T**achycardia (murmur) and **T**achypnea, **S**tridor (*Refer to Symptoms of Hypoxia in an Infant "GRUNTS" for more specifics in the Cardiac section.*)

"**HYPOGLYCEMIA**" frequently occurs in the first few hours of life secondary to the use of energy to establish respirations and maintain body heat. Newborns of mothers who have diabetes mellitus, may be small or large for gestational age, are typically less than 37 weeks of gestation, or greater than 42 weeks of gestation are at risk for hypoglycemia and should have a serum glucose drawn within the first 2 hours of life. They may present with the "**JITTERS**".

Jitteriness, **I**ncreased high-pitched cry, lethargy, **T**witching, **T**he heel stick blood glucose level < 40 mg/dL, **E**ye rolling, **R**espirations irregular, **S**eizure.

Treat hypoglycemia immediately by administering 5% Dextrose in Water intravenously if the infant is not able to tolerate po feedings.

The neonate must be assessed for signs and symptoms of "**HYPOTHERMIA**". Neonates are at risk for heat loss due to their large body surface related to body mass and decreased body fat. They also do not have the shivering mechanism present at birth. Normal temp is 97.5 to 99 degrees F. Decreased body temp will increase oxygen demand and increase utilization of blood glucose. This can lead to metabolic acidosis. Signs of hypothermia are outlined in "**TEMP**".

- **T** **T**emp: Axillary (Should be at 36.5° to 37.2° C (97.7 to 98.9° F)
- **E** **E**valuate client's color for cyanosis
- **M** **M**aintain client's Temperature & keep warm by covering head with a cap; no procedures until T stable
- **P** **P**ulse, RR–Ongoing evaluation for tachycardia/tachypnea

"**HEMORRHAGE**"–May result from a complication of improper cord care if the cord clamp is not tight enough.

I CAN TESTING HINT: It is normal for the neonate to experience apnea for 10 seconds or present with acrocyanosis. It is NEVER expected for the neonate to present with "GRUNTS", "JITTERS", HYPOTHERMIA, OR HEMORRHAGING!

THE 4 Hs

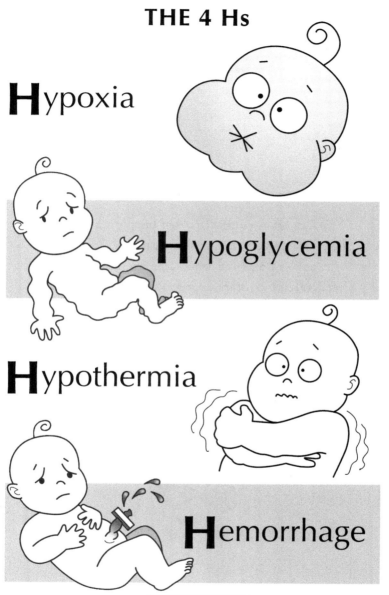

"You can train yourself to see people's strengths. Start focusing on those good qualities. Your entire outlook is poisoned when you operate out of a critical spirit. Start appreciating that person's strengths and learn to downplay the weaknesses."

JOEL OLSTEEN

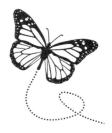

DIETS

Foods High in Folic Acid

Several conditions require a client to eat a diet high in folic acid. Some examples of these are iron deficiency anemia, chronic alcohoism, pregnancy and malnutritional anemia. Here is a visual to help you remember those foods high in Folic Acid.

FOLIC ACID

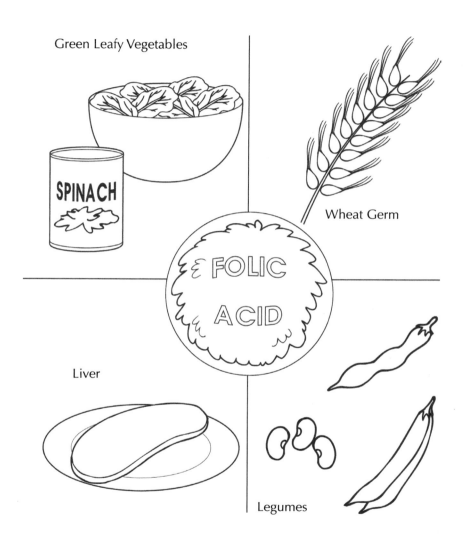

Foods High in Iron

What type of clients need to be on a diet high in iron? If you indicated any of the following, you are right. Clients with hemodilutional anemia who are pregnant, poor dietary intake of iron, surgery of gastrointestinal tract, problems with absorption and clients on IV therapy for 10 days or more need to be on a diet high in iron.

The foods which are high in iron are organ meats (think about an organ that plays music), red meats, fish, green leafy vegetables, raisins (the California Raisin), sunflower seeds and legumes.

IRON

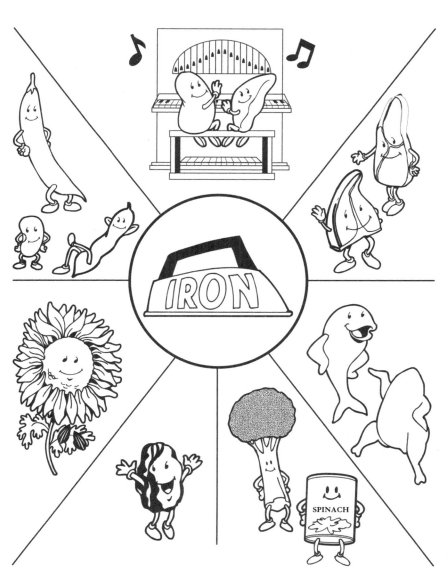

Foods High in Protein

Foods high in protein can easily be remembered if you recall the jingle *Happy To Consume My Calories Sanely*. **H**amburger, **T**una, **C**hicken, **M**ilk, **C**ottage Cheese and **S**oy Beans are high in protein.

PROTEIN

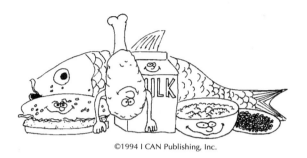

©1994 I CAN Publishing, Inc.

Happy = **H**amburger

To = **T**una

Consume = **C**hicken

My = **M**ilk

Calories = **C**ottage Cheese

Sanely = **S**oy Beans

Foods High in Potassium

An easy way to remember foods high in Potassium (K^+) is the **ABC Fruit** and **Veggie Plate**. Apples, Bananas, Cantaloupe (melons) and Citrus such as orange juice are high in K^+. Asparagus, Broccoli and Carrots are also high in potassium. Another vegetable to remember that is high in potassium is the potato! Teach clients about the **ABC Fruit** and **Veggie Plate,** especially those clients who are taking diuretics.

Clients with severe burns, others who have hypersecretion of the adrenal cortex or on long term steroid therapy will benefit from these foods.

K FOODS =
ABC FRUIT/VEGGIE PLATE

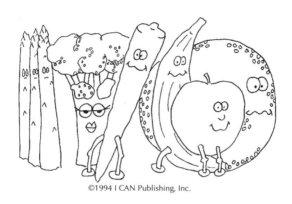

FRUITS
Apples
Bananas
Cantaloupe

VEGGIES
Asparagus
Broccoli
Carrots

Foods High in Sodium

The all-American **HOT DOG**–your way to remember foods that are high in salt (sodium). What is the first thing you must have for a hot dog? A wiener of course. Can't have a hot dog without a wiener and what is a wiener? It's processed meat in a tube that is high in salt.

Now, imagine walking through the delicatessen with us, looking up and seeing all of those tubes of meat hanging from the ceiling. Pressed ham, salami, bologna–all high in salt. Next we need a bun for the wiener. Of course, we put baking soda in our bread to make it rise (soda is salt). Next, comes ketchup which is processed tomatoes that are high in salt. Some folks will mess up a perfectly good hot dog with pickles! Did you ever make pickles? You throw cucumbers into brine (salt water). Those who have to have a chili dog, open a can of chili. Canned foods are usually high in salt. Then of course some of our German friends must have sauerkraut on their dogs which is also high in salt. So, to remember those foods high in sodium, all you have to know is **HOT DOG**!

FOODS HIGH IN SODIUM

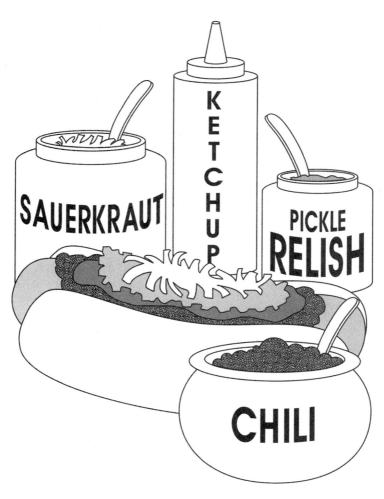

Low-Residue Diet

Daddy had some sort of rectal surgery or diarrhea that makes it a necessity for him to sit on his pillow. Low residue diets are used to reduce fiber and slow bowel movements. Clients with Crohn's disease and colitis may benefit from this particular diet. Here's an easy way to remember the low residue diet.

- **L**   **LIMITED FAT AND FRIED FOODS**
- **O**   **ZERO MILK**
- **R**   **REAL FRESH FISH / UNSEASONED GROUND MEAT**
- **E**   **EGGS BOILED,** not fried
- **S**   **STRAINED FOODS**

As you can see for yourself, this diet is NO FUN for Daddy!

LOW-RESIDUE DIET

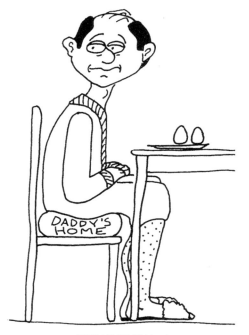

L imited fat

O zero milk

R eal fresh fish/ground meat

E ggs boiled

S trained foods

Celiac Disease Diet

Celiac Disease is an inborn error in metabolism of barley, rye, oat products, and wheat causing malabsorption of some nutrients. Some clients who have gastritis complain of diarrhea, abdominal pain, and bloating.

This diet is known as a gluten-free diet and helps relieve the symptoms. In order to assist you to remember this diet, think of the intestinal flora like the BROW over your eye.

- **B** BARLEY
- **R** RYE
- **O** OATS
- **W** WHEAT

Remember, corn and rice may be substituted for grains in the diet.

CELIAC DIET

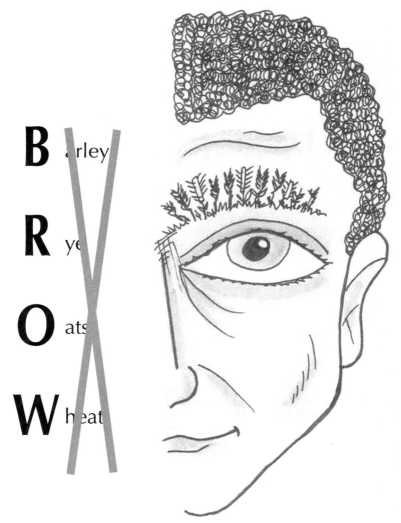

B arley
R ye
O ats
W heat

©2004 I CAN Publishing, Inc.

"We cannot always control our thoughts, but we can control our words, and repetition impresses the subconscious, and we are then master of the situation."

FLORENCE SCOVEL SHINN

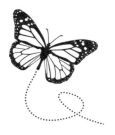

PSYCHOSOCIAL INTEGRITY

Therapeutic Communication

Therapeutic interaction takes place when **TRUST** is established. Think of joining hands with someone special to you. The letters in **TRUST** help us remember the dynamics of therapeutic communication. *Listening is one of our best assessment tools for this section.*

T **TRY EXPRESSION**–Encourage the exploration of thoughts, perceptions, feelings, and actions. Use broad openings and ask open ended questions.

R **REFLECTION OF WORDS**–Confirms to the person that you are actively listening. For example, "I am really mad at my mother for grounding me." "You sound angry because you were grounded."

U **USE OF SILENCE**–Just sit and allow the person to make the next response.

S **SETTING LIMITS**–What type of people may need to have limits set? People with personality and substance abuse disorders, affective disorders, children and spouses.

T **TIME WITH CLIENT**–Taking time with the client allows them to know that you care even if they refuse to communicate.

TRUST

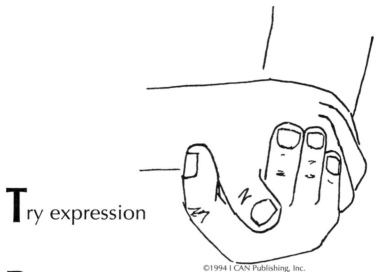

Try expression

Reflection of words

Use of silence

Set limits

Time with client

Communication Strategies For Test Questions

THERAPEUTIC	HYPOMANIA (DEPRESSION)	SUICIDE	MANIC
Try expression **R**eflect **R**apport **U**se silence **S**et limits **T**ime with client	**S**it with client even if silent; practice social skills through role playing if client needs help. **E**xamples vs. asking questions. For example: "I noticed you participated in the meeting today." versus, "Did you attend the meeting?" **L**ong sentences out! Give short, concerte sentences due to problems with focusing. **F**ocus on safe and structured environment. Provide client with a written schedule to provide structure.	**S**leep/rest!!! Self-worth is so important. Show you care! **A** one-one relationship; close observation. Assess if client has a plan to hurt self. Is there an increase in energy level? **F**ocus on removing harmful objects. **E**xecute a contract not to hurt self. Encourage expression of feelings.	**C**alm approach; concise explanations. **A**void power struggles; do not react personally to client's comments; avoid competitive activities. **L**isten to and act on legitimate client concerns; set limits. **M**anipulative behaviors are not reinforced. **S**timulation ↓; quiet room.

Communication Strategies For Test Questions *(cont'd.)*

DELUSIONAL	AGGRESSIVE	POST-TRAUMATIC STRESS	COGNITIVE DISORDERS
Reinforce/clarify **REALITY!** **E**ncourage social interaction. **TRUST!** **A**void arguing with client during a hallucination; acknowledge experience, but do not share in the experience. **L**isten to client; protect from injury when he/she hears "voices" or experiences a "vision".	**S**peak softly, slowly. **A**void asking, "Why"; ask, "What is bothering you?" **F**ew instructions at 1 time. **E**valuate environment for safety. **T**ry to get client to verbalize feelings. **Y**ou should position yourself near the door.	**A**ctive Listening. **A**ssess for suicide. **A**ssist client to develop objectivity about event. **A**ctive problem solving regarding how to handle anger, anxiety, & feelings about event. **A**ctive with group therapy.	**R**oute (Structure) **R**einforcement **R**epetitions **R**eality **R**emoving rugs, cords, etc. **R**eminiscence/Review of life **R**einforce Reality

I CAN TESTING HINT: "*Communication Strategies for Test Questions*" have been developed after working with thousands of nursing students and graduates who have consistently stated, "*We are confused on how to answer questions regarding communication. How do we respond to different clinical situations?*" The chart above starts with the clinical presentation (i.e., depression, suicide, etc.). The larger box reviews the strategy for answering "communication" questions. This chart has evolved with the input from students just like YOU who are now RNs, and have successfully passed the NCLEX®! You CAN do this!!!

Conditions That Must Be Reported As Required By The Law

This technique has been developed to assist you in knowing how to "*Comply with state and/or federal regulations on reporting client conditions (Communicable disease, Abuse, Animal bites, Accidents resulting in death, gunshot/knife wounds, evidence of neglect)*".

This standard can be easily remembered by the "**Banged up Bird**" on the right page. The poor bird has a **black eye from abuse, a hole from a gunshot wound, trying to catch the communicable disease**, and with all that going on he certainly has **evidence of being neglected**.

These are exceptions to privacy requirements, since some information is required by law to report. "**CAGE**" will assist you in organizing these client conditions.

I CAN TESTING HINT: When answering test questions, the key to remember is the importance to report any of these conditions. Of course, if the client is hemorrhaging from a gunshot wound, then it is the priority to intervene with the immediate physiological needs first. Reporting is a law!

CAGE

C ommunicable diseases

A buse; animal bites; accidents resulting in death

G unshot/knife wounds

E vidence of neglect

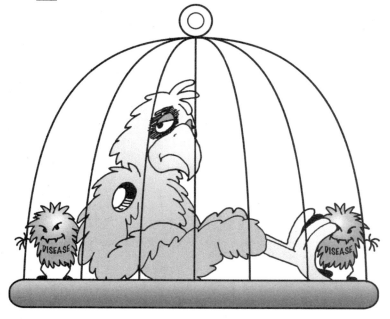

Documentation Guidelines For Suspected Abuse

In being an advocate for the clients, it is important for the nurse to assess for abuse and/or neglect and intervene as appropriate. The key to being an advocate and answering questions about the client who has experienced abuse is to provide a "SAFE" environment for the client. We reviewed previously what conditions must be reported: (**C**ommunicable disease, **A**buse, **A**nimal bites, **A**ccidents resulting in death, **G**unshot/knife wounds, **E**vidence of neglect)". Now, we need to review how to keep the client "SAFE" and guidelines for documentation of the "**ABUSE**".

Safe environment and self-protection.

ABUSE: Know the legal responsibilities in regard to state practice acts and abuse. Know guidelines for documentation if abuse is suspected.

Familiar with available community resources such as crisis hotlines, support groups, parent effectiveness educational groups; primary prevention-education regarding the risks for abuse; secondary prevention-screening activities to identify victims of abuse and interventions to stop it; and tertiary prevention-counseling, emergence treatment that goes on in shelters to support victims and rehabilitate these clients.

Education of parents regarding normal growth and development of children; the role of setting realistic expectations; education for family members of older clients to identify community support; education for spouses or intimate partner abuse.

If a client is a victim of suspected "**ABUSE**", then it is the legal responsibility for the nurse to follow specific guidelines with documentation. This is both a legal issue and an NCLEX® standard. The first step with any nursing process is to assess. These **assessments** must be very specific….location, size, shape of bruise, lacerations. If possible, a photograph of the client would demonstrate the external injuries. Remember, a client's or parent's permission prior to photographing the client is a must! If possible, **use and describe the objective** assessments on an anatomic diagram. **Evaluate** and review the characteristics and location of this pain. When the client is attempting to describe the abuser, **be exact with their words**. The nurse should NEVER promise not to tell what client shares, since it is a LEGAL responsibility to report abuse. If a promise is made, then trust is violated! The nurse should ALWAYS take any report of potential abuse seriously! **Specific quotations** from the client may need hospital security support. If the client is able to describe the events prior to the abuse, then include the date, time, and location of the event as described by the client. Document the sequence of events prior to the abuse. If other people were close to the victim during the abuse, then list these individuals in the documentation. If the abuse was with a child, then clearly assess and document the parent and child interaction.

While the priority of care is to maintain safety for this abused client in addition to meticulous documentation, it is also very important to NEVER say anything that would sound like the client is being blamed for this situation! The role of the nurse is to be an advocate for clients, promoting a trusting relationship while providing "SAFE" care!

ABUSE

A ssessment

B e exact with words from client

U se and describe objective assessments

S pecific quotations

E valuate pain

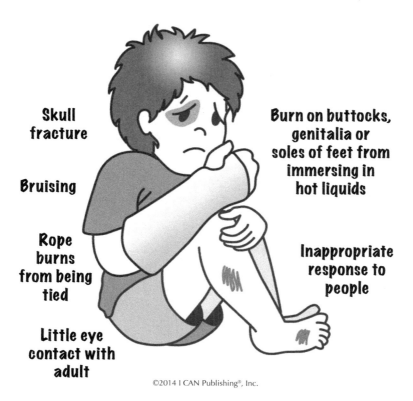

Anorexia

Anorexia is a very difficult eating disorder to overcome. The person suffering from it simply won't eat even though one coaxes and encourages. These clients are very compulsive and controlling. They strive for perfection in every facet of their life, work, school, relationships, and body. Because of their lack of subcutaneous fat, they become amenorrheic. Most anorexics are excessive exercisers, often runners. Through exercise, they burn up the few calories that they consume. Anorexics get in severe trouble when they become so malnourished that their electrolytes become unbalanced. Electrolyte imbalance, particularly hypokalemia, is a frequent cause of death in this very serious disease.

Persons with anorexia who are very thin and experiencing complications will be hospitalized until they become stable, show physiological improvement, and demonstrate weight gain. Nursing care then focuses on reversing the malnutrition, improvement in family dynamics, and individual psychotherapy. The overall goals include weight gain, development of a positive self-image, and supportive family interactions. *Weight and electrolyte balance are our best assessment tools for this issue.*

ANOREXIA

S imply won't eat

T ype A personality

A menorrhea

R un–extreme exercise

V icious cycle–lifetime

E lectrolyte imbalance; (low–blood hemoglobin test)
  ↓ Na
  ↓ K
  ↓ Ca
  ↓ Cl

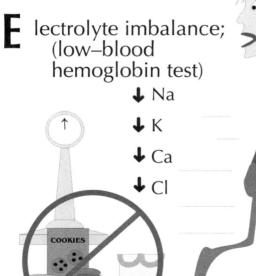

Bulimia

S   **SHOVE IT IN.** Bulimics eat large amounts of food at one time. Their intake is much more than most people can imagine.

T   **TOOTH ENAMEL IS DESTROYED.** Their tooth enamel becomes destroyed from gastric acid in the mouth when vomiting.

U   **UPCHUCK.** Bulimics purge in a number of ways including laxative abuse and use of diuretics, but the most common is vomiting.

F   **FULL WEIGHT.** Clients suffering from bulimia are usually not exceptionally thin, but maintain a normal or full weight.

F   **FEAR OF FAT.** A basic issue of the disease is an extreme fear of fat.

Hospitalization for bulimia is required if complications, such as electrolyte imbalance or cardiac symptoms, occur. Nursing care is similar to that for anorexia nervosa focusing on adequate nutrition and individual and family psychotherapy.

Expected outcomes include adequate balanced food and fluid intake, healthy mucous membranes and skin, maintenance of normal weight, and absence of binge eating and purging.

Bulimics do ingest a lot of S T U F F.

BULIMIA

S hove it in

T ooth enamel is destroyed

U pchuck

F ull weight

F ear of fat

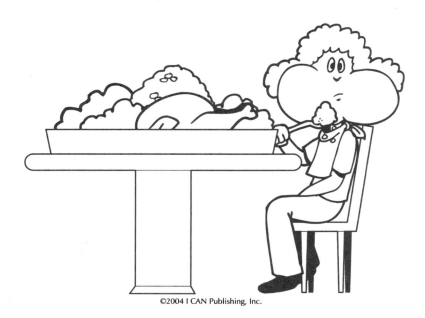

Interventions For Anxiety

ANXIETY! Welcome to nursing school! Would you agree? Perhaps we should say, "Welcome to life!" Before we can successfully help our clients deal with their anxiety, we need to remain **CALMER** ourselves.

- **C**   **CALM**–Create a comfortable, calm environment for relaxation. A quiet room with soft music may help enhance this feeling.

- **A**   **AWARENESS OF ANXIETY**– Identify and describe feelings. Modify stress producing situations.

- **L**   **LISTEN**–Listen to both client and to yourself. Implement "TRUST." Protect the defenses and coping mechanisms.

- **M**   **MEDICATIONS**–When all else fails, use those drugs. A memory tool for anti-anxiety medications is on the next page.

- **E**   **ENVIRONMENT**–Walking, crying, working and concrete tasks may help moderate anxiety. Safety is paramount if meds have to be used.

- **R**   **REASSURANCE**–Implement "TRUST."

INTERVENTIONS FOR ANXIETY

C alm

A nxiety-aware

L isten

M eds—Lexapro, Klonopin, Ativan, Xanax, Cymbalta, Buspar, and Valium

E nvironment

R eassurance

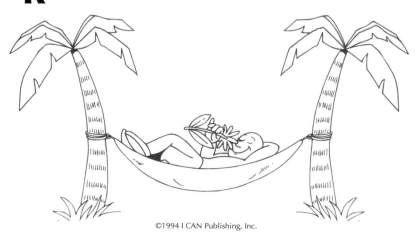

Anti-Anxiety Medications

Clients who are anxious may feel like they are going "**BATS**." These **BATS** will assist you in remembering these anti-anxiety medications.

B   **BETA ADRENERGIC BLOCKERS** may be used for a rapid heart rate.

BENZODIAZEPINES such as alprazolam (Xanax), chlordiazepoxide (Librium), diazepam (Valium), lorazepam (Ativan) and others decrease anxiety by depressing the limbic and subcortical central nervous system.

A   **ANTIHISTAMINES** such as hydroxyzine (Atarax) may decrease anxiety if the client is a potential abuser of benzodiazepines.

T   **TRICYCLICS** and MAO inhibitors may be used for panic attacks.

S   **SSRIs** (serotonin selective reuptake inhibitors) may be effective in managing anxiety.

ANTI-ANXIETY MEDICATIONS

B eta adrenergic Blockers
enzodiazepines

A ntihistamines—COPD or potential abuse of benzodiazepines

T ricyclics and MAO inhibitors for panic attacks

S SRIs

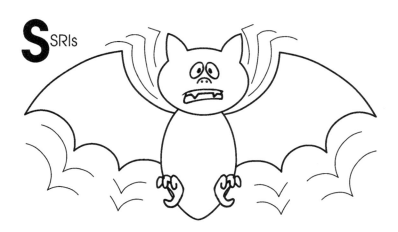

©1997 I CAN Publishing, Inc.

Symptoms of Depression

People that become depressed become very worried about themselves. They realize that they feel terrible and may feel trapped in these feelings. **IN SAD CAGES** will help you remember the symptoms and concerns of the depressed client.

- **I**   **INTEREST** is lacking in most everything. They may feel lethargic. Libido may be decreased and they are commonly apathetic. They may experience despair.
- **N** **NO SELF ESTEEM**

- **S** **SLEEP** is hard to come by. They often have several hours of sleep and then awaken with the inability of going back to sleep. Real rest is often hopeless which may add to the depression. Some people may want to sleep all the time. They are so depressed they do not want to get out of bed.
- **A** **APPETITE** is very often depressed. Food doesn't look good or taste good.
- **D** **DEPRESSED** people can become very tearful. They no longer smile and have a "flat affect" or no expression on their face.

- **C** **CONCENTRATION** is often lacking. They may not be able to do their jobs or maintain their relationships due to the depression.
- **A** **ACTIVITY** is decreased. They may become "couch potatoes" and refuse to participate in routine activities. Exercise may be an activity that they can no longer perform.
- **G** **GUILT** may bring a very negative view of self, world, and future.
- **E** **ENERGY** level is decreased. They may have a poverty of ideas and turn their aggressive feelings inward.
- **S** **SUICIDE** precautions are mandatory. Maintaining a safe environment and negotiating a contract with them may be life saving.

SYMPTOMS OF DEPRESSION

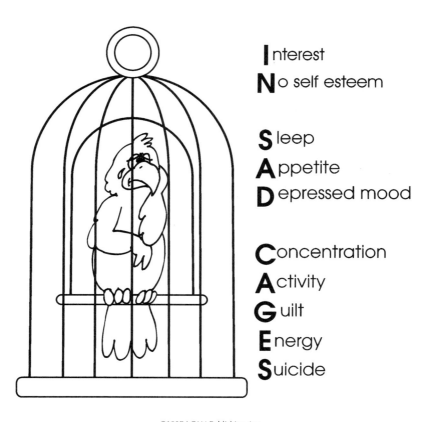

Management of Depression

The depressed client may think of suicide. The presence of a suicidal plan, including specifics related to the method, indicates a potential risk. Harmful environment (windows in a tall building) and harmful objects (razors, knives, automobiles, etc.) should be carefully removed until the client gets in a better place. A structured environment usually works best due to their impairment in decision making.

Food may play an important role in severe depression. Some clients "stuff their feelings" and gain large amounts of weight, while others have no appetite at all and lose substantial weight. They may lose interest in food and activities surrounding their life. We can encourage participation in activities that promote a sense of accomplishment, in addition to other tasks to help increase their interest in life.

Depression, no energy, lack of self-esteem, and little concentration, often lead to decreased bathing, inappropriate attire, and decreased interpersonal friendships. Clients need friends and family at this point. We can listen, continue to establish trust, and convey a kind, pleasant concern, to help promote a sense of dignity and self-worth.

The risk for suicide is a safety issue for the client. Meticulous assessment, documentation, consultation, and necessary referrals are imperative to maintaining client safety and avoiding legal liabilities.

SUICIDE

S uicide precautions

U nusual eating

I nterest lacking, apathetic

C oncentration decreased

I nterpersonal relationships suffer

D epressed mood

E nergy/activity altered
steem depleted

Antidepressant Medications: Tricyclic Antidepressants

Tina Tricycle is sitting on the curb because she is taking new antidepressants and should not drive heavy machinery. She may need to take her medication at night so she won't be too sleepy. Notice the number 3 on her tricycle. This will remind you that it takes approximately 3 weeks for the tricyclic antidepressants to achieve a therapeutic level. Her big **HAT** will help you remember some of the undesirable effects that she may experience while on this drug.

Tina must be taught that her compliance is vital to maintain a therapeutic level. She also must know that some herbs such as St. John's Wort may cause drug/drug interactions.

Tina should not take MAO inhibitors while she is taking tricyclics. Tina wants this medicine to improve her sad face and her interest in riding her tricycle.

TINA TRICYCLE

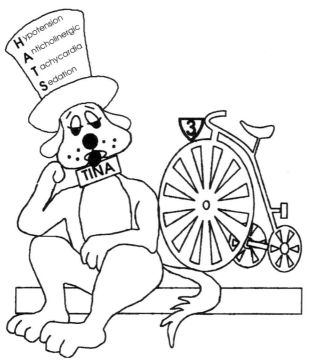

©2001 I CAN Publishing, Inc.

Trimipramine

Imipramine

Nortriptyline

Amitriptyline

Monoamine Oxidase (MAO) Inhibitors

A few examples of these antidepressant medications are Marplan, Nardil and Parnate. They are given to inhibit the enzyme, monoamine oxidase, which breaks down norepinephrine and serotonin, increasing the concentration of these neurotransmitters. To assist you in reviewing the foods to stay away from while on these medicines, refer to the king on the next page or think of a tyrant (representing tyramine).

At 4:30 P.M. he goes into his study, and sits down to an ice cold mug of BEER, 2 glasses of WINE, and a platter of aged CHEESE. Later on in the evening, he goes into his dining room for a plate of LIVERS, home-made steaming hot YEAST ROLLS, a bowl of FIGS, a glass of COLA, and a large piece of CHOCOLATE pie. In the middle of the table, there are 7 bottles of OVER-THE-COUNTER COLD MEDICINES. Tyramine is in most of these.

If the client takes tyramine (or any of these foods or meds), while on the MAO, it will cause a HYPERTENSIVE CRISIS. This will be characterized by increased temperature, tremors, tachycardia and a marked elevation in the blood pressure.

Watch for strokes!

MONOAMINE OXIDASE (MAO) INHIBITORS

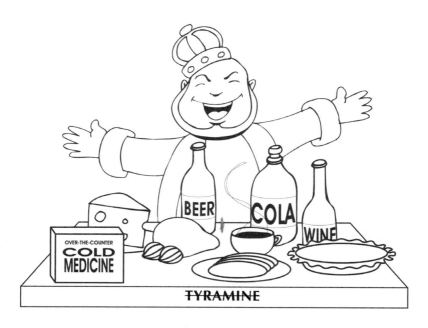

Bipolar Disorder

This psychiatric challenge is very well named. Our clown is interestingly dressed on one side and quite shabbily dressed on the other. Unless these folks are treated, their behavior is at opposite ends of the pole. Sometimes they will be so UP that they are manic, and other times they are so DOWN in the dumps that they're ready to kill themselves.

When they are **UP**, they may think they are Elvis or some other magnificent person. They may think this 24 hours a day. They don't have time to rest, eat or sleep. Try giving them finger foods and providing noncompetitive activities to decrease their hyperactivity. Setting limits, being firm and helping them stay on Lithium may be the best approach. Lithium works best when there is a sodium balance, so try to find them something to do besides play football which is sure to make them sweat. (Besides, this is competitive–Talk about hyper!)

When they are **DOWN**, it's hard to please them. Everything is negative, nothing is right. They still do not eat or sleep well because they are too depressed. Suicide is a common problem. Maintain Lithium at 0.5-1.5 mEq/L. Report any assessment which will alter the sodium level. Other medications currently used to treat this process may include anticonvulsants, antipsychotics, and benzodiazepines.

GOOD LUCK!

BIPOLAR DISORDER

Mood elevated

A grandiose delusion

Need for sleep, eat ↓

Inappropriate

Clanging, loud, vulgar

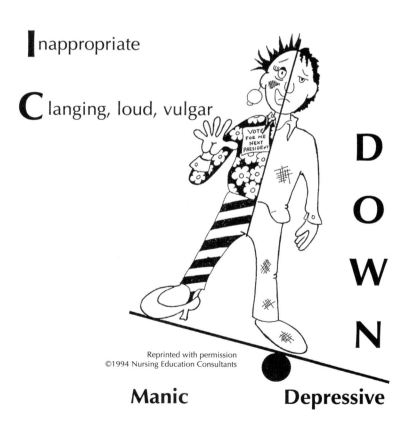

D
O
W
N

Manic   Depressive

Lithium

Lithium is used for the manic episode in biplolar disorder. It acts to lower concentrations of norepinephrine and serotonin by inhibiting their release. Maintenance lithium serum levels should be between 0.6–1.2 mEq/Liter. Blood tests need to initially be done weekly. Maintenance blood levels should be done one time per month. Lithium should be taken the same time each day preferably with meals or milk. Do not crush, chew, or break the extended-release or film coated tablets.

Laboratory studies of the **thyroid** hormone and periodic palpation of the thyroid gland should be a part of preventive therapy. Report signs of hypothyroidism. Symptoms are reversible when lithium is discontinued and supplemental thyroid is provided.

Polyuria or **incontinence**, mild **thirst**, fine **hand tremors** or jaw tremors may occur in early treatment of mania or sometimes persist throughout therapy. Usually however, symptoms subside with temporary reduction of dose. A neuromuscular reaction is **unsteady gait**.

Encourage a diet containing normal amounts of salt and a fluid intake of 3 liters per day. Assess clients who are high risk to develop toxicity such as postoperative, dehydration, hyperthyroidism, renal disease, or those clients taking diuretics.

You will find LITHIUM on Monitoring Lab Values by the Magic 2s.

Lithium was the first mood stabilizing drug approved by the U.S. Food and Drug Administration and is probably the most common drug used for bipolar disorder (see next page). Valproic acid (Depakote) and carbamazepine (Tegretol) are anti-convulsant drugs, yet also have a mood stabilizing effect. These drugs may be combined with Lithium or with each other for maximum effectiveness.

DRUG FOR MANIC CLIENT

L evels

I ncontinence

T hirst
hyroid

H and tremors

I ncrease fluids

U nsteady

M anic
orton's Salt

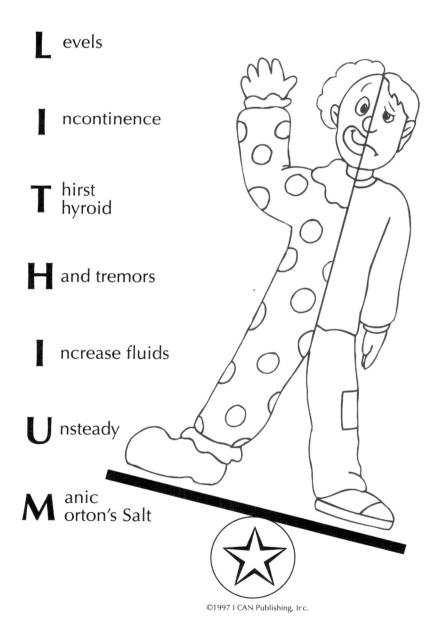

Schizophrenia

The schizophrenic disorders are **HARD** to deal with. Their behavior is often maladaptive and involves alterations in thinking, moods, feelings, perceptions, communication patterns and interpersonal relationships.

The schizophrenic client has a **HARD** time with relationships and a **HARD** time with the establishment of trust. The word "**HARD**" may help you remember the characteristic dimensions of schizophrenia. It's **HARD** being schizophrenic and it's HARD (challenging) providing nursing care. "**TIME**" will assist you in remembering the nursing care for these clients. Remember, these clients may lose the concept of "**TIME**", so we need to take "**TIME** "when providing care to our clients.

The positive symptoms of schizophrenia are most easily identified symptoms. These include examples of behavior such as **delusions, hallucinations, alteration in speech**, and behavior that are seen as bizarre for the client such as walking in a zig-zag line or backwards in a continuous manner. **Negative symptoms** are more difficult to treat successfully. These include **affect, alogia, avolition, anhedonia, anergia**. **Affect** is typically a facial expression that does not change and may be flat. **Alogia** presents with an alteration (lack of) speech or thought. This behavior would result in the client only mumbling in response to a question from a family member. The behavior of **avolition** presents with the client participating in clearing the table after breakfast, but is unable to move on to the next task without reminding or prompting. There is a lack of motivation in personal hygiene in addition to activities. Clients with **anhedonia** experience a lack of joy or happiness. There is an indifference in the client's response to experiences or things that frequently make others happy. An example would be if the client saw their newborn grandchild for the first time and responded with a blank stare. **Anergia** is a lack of energy. **Real problems with cognitive symptoms** make it difficult for the client to think resulting in poor decision-making, problem-solving, and memory deficits. This makes it difficult for the client to live independently. Another group of examples of behavior is the dimension of **depressive symptoms**. These would result in the client presenting with symptoms of hopelessness and/or suicidal ideation.

The nurse said to the person with schizophrenia, *"It's time for lunch."*
He said, *"I'm DEAD. Dead folks don't eat."*
She said, *"It's time for meds."*
He said, *"Dead folks don't take meds."*
She said, *"Time for a bath."*
You guessed it. *"Dead folks don't bathe either."*
How to prove to him that he was not dead? She had a great idea! She asked, *"Do dead folks bleed?"*
"Of course dead folks don't bleed," he answered.
She went after her needle and syringe and took some blood from his arm, held it up proudly and said, *"SEE!"* He said, *"I'll be damned, dead folks do bleed."*

The moral to this story is that they cannot be reasoned with and the nursing care is **HARD**, but we must take **TIME** when providing care to our clients!

I CAN TESTING HINT: This is a great concept for answering a question evaluating "Select all that apply" regarding the positive or negative symptoms of schizophrenia.

SCHIZOPHRENIA

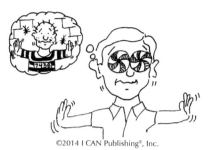

H allucinations, delusions, alterations in speech—Positive symptoms

A ffect, alogia, avolition, anhedonia, anergia—Negative symptoms

R eal problems with cognitive symptoms—Due to problems with thinking, it makes it difficult to live independently (i.e., Decision making/problem-solving abilities are poor, memory deficits, etc.).

D epressive symptoms – Suicidal ideation, hopelessness

T rust (therapeutic communication): Establish trust, accept/support feelings, etc. (Refer to COMMUNICATION STRATEGIES FOR TEST QUESTIONS)

I ndependence: Encourage independence with personal hygiene, but assist as needed. Avoid encouraging a dependent relationship. Structure time for activities in order to limit time for withdrawal.

M edications: Teach family the importance of medication compliance.

E nvironment safe and support self-esteem: Provide safe and secure environment; encourage client to identify positive characteristics about self.

Undesirable Effects of Antipsychotic Drugs

People that take antipsychotic drugs may have a different **STANCE**. They may shuffle their feet or have other unusual symptoms while taking these mood-altering drugs. **STANCE** will help you remember many of these undesirable effects.

- **S** **SEDATION**, sleepiness and **SUNLIGHT SENSITIVITY** are common with these drugs. Often they are not able to drive.

- **T** **TARDIVE DYSKINESIA** is an irreversible effect that changes the stance because it changes the head.

- **A** **ANTICHOLINERGIC** effects can make the client's mouth dry and can cause constipation. **AGRANULOCYTOSIS** is an undesirable effect. Report sore throats or signs of sepsis.

- **N** **NEUROLEPTIC MALIGNANT SYNDROME** may occur.

- **C** **CARDIAC EFFECTS** of orthostatic hypotension are common.

- **E** **EXTRAPYRAMIDAL** effects such as pill rolling and akathesia may occur.

UNDESIRABLE EFFECTS OF ANTIPSYCHOTICS

S edation
Sunlight sensitivity

T ardive dyskinesia

A nticholinergic
Agranulocytosis

N euroleptic malignant syndrome

C ardiac arrhythmias (orthostatic hypotension)

E xtrapyramidal (akathesia)

©2001 I CAN Publishing, Inc.

Alcoholism

One of the goals during the long-term rehabilitation is to assist client in identifying alternate coping mechanisms. "**COPES**" is the key in reviewing the priority nursing plans.

C   **COPING MECHANISMS**–Encourage client to develop alternative coping mechanisms other than alcohol to deal with stress. The client must be responsible for sobriety.

O   **ORIENT TO COMMUNITY RESOURCES**–Refer clients to available community resources such as Alcoholics Anonymous (AA), Alanon and Alateen. Abuse of spouses or children often occur while the client is drinking. Notify appropriate protection services for suspected child, spouse, or elder abuse.

P   **PLAN** may include antabuse. Antabuse is a drug used by a willing client as a deterrent that will make the client violently ill (flushing, hypotension and nausea and vomiting if he takes it and drinks alcohol). The nurse should always know when the client had the last drink before she administers this drug. Never administer any medications or substances with alcohol in them (i.e., cough syrup, mouth wash, shaving cream, etc.) while the client is taking antabuse.

E   **ENCOURAGE DIET**–Vitamin B complex is often used for the alcoholic client with delerium tremens and for the treatment of peripheral neuritis. Alcoholics often have avitaminosis because they drink instead of eat. Folic acid deficiency can lead to obstetrical complications.

S   **SEIZURES**–Delerium Tremens usually occur within 48 hours after cessation of drinking. Picking at the bed covers, tremors of hands, anxiety, nausea, hypertension and nightmares followed by seizures may cause an emergency.

ALCOHOLISM

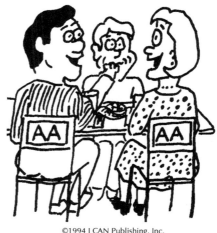

©1994 I CAN Publishing, Inc.

C oping mechanisms

O rient to community resources

P lan may include antabuse

E ncourage vitamin B, folic acid

S eizures

Abstinence Maintenance Following Detoxification
"BEAT" Addiction Again, by Way of Revia!

Several plans are important for assisting the client with an alcohol addiction during the long-term rehabilitation. If the client does fail, do not reprimand or give negative feedback for the failure. The goals of the nurse are to set limits, be supportive, and remain nonjudgmental. When the nurse is implementing the plan of care for this client, the priority is assisting the client to "**ERASE**" the addiction.

- **E** **E**ncourage client to develop coping mechanisms rather than using alcohol.
- **R** **R**emain nonjudgmental; responsibility for sobriety belongs to client.
- **A** **A**void sympathy; clients will rationalize and manipulate behavior.
- **S** **S**et limits on behavior in a kind but firm manner.
- **E** **E**ncourage participation in social groups and activities; encourage and refer to community resources such as Alcoholics Anonymous (AA), etc.

The next part of the plan to "**BEAT**" the addiction is to promote adherence to the prescribed therapeutic regimen. Refer to the right page as we review the opioid antagonist, **Revia**, which will decrease the craving for alcohol. "**Re**" means "*again*"! Our goal is for the client to be able to again experience energy when rising in the AM, and enjoy the many gifts of life such as the sun rising and setting.

The "**V**" symbolizes two paths for the client. If the client chooses the left path, the road less traveled (*the one to hard work*), then the goal to beat the addiction can be fulfilled. If the client chooses the other path, then the addiction will continue. The client, however, does not have to take this journey alone. "**Via**" means "*by way of*", so in other words, the client can have help to "**BEAT**" the addiction again, "*by way of Revia*".

As with any medication, SAFE administration is of paramount importance to assist in achieving successful outcomes for the client. One of the first concerns for clients taking this drug is to use with caution if there is a history of a **B**leeding disorder such as hemophilia, hepatic, or renal impairment. **E**ducate client to avoid any alcohol containing products such as mouthwash, cough syrups, etc. **A**ddiction to alcohol or narcotics is the indication to take this medication. Client needs to be taught to **T**ake tablet with a full glass of water and food to decrease stomach upset. Recommend client carry an ID card or wear a medical alert bracelet indicating the use of naltrexone (Revia), in case of an emergency. Overdose symptoms may include nausea, stomach pain, dizziness, or seizure (convulsions). Notify healthcare provider. For additional information regarding Revia, refer to the book *Pharmacology Made Insanely Easy, 4th edition*, by Manning & Rayfield; published by I CAN Publishing®, Inc. (www.icanpublishing.com).

REVIA

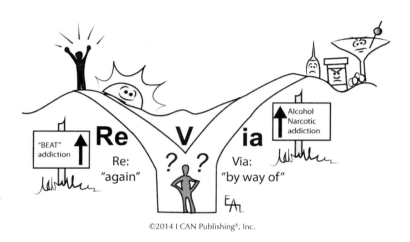

"BEAT" addiction again, by way of Revia!

B leeding disorder, Hepatic or Renal impairment —use with caution

E ducate to avoid alcohol containing products (mouthwash, cough syrups...)

A ddiction to alcohol or narcotics is the indication to take this medication

T ake tablet with a full glass of water and food to decrease stomach upset

Abstinence Maintenance Following Detoxification Antabuse "Ant-Abuse"

Disulfiram (**ANT-ABUSE**) is used to promote adherence to prescribed therapeutic plans. Disulfiram is a drug taken with alcohol will result in nausea, vomiting, weakness, sweating; hypotension, palpitations; and flushed face.

Refer to the previous left page reviewing the plans to help "ERASE" and *"BEAT" Addiction Again, by Way of Revia*! The plans to "ERASE" the addiction are relevant to any client with an addiction who needs assistance with abstinence maintenance (following detoxification).

The different component of care in this plan is managing the drug, "**ANT-ABUSE**". Refer to the right page as we review our dear little ants that chose not to stick with the plan for the management of their alcoholism. The ant on the left decided to go ahead and drink some alcohol, and then quickly proceeded to the toilet to "**BARF**"! The choice to drink alcohol when taking disulfiram is indeed "**ANT-ABUSE**"! This is why it is an aversion therapy. *No type of enjoyment is worth vomiting (barfing) for! Do you agree?*

When taking this medication, the client needs to be informed of the importance of wearing a **B**racelet that is a medical alert indicating the undesirable effects from this medication may include nausea, vomiting, weakness, sweating, and/or liver toxicity. **A**cetaldehyde syndrome may progress to respiratory depression, cardiovascular suppression, seizures, and death. Review with the client that the medication effects may persist for 2 weeks after the discontinuation of the disulfiram. **R**emind client to avoid products containing alcohol (e.g., mouth wash, cough syrup, after shave, etc.). Clients need to be encouraged to **F**ollow a 12 step self-help program focusing on guidance, education, and the sharing of experiences that are unique to the individual.

The desired outcome for clients taking "**ANT-ABUSE**" will be that they will stick to the plan, and not to go off like the ants on the right page did to sneak some alcohol. The clients will be successful in abstinence from alcohol and participate on a regular basis in a self-help group.

ANT-ABUSE

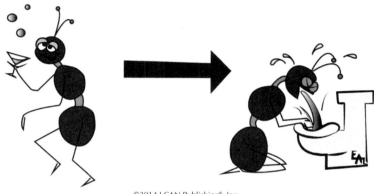

B racelet—medical alert bracelet should be worn; (UE; N/V, weakness, sweating, liver toxicity)

A cetaldehyde syndrome may occur. Watch for: respiratory arrest, cardiovascular suppression, seizures, death

R emind client to avoid products containing alcohol (e.g., mouth wash, cough syrup, after shave)

F ollow up with a 12 step self-help program

Difference In Delirium And Dementia

Delirium is a cognitive disorder that is typically secondary to another physiologic process. The clinical assessment findings usually develop over a short period of time. Once the physiological cause has been treated, the symptoms typically fluctuate and are often reversible and temporary. Refer to the right page for an easy way to remember the difference. **The FTD florist is quick delivery and response. This is the same as delirium; quick onset and delivery.**

Dementia, however, is a cognitive disorder characterized by the loss of intellectual abilities to such an extent that occupational and social skills are affected in a negative manner. It affects the *judgment, affect, ability to remember, think, and orientation*. Most of the time the disorder is progressive and is irreversible.

"**ACUTE** "will assist you in remembering priority information for delirium and "**DEMENTIA**" will assist you in remembering priority information for a client with dementia. The right page says it all: *delirium is like the FTD florist with "quick delivery and quick return"*. *"CEMENTIA" rhymes with dementia and is slow to develop (just like after cement dries, it is irreversible)*.

Delirium is "**ACUTE**"
- **A** Assess for contributing factors
- **C** Clouded state of sensorium or state of consciousness; disorientation
- **U** U must consider SAFETY! (non-stimulating environment; low bed position; no cigarettes, matches, lighters, sharp objects)
- **T** The side rails should be padded if client has a seizure disorder
- **E** Etiologic factors: meningitis, encephalitis, respiratory and urinary infection, hypoglycemia, **dehydration**, vomiting, hypoxia, **drug intoxication and withdrawal**, pain and sleep deprivation, head trauma

"**DEMENTIA**"
- **D** Dementia disrupts the final stage of family development (*retirement, generativity, etc.*)
- **E** Exaggeration of previous personality traits
- **M** Mini-Mental Examination–shows disorientation and lack of self recall
- **E** Events and activities of 10 years ago client can recall, but not 10 minutes ago
- **N** Note: avoid dependence; establish routine for activities of daily living; do NOT isolate from others
- **T** The R's are important for these clients: *Repetition, Routine, and Reinforcement*
- **I** Irreversible cerebral atrophy and neuritic plaques. Interaction with client: speak slowly and in a face-to-face position if client also has a hearing loss. Shouting causes distortion of high-pitched sounds.
- **A** Alzheimer's Disease: Loss of memory, intellectual functioning, orientation, affective regulation, motor coordination, and personality, with eventual loss of bowel and bladder control to the point of incapacitation

DELIRIUM AND DEMENTIA

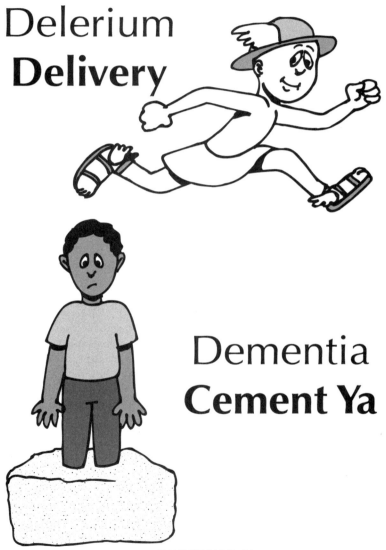

Dementia

"**The Slow House of Alzheimer's**" tells the story of Poppa, who came to live with his son, but was so confused. The first night Son found Poppa a mile down the road in his pajama shirt and boxer shorts. He had fallen and his leg was bleeding. Poppa was "going to the house" (4 states away). To protect him, Son put a chair in front of his bedroom door, so that when he got up in the middle of the night he would be heard. Poppa would have gone nuts if he had been restrained. Barriers are much safer and more humane.

Son's wife could not wait to take Poppa to the cafeteria dining room so he could choose his own food, but Poppa stood there and stood there. Son's wife had to choose his food because decisions were impossible. The bathroom was a problem. Poppa had used the "out of doors" when he was a boy and his memory had regressed. It was easier to schedule his elimination than to embarrass the neighbors. Unfortunately the schedule was not always accurate and sometimes there were embarrassing wet clothes.

This story is a common one for people with dementia. **"The Slow House of Alzheimer's"** will help you remember the symptoms of **lost and wandering, confusion, decision difficulty, incontinence** and **confinement for safety**.

These changes are often progressive and irreversible. The cardinal rule for the geriatric population is do not push too fast (go slowly). It is important to reorient Poppa to the current **reality**. Objects such as clocks and calendars may help. Poppa's self-esteem may benefit through **reminiscing**. He may be able to recall events 10 years ago, but not 10 minutes ago. Poppa needs to be encouraged to remain **independent** as long as possible. Avoid dependency. Develop a plan for activities of daily living and remember consistency is important. As Poppa has illustrated, safety is very important. Due to sundowners and the increase risk of wandering and falling, **safety** precautions may become a high priority for these clients.

Remember, the difference between dementia (Alzheimer's) and delirium is that dementia is progressive and irreversible. Delirium or acute confusion state can result from sepsis, drug drug interactions, fluid and electrolyte imbalances, etc.

THE SLOW HOUSE OF ALZHEIMER'S

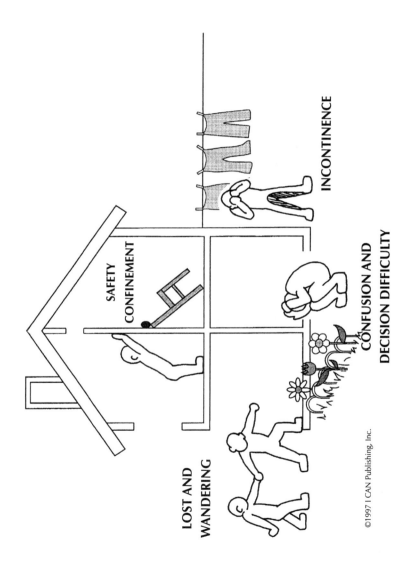

Combative Client

Many people feel they put combat boots on the minute they get up in the morning, but we are referring to the client who is out of control. This may include folks that are real mad, manics, alcoholics, dementias and personality disorders just to name a few. It does not matter what the etiology is; the concept of "**COMBAT**" is still the same.

C   **CONTROL IMMEDIATE SITUATION**–Get their attention. Remove harmful objects. Maintain distance between self and client. Remain neutral.

O   **OUT OF SITUATION**–Remove client from the environment to de-escalate combative behavior.

M   **MAINTAIN CALM**–Do not hurry. Channel the agitated behavior.

B   **BE FIRM AND SET LIMITS**–Be consistent and prevent overt aggression.

A   **AVOID RESTRAINTS**–Use restraints as a last intervention.

T   **TRY CONSEQUENCES**–Positive consequences for positive behavior.

COMBATIVE CLIENT

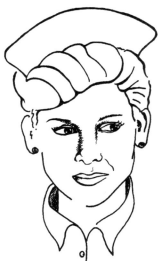

Control immediate

Out of situation

Maintain calm

Be firm/set limits

Avoid restraints

Try consequences

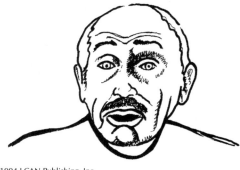

©1994 I CAN Publishing, Inc.

Post-Traumatic Stress Syndrome

Post-Traumatic Stress Syndrome is severe anxiety which results form a traumatic experience (e.g., rape, incest, war, etc.). The level of anxiety is proportional to the perceived degree that is experienced by the client.

The anxiety is manifested in symptomatic behavior that can occur whenever there is a visible reminder of the trauma or event at night during a nightmare. "**NITE**" will assist you in organizing how the client might experience the anxiety.

N Nightmare
I Intrusive thoughts
T The flashback of the experiences
E Emotional detachment

The client's response to the anxiety may be shock, anger, panic, or denial. More self-destructive behaviors may occur such as substance abuse or suicidal ideations.

The plan for these clients includes the "Six As:"

Active Listening!

Assess suicide risk!

Assist client to develop objectivity about the event and problem-solve regarding alternative strategies for handling anxiety and feelings related to the event.

Active with group therapy and other clients who have also experienced traumatic events.

Administer antianxiety and antipsychotic meds as prescribed, so as to manage behavior and provide rest!

Advocate for the client!

The role of the nurse is to be the advocate for the client by providing a consistent and nonthreatening environment. If client is at risk for suicide, implement suicidal precautions. Nonjudgmental acceptance and being there for the client by actively listening will go a long way in proving a safe and supportive environment!

POST-TRAUMATIC STRESS SYNDROME

Nightmare

Intrusive thoughts

The flashback of the experiences

Emotional detachment

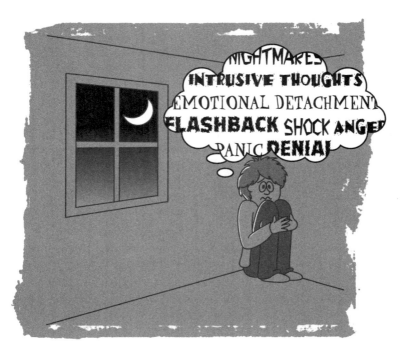

Cultural Aspects

Our world grows smaller as we visit and work in countries other than our own and as people from other cultures come to the United States to live and work. We are grateful to have had the opportunity to work with international nurses that have assisted us with using the word **SPIRIT** to bring together the commonalities in many of our cultures.

- **S** **SOUL FOOD**–foods that are comfort foods for us are important to or forbidden by our culture or religion. Example–Many people of Italian descent love pasta, but when diagnosed with diabetes may have to severely limit pasta intake.

- **P** **PRODUCTS** such as blood products, have different connotations to different cultures and religious groups. For example, the Jehovah's Witness Religion chooses to refuse blood and blood products. Alternative fluids and autologous transfusions may be acceptable

- **I** **INTERACTIONS** in communication differ with many cultures. For example, South African people may love to entertain with song and dance while many Asians are shy and reserved. Native Americans may be offended with direct eye contact while American businessmen may be offended it there is no direct eye contact. Interpreters may need to be utilized to have effective communication when people are ill.

- **R** **RITUALS** are a part of every culture, births, weddings, and funerals are time-honored events in most all cultures and may have any rituals associated with them. For example, some cultures choose to burn the umbilical cord when if falls off the infant to "keep the sins of the mother from being visited on the baby."

- **I** **IN TRANSITION** from the body of life to the spiritual life is especially important for nurses. For example, Moslem men should be cared for after death only by another man.

- **T** **TEACHING** healthcare promotion and prevention of illness may be challenging to many cultures that may value voodoo, Chinese herbs, medicine men and other kinds of treatment. Our nursing goal is to determine the cultural issues so that we can increase compliance with healthcare without offending global cultures while valuing their practices.

CULTURE

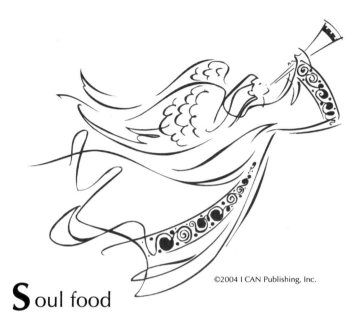

Soul food

Products (blood)

Interactions (communication)

Rituals

In transition

Teaching

"You will find that it is necessary to let things go;
simply for the reason that they are heavy."

UNKNOWN

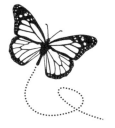

LABORATORY VALUES

The Magic 2s

The magician is pulling the prescription drugs out of his magic hat and reminding you that you can use the "MAGIC 2s" as a way to remember the toxicity level. These are the medications most commonly monitored for therapeutic dosage.

MONITORING DRUGS BY THE MAGIC 2s

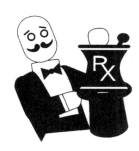

Drug	Range	Toxicity
Digitalis	.5-1.5	**2**
Lithium	.6-1.2	**2**
Aminophylline (Theophylline)	10-20	**20**
Dilantin	10-20	**20**
Acetaminophen	1-30	**200**

© 1997 I CAN Publishing, Inc.

The Magic 4s

Sometimes it's hard to remember those electrolyte extracellular levels; however, we MUST because they affect the heart as recorded by the EKG. The digit **4** can be magic in helping to remember. Even though not electrolytes, the hemoglobin and hematocrit can also be remembered using a **4**. For example if the hemoglobin is **14** the hematocrit will be **4**2. The pH, pCO_2, and HCO_3, may also be difficult to remember until you review the **MAGIC 4s**.

THE MAGIC 4s

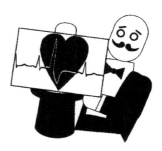

Electrolyte	Range	Magic 4
K	3.5–5.5	**4**
Cl	98–106	10**4**
Na	135–145	1**4**0
pH	7.34–7.45	7.**4**0
pCO_2	35–45	**4**0
HCO_3	22–26	2**4**

©1997 I CAN, Inc.

REFERENCES

Center for Disease Control and Prevention: *2007 Guideline for isolation precautions: preventing transmission of infectious agents in healthcare settings*. Retrieved from http://www.cdc. gov/hicpac/2007ip/2007isolationprecautions.html

Department of Health & Human Services. *Understanding HIPAA Privacy* (n.d.). Retrieved from http://www.hhs.gov/ocr/privacy/hipaa/understanding/consumers/index.html

Eliopoulos, C. (2009). Gerontological nursing. (7th ed). Philadelphia, PA: Lippincott Williams & Wilkins.

Ignatavicius, D. D., & Workman, M. L. (2013). *Medical-surgical nursing: Patient-centered collaborative care* (7th ed.). St. Lous, MO: Saunders.

National Council of State Boards of Nursing. *2012 NCLEX® Examination Candidate Bulletin*. https://www.ncsbn.org/2012_NCLEX_Candidate_Bulletin.pdf

NCSBN. (2012). *2011 RN Practice Analysis: Linking the NCLEX-RN® Examination to Practice* (Vol. 53). https://wwwncsbn.org/12_RN_Practice_Analysis_Vol53.pdf

NCSBN. 2012. *Proposed 2013 NCLEX-RN® Test Plan*. National Council of State Boards of Nursing Annual Meeting, August, 2012.

Manning, L. & Rayfield, S. (2013). *Pharmacology made insanely easy* (4th ed.). Duluth, GA: I CAN Publishing, Inc.

Potter, P., & Perry, A. (2012). *Fundamentals of nursing* (8th ed.). St. Louis, MO: Mosby.

INDEX

Note: italicized page numbers refer to images.

A

Abstinence Maintenance Following Detoxification 536, *537*, 538, *539*
Abuse, documentation guidelines for suspected 508, *509*
Accuracy of Orders 36, *37*
Ace Inhibitors 138, *139*
Acetaminophen Overdose 294, *295*
Acid-Base Balance
 Acid-Base 178, *179*, 184, *185*
 Acid-Base Compensatory Mechanisms 182, *183*
 Acid-Base Status 180, *181*
 Shock 186, *187*, 188, *189*
Addison's Disease 260, *261*
Adolescent (13 to 18 Years) 440, *441*
Airborne Precautions 64, *65*
Alcoholism 534, *535*
Anaphylactic Reactions 90, *91*
Ancillary Personnel Limitations 22, *23*
Anesthesia, regional 478, *479*
Anorexia 510, *511*
Antacids 274, *275*
Anti-Anxiety Medications 516, *517*
Anticholinergics 272, *273*
Anticoagulants 362, *363*
Antidepressant Medications
 Monoamine Oxidase (MAO) Inhibitors 524, *525*
 Tricyclic Antidepressants 522, *523*
Antipsychotic Drugs 532, *533*
Anxiety 514, *515*
Applications of Heat and Cold 96, *97*
Arterial Vascular Disease 158, *159*
Arthritis 304, *305*
Assessments After Any Test That Ends in "Scopy" 174, *175*
Assignment of Rooms 54, *55*
Asthma 196, *197*
Atrial Dysrhythmias 146, *147*
Autonomic Dysreflexia 364, *365*

B

Basal Cell Carcinoma 394, *395*
Bell's Palsy 354, *355*
Benign Prostate Hypertrophy 414, *415*
Beta$_2$-Adrenergic Agonists 198, *199*
Beta Blockers 140, *141*
Beta Strep 86, *87*
Bipolar Disorder 526, *527*
Botox 358, *359*
Breath Sounds 166, *167*
Bulimia 512, *513*
Burns 398, *399*

C

Calcium Channel Blockers 142, *143*
Cane Walking 318, *319*
Cardiac Dysrhythmias 146–151
 Atrial 146, *147*
 Heart Blocks 150, *151*
Cardiac Management 136, *137*
Cardiac Sounds 112, *113*

Cardiac System 104–163
Cardiovert 148, *149*
Care of Client
  Standard Precautions in all settings 60, 61
Celiac Disease Diet 498, *499*
Centesis 172, *173*
Central Venous Pressure 152, *153*
Chest Drainage, Water-Sealed 202, *203*
Chronic Obstructive Pulmonary Disease (COPD) 192, *193*
Chronic Renal Failure (Lab Changes) 232, *233*
Cirrhosis 292, *293*
Client Education 424, *425*
Clostridium Difficile 72, *73*, 74, *75*
Cold, applications of 96, *97*
Colostomy 278, *279*
Combative Client 544, *545*
Communication Strategies For Test Questions 504, 505
Conditions That Must Be Reported As Required By The Law 506, *507*
Congenital Heart Disease 126, *127*
COPD 192, *193*
  Interventions For 194, *195*
Cost Effectiveness 32, *33*
Cover Your Assets 38, *39*
Cranial Nerves 334, *335*
Cranial Nerves (3, 4, 6, and 8) 332, *333*
Crohn's Disease 276, *277*
Crutch Walking 314, *315*, 316, *317*
Cultural Aspects 548, *549*
Cushing's Disease/Syndrome 258, *259*
Cyanotic Heart Defects 122, *123*
Cystic Fibrosis 200, *201*

D

Defibrillate 148, *149*
Delegation 20, 21
  Ancillary Personnel Limitations 22, *23*

Do Not Delegate What You Can "Teach" 30, *31*
Floating Nurses Between Units 26, *27*
Graduate Nurse 28, *29*
UAP, Tasks to be Delegated 24, *25*
Delirium 540, *541*
Dementia 540, *541*, 542, *543*
Depression 518, *519*, 520, *521*
Diabetes Insipidus 244, *245*
Diabetes Mellitus 252, *253*
Diagnostic Procedures 114, *115*
Diagnostics For
  Cardiac System 116, *117*
  Endocrine System 240, *241*
  Gastrointestinal System 264, *265*
  Hematology 402, *403*
  Hepatic And Biliary System 288, *289*
  Ophthalmic and Hearing 370, *371*
  Integumentary System 386, *387*
  Maternity Client 454, *455*
  Musculoskeletal System 300, *301*
  Neurological System 324, *325*
  Renal System 230, *231*
  Respiratory System 170, *171*
Dialysis 236, *237*
Diarrhea, infant with severe 266, *267*
Diets
  Celiac Disease 498, *499*
  Foods High in Folic Acid *486*, *487*
  Foods High in Iron 488, *489*
  Foods High in Potassium 492, *493*
  Foods High in Protein 490, *491*
  Foods High in Sodium 494, *495*
  Low Residue Diet 496, *497*
Dilantin 348, *349*

Disaster Plan 98, *99*
Discharge 44, *45*
Diverticular Disease 286, *287*
Donning PPE 80, *81*
Droplet Precautions 70, *71*
Dumping Syndrome 280, *281*
Dysrhythmias
   Atrial 146, *147*
   Heart Blocks 150, *151*

E
Ear Drops 380, *381*
Eight Rights to Medication Administration 48, *49*
Elevated Liver Enzymes 290, *291*
Endocrine System 240–261
   Diagnostics for 240, *241*
Equipment 92, *93*

F
Fall Risk 88, *89*
Fetal Heart Decelerations 466, *467*
   Early (head compression) 468, *469*
   Late (uteroplacental insufficiency) 472, *473*
   Late (Uncoil) 474, *475*
   Variable (cord compression) 470, *471*
Fever 84, *85*
Fluid Volume Status 210, *211*
   Fluid Shifts 212, *213*
   Hypercalcemia 222, *223*
   Hyperkalemia 218, *219*
   Hypernatremia 214, *215*
   Hypocalcemia 224, *225*
   Hypokalemia 220, *221*
   Hyponatremia 216, *217*

G
Gastric Reflux 270, *271*
Gastrointestinal System 264–297
Geriatrics (85 Years and Over) 448, *449*, 450, *451*
Gestational Diabetes 464, *465*
Glasgow Coma Scale 330, *331*
Glaucoma 374, *375*, 376, *377*
Gout 308, *309*
"Grams"
   Priority Care After 120, *121*
   Priority Care Prior to 118, *119*
Growth and Development 426, *427*
   Adolescent (13 to 18 Years) 440, *441*
   Geriatrics (85 Years and Over) 448, *449*, 450, *451*
   Infancy 430, *431*
   Middle Adulthood (40 to 60 years) 444, *445*
   Older Adulthood (60 to 85 Years) 446, *447*
   Preschool (4 to 5 Years) 436, *437*
   School Age (6 to 12 Years) 438, *439*
   Toddler (1 to 3 years) 432, *433*
   Young Adulthood (19 to 40 Years) 442, *443*

H
Hand Hygiene 56, *57*
Health Promotion 422–453
Hearing Impairment 382, *383*
Heart Blocks 150, *151*
Heart Failure 132, *133*
Heat, applications of 96, *97*
Hematology 402–411
Hemodynamics (The 6s) 152, *153*
Hemodynamics (The 12s) 154, *155*
HIPAA 16, *17*
Hydrocephalus 328, *329*
Hypercalcemia 222, *223*
Hyperkalemia 218, *219*
Hypernatremia 214, *215*
Hypertension, pregnancy-induced 460, *461*
Hyperthyroidism 246, *247*
Hypocalcemia 224, *225*
Hypoglycemia 256, *257*
Hypokalemia 220, *221*
Hyponatremia 216, *217*
Hypothyroidism 250, *251*
Hypoxia In An Infant 128, *129*

I

Identification, client 52, *53*
Immobility 312, *313*
Immunizations 452, *453*
Impetigo 388, *389*
Inadequate Peripheral Artery Perfusion 160, *161*
Increased Intracranial Pressure 340, *341*
Infancy 430, *431*
Infection Control Precautions
   Airborne 64, *65*
   Clostridium Difficile 72, *73*, 74, *75*
   Contact Precautions 72, *73*
   Droplet Precautions 70, *71*
   Hand Hygiene 56, *57*
   Methicillin-Resistant Staphylococcus Aureus (MRSA) 76, *77*
   Positive Pressure 78, *79*
   Room Assignments 54, *55*
   Sequence for Donning PPE 80, *81*
   Sequence for Removing PPE 82, *83*
   Standard Precautions 58–63
   Transmission-Based 62, *63*
   Varicella (Chickenpox) 68, *69*
   Viral Infections 66, *67*
Infor Matics 10, *11*
Informed Consent 14, *15*
Insulin 254, *255*
Integumentary System 386–399

K

Kawasaki Disease 130, *131*
Kidney Disease (Chronic Renal Failure/CRF) 234, *235*

L

Labor and Delivery
   Decelerations
     Early (head compression) 468, *469*
     Late (uteroplacental insufficiency) 472, *473*
     Late (Uncoil) 474, *475*
     Variable (cord compression) 470, *471*
   Pitocin 476, *477*
Laboratory values 552, *553*, 554, *555*
Legal Aspects 18, *19*
Leukemia 408, *409*
Lice 390, *391*
Lithium 528, *529*
Low-Residue Diet 496, *497*
Loop Diuretics 144, *145*
Lung Sounds 190, *191*

M

Magnesium Sulfate Toxicity 462, *463*
Malignant Melanoma 396, *397*
Management 2–49
Management: Safety 34, *35*
Maslow's Hierarchy 4
Mastectomy 416, *417*
Medications
   Ace Inhibitors 138, *139*
   Acetaminophen 294, *295*
   Allopurinol (Zyloprim) 308, *309*
   Anesthesia, Regional 478, *479*
   Antacids 274, *275*
   Anti-Anxiety Medications 516, *517*
   Anticholinergics 272, *273*
   Anticoagulants 362, *363*
   Antidepressant Medications 522–525
   Antipsychotic Drugs 532, *533*
   $Beta_2$-Adrenergic Agonists 198, *199*
   Beta Blockers 140, *141*
   Botox 358, *359*
   Calcium Channel Blockers 142, *143*
   Dilantin 348, *349*
   Insulin 254, *255*
   Lithium 528, *529*
   Loop Diuretics 144, *145*

Magnesium Sulfate 462, *463*
Nephrotoxic Drugs in the Renal System 228, *229*
Nonsteroidal Anti-Inflammatory Drugs (NSAIDs) 306, *307*
Pitocin 476, *477*
Tylenol 294, *295*
Men & Women's Care / Cancer 414–419
Meningitis 342, *343*, 344, *345*
Meningocele/Omphalocele 326, *327*
Methicillin-Resistant Staphylococcus Aureus (MRSA) 76, *77*
Middle Adulthood (40 to 60 years) 444, *445*
Miotics 378, *379*
Monoamine Oxidase (MAO) Inhibitors 524, *525*
Multiple Myeloma 410, *411*
Musculoskeletal System 300–321
Myasthenia Gravis 352, *353*

N

Neonate Assessments: "The 4 Hs" 482, *483*
Nephrotoxicity (drugs) in the Renal System 228, *229*
Neurological Checks 336, *337*
Neurological System 324–367
New Graduate 28, *29*
Nonsteroidal Anti-Inflammatory Drugs (NSAIDs) 306, *307*
Nurses Who Float 26, *27*
Nursing Process 4

O

Obesity 428, *429*
Older Adulthood (60 to 85 Years) 446, *447*
Open Angle Glaucoma 374, *375*, 376, *377*
Osteoporosis 302, *303*

P

Pancreatitis 296, *297*

Parasitic Infestations: Pediculosis 390, *391*
Parkinson's Disease 350, *351*
Peptic Ulcer Disease 268, *269*
Peripheral Vascular Disease: Arterial Versus Venous 158, *159*
Peripherally Inserted Central Catheter Care 156, *157*
Physical Assessment 104, *105*
Pitocin 476, *477*
Poison Control 434, *435*
Polycythemia 406, *407*
Postpartum Assessment 480, *481*
Post-Traumatic Stress Syndrome 546, *547*
Post-Operative GI Assessment 284, *285*
PPE
  Donning 80, *81*
  Removing 82, *83*
Precautions
  Airborne 64, *65*
  Standard 58–61
  Transmission-Based 62, *63*
Pregnancy
  Danger signs 458, *459*
  Decelerations 466–475
  Gestational Diabetes 464, *465*
  Hypertension 460, *461*
  Normal discomforts during 456, *457*
Preschool (4 to 5 Years) 436, *437*
Prevention, levels of 422, *423*
Prioritizing 2–7
Priority Topics for Teaching, Nursing Personnel 46, *47*
Psychosocial Integrity 502–549
Pulmonary Artery Wedge Pressure 154, *155*
Pulmonary Edema 176, *177*

R

Radium Implants 418, *419*
Raynaud's Phenomenon 162, *163*
Reduce Cardiac Workload 134, *135*

Referrals 42, *43*
Regional Anesthesia 478, *479*
Renal System
  Diagnostics for 230, *231*
  Dialysis 236, *237*
  Lab Changes with Chronic Renal Failure 232, *233*
  Renal Failure, chronic 234, *235*
  Renal Pathology 226, *227*
Report, Provide and/or Receive 12, *13*
Respiratory System 166–207
  Respiratory Medications: Beta$_2$-Adrenergic Agonists 198, *199*
Restraints 94, *95*

S
Safe Use of Equipment 92, *93*
SBAR 12, *13*
Schizophrenia 530, *531*
School Age (6 to 12 Years) 438, *439*
"Scopy," Assessments After Any Test That Ends in 174, *175*
Seizures 346, *347*
Sensory Perception 370–383
Shock 186–189, 338, *339*
SIADH 242, *243*
Sickle Cell Anemia 404, *405*
Skin Integrity 392, *393*
Spinal Cord Client 360, *361*
Standard of Care 40, *41*
Stethoscope 106, *107*
Stroke 366, *367*

T
Teaching (Priority Topics for nursing personnel) 46, *47*
Test Questions, Communication Strategies For 504, *505*
Test Questions, Prioritization Strategies 4, 5
Tetralogy of Fallot 124, *125*
Therapeutic Communication 502, *503*

Thyroid
  Hyperthyroidism 246, *247*
  Hypothyroidism 250, *251*
Thyroidectomy 248, *249*
Toddler (1 to 3 years) 432, *433*
Traction 310, *311*
Transmitted Voice Sounds 168, *169*
Transurethral Resection of the Prostate (TURP) 414, *415*
Trending 8, 9
Triage 100, *101*
Trigeminal Neuralgia (Tic Douloureux) 356, *357*
Tuberculosis 206, *207*
Tubes 282, *283*
Tylenol (Acetaminophen) Overdose 294, *295*

U
UAP Tasks 24, *25*
Ulcerative Colitis and Crohn's 276, *277*

V
Varicella (Chicken Pox) 68, *69*
Ventilator Care 204, *205*
Viral Infections 66, *67*
Visual Changes 372, *373*
Vital Signs 108, *109*
Vital Sign Values 110, *111*

W
Walker 320, *321*
Water-Sealed Chest Drainage 202, *203*

Y
Young Adulthood (19 to 40 Years) 442, *443*